Advanced Electrochemical and Opto-Electrochemical Biosensors for Quantitative Analysis of Disease Markers and Viruses

Advanced Electrochemical and Opto-Electrochemical Biosensors for Quantitative Analysis of Disease Markers and Viruses

Editors

Najmeh Karimian
Federico Polo
Paolo Ugo

MDPI • Basel • Beijing • Wuhan • Barcelona • Belgrade • Manchester • Tokyo • Cluj • Tianjin

Editors
Najmeh Karimian
University Ca' Foscari of Venice
Italy

Federico Polo
University Ca' Foscari of Venice
Italy

Paolo Ugo
University Ca' Foscari of Venice
Italy

Editorial Office
MDPI
St. Alban-Anlage 66
4052 Basel, Switzerland

This is a reprint of articles from the Special Issue published online in the open access journal *Biosensors* (ISSN 2079-6374) (available at: https://www.mdpi.com/journal/biosensors/special_issues/opto_biosensors).

For citation purposes, cite each article independently as indicated on the article page online and as indicated below:

LastName, A.A.; LastName, B.B.; LastName, C.C. Article Title. *Journal Name* **Year**, *Volume Number*, Page Range.

ISBN 978-3-0365-4499-1 (Hbk)
ISBN 978-3-0365-4500-4 (PDF)

Contents

About the Editors . . . vii

Najmeh Karimian, Federico Polo and Paolo Ugo
Advanced Electrochemical and Opto-Electrochemical Biosensors for Quantitative Analysis of Disease Markers and Viruses
Reprinted from: *Biosensors* **2022**, *12*, 296, doi:10.3390/bios12050296 . . . 1

Syed Akif Raza Kazmi, Muhammad Zahid Qureshi and Jean-Francois Masson
Drug-Based Gold Nanoparticles Overgrowth for Enhanced SPR Biosensing of Doxycycline
Reprinted from: *Biosensors* **2020**, *10*, 184, doi:10.3390/bios10110184 . . . 5

Rebeca M. Torrente-Rodríguez, Cristina Muñoz-San Martín, Maria Gamella, María Pedrero, Neus Martínez-Bosch, Pilar Navarro, Pablo García de Frutos, José M. Pingarrón and Susana Campuzano
Electrochemical Immunosensing of ST2: A Checkpoint Target in Cancer Diseases
Reprinted from: *Biosensors* **2021**, *11*, 202, doi:10.3390/bios11060202 . . . 19

Marcin Gwiazda, Sheetal K. Bhardwaj, Ewa Kijeńska-Gawrońska, Wojciech Swieszkowski, Unni Sivasankaran and Ajeet Kaushik
Impedimetric and Plasmonic Sensing of Collagen I Using a Half-Antibody-Supported, Au-Modified, Self-Assembled Monolayer System
Reprinted from: *Biosensors* **2021**, *11*, 227, doi:10.3390/bios11070227 . . . 33

Neda Rafat, Paul Satoh and Robert Mark Worden
Electrochemical Biosensor for Markers of Neurological Esterase Inhibition
Reprinted from: *Biosensors* **2021**, *11*, 459, doi:10.3390/bios11110459 . . . 53

Maliana El Aamri, Ghita Yammouri, Hasna Mohammadi, Aziz Amine and Hafsa Korri-Youssoufi
Electrochemical Biosensors for Detection of MicroRNA as a Cancer Biomarker: Pros and Cons
Reprinted from: *Biosensors* **2020**, *10*, 186, doi:10.3390/bios10110186 . . . 73

Patrick Severin Sfragano, Giulia Moro, Federico Polo and Ilaria Palchetti
The Role of Peptides in the Design of Electrochemical Biosensors for Clinical Diagnostics
Reprinted from: *Biosensors* **2021**, *11*, 246, doi:10.3390/bios11080246 . . . 119

Laura Fabiani, Veronica Caratelli, Luca Fiore, Viviana Scognamiglio, Amina Antonacci, Silvia Fillo, Riccardo De Santis, Anella Monte, Manfredo Bortone, Danila Moscone, Florigio Lista and Fabiana Arduini
State of the Art on the SARS-CoV-2 Toolkit for Antigen Detection: One Year Later
Reprinted from: *Biosensors* **2021**, *11*, 310, doi:10.3390/bios11090310 . . . 139

About the Editors

Najmeh Karimian

Najmeh Karimian, a Research Fellow, holds a PhD in Analytical Chemistry from Ferdowsi University of Mashhad, Iran. To date, she has spent the majority of her career at Ca' Foscari University of Venice, Italy. During her PhD studies, she joined the Biosensors and Bioelectronics Centre at Linköping University in Sweden as a visiting researcher, where her work focused on the development of chemo-/biosensors based on molecularly imprinted polymers. In 2015, she was awarded a Postdoctoral Researcher Fellowship by the Department of Molecular Sciences and Nanosystems at University Ca' Foscari of Venice in Italy, where she developed her research on the fabrication and evaluation of nanoelectrode ensembles (NEEs) as sensing platforms. Her research interests lie in the area of development of electrochemical chemo-/biosensors for environmental, clinical, and food analyses.

Federico Polo

Federico Polo (Associate Professor) obtained his Laurea in Industrial Chemistry in 2003 and PhD in Chemical Sciences in 2007 at the University of Padova. During his PhD studies, he was a visiting student at the Georgia Institute of Technology (USA). He then served as a postdoctoral fellow at Georgia Institute of Technology (USA), Westfälische Wilhelms-Universität Münster (Germany), and University of Padova. In 2015, he was appointed Senior Scientist at Centro di Riferimento Oncologico-IRCCS in Aviano, Italy. In 2018 he was appointed Assistant Professor at Ca' Foscari University of Venice. In 2021, he was appointed Associate Professor at Ca' Foscari University of Venice. In addition, he was a visiting scholar at the University of Connecticut (USA) and Université de Montréal (Canada). His research area focuses on molecular electrochemistry and electron transfer mechanism in molecular model systems based on donor/acceptor redox moieties connected by a peptide bridge. His current scientific interests and activities in the field of molecular electrochemistry concern electron transfer mechanisms and electrogenerated chemiluminescence, electroluminescent devices, and biosensing platforms for precision medicine.

Paolo Ugo

Paolo Ugo is a former Professor of Analytical and Bioanalytical Chemistry and currently honorary Senior Researcher at Ca' Foscari University of Venice (Italy). Paolo earned his doctorate degree in Industrial Chemistry in 1980. After working for two years in a pharmaceutical company, he started his academic carrier as Assistant Professor of Analytical Chemistry at the University of Venice in 1983. In 1987–1988, he was a visiting associate at the California Institute of Technology, Pasadena. Prof. Ugo has been the coordinator of research projects concerning electrochemistry, chemical sensors, and biosensors for environmental, food, and health control, collaborating actively with several research institutions in Italy and abroad. He has authored 160 peer-reviewed scientific research articles and served as guest editor for various special issues of international journals on topics related to electroanalytical chemistry and biosensors.

biosensors

MDPI

Editorial

Advanced Electrochemical and Opto-Electrochemical Biosensors for Quantitative Analysis of Disease Markers and Viruses

Najmeh Karimian [1,*], Federico Polo [1,2] and Paolo Ugo [1]

1 Department of Molecular Sciences and Nanosystems, University Ca' Foscari of Venice, Via Torino 155, 30172 Mestre-Venezia, Italy; federico.polo@unive.it (F.P.); ugo@unive.it (P.U.)
2 European Centre for Living Technology (ECLT), Ca' Bottacin, Dorsoduro 3911, 30124 Venice, Italy
* Correspondence: najmeh.karimian@unive.it

Instrumental laboratory methods for biochemical and chemical analyses have reached a high level of reliability with excellent sensitivity and specificity. However, the complex sample preparation, the need for trained personnel as well as the use of sophisticated and expensive instrumentation still represent a drawback. Despite the indispensability of laboratory methods that guarantee excellence with regard to their analytical reliability, the need to carry out quantitative analyses for large-scale and rapid screening purposes has prompted the development of novel analytical tools, such as biosensors, capable of providing accurate and precise analytical information at low cost, ease of use and applicability for decentralized monitoring and point-of-care testing [1,2]. The recent global health crisis caused by the COVID-19 pandemic has further alerted the world to the urgent need for rapid and reliable analytical devices, which are suitable for the detection of biologically active components of clinical relevancy.

Especially for the case of immunological tests, this recent experience has highlighted the gap between, e.g., classical ELISA, which provides quantitative and reliable responses, although it must be performed in a centralized laboratory by trained personnel, and strip lateral flow tests with visual detection, suitable for decentralized use, although capable to provide only qualitative information, sometimes with not ideal sensitivity and specificity. New analytical devices are therefore highly sought to fill this gap, which must combine the capability of providing quantitative instrumental responses with fast and user-friendly applicability.

The advantages of electrochemical and optical biosensors (low cost and easy transduction) are nowadays complemented in terms of improved sensitivity by combining electrochemistry (EC) with optical techniques such as electrochemiluminescence (ECL), EC/surface-enhanced Raman spectroscopy (SERS) and EC/surface plasmon resonance (SPR) [3]. Despite recent impressive technological progress in this area, there are still pitfalls that must be overcome to progress towards real world applicability. To this goal, biosensors need to become self-contained and usable automatically or semi-automatically, while guaranteeing precise chemical information and analytical reliability. Hopefully, advances to reach these difficult tasks can derive from the continuous development and application of informatics tools, such as machine learning-based methodologies [4,5]. However, progress in the design of the biosensors' architecture will also be crucial.

The present Special Issue focuses on some of the abovementioned challenges, while proposing novel approaches and exploring new applications in electrochemical, optical and opto-electrochemical biosensors. In particular, the focus is on the quantitative detection of disease markers and viruses. To this aim, this Special Issue presents both original research articles and authoritative review papers.

Interesting features of SPR sensors include label-free detection, high sensitivity, real-time monitoring and applicability to raw sample [6,7]. In their contribution to this Spe-

Citation: Karimian, N.; Polo, F.; Ugo, P. Advanced Electrochemical and Opto-Electrochemical Biosensors for Quantitative Analysis of Disease Markers and Viruses. *Biosensors* **2022**, *12*, 296. https://doi.org/10.3390/bios12050296

Received: 26 April 2022
Accepted: 29 April 2022
Published: 4 May 2022

cial Issue, Masson and coworkers present the new possibility of exploiting SPR to develop a so-called doxy-AuNPs-based SPR biosensor for the fast and sensitive detection of doxycycline [8]. Indeed, the authors demonstrate that the drug doxycycline can tune the formation of Au nanoparticles to enhance the response of a SPR biosensor to this drug. Among other interesting features, it is worth mentioning that the resulting SPR signal scales directly with the concentration of doxycycline, contrary to the usual SPR-based immunosensors which, being based on competition assays, result in a progressive lowering of the response while increasing the analyte concentration.

In their article, Campuzano, Pingarron and coworkers [9] present a novel amperometric immunosensor for the determination of ST2, a member of the interleukin 1 receptor family. ST2 has well-known relations with inflammatory and other diseases so that high levels of sST2 are found in the serum of patients suffering from several disorders. The proposed method is based on a sandwich immunoassay with electrochemical detection, using a disposable screen-printed carbon electrode. Magnetic immunoconjugates are built on the surface of carboxylic acid-microsized magnetic particles. Captured ST2 is finally sandwiched by a biotinylated secondary antibody conjugated with a streptavidinated peroxidase. The sensor shows interesting selectivity and sensitivity, allowing the determination of soluble ST2 in plasma samples from healthy individuals and patients diagnosed with pancreatic ductal adenocarcinoma (PDAC), with the advantage of a relatively short analysis time (45 min). The good correlation of the obtained results with those provided by classical ELISA demonstrates the potential of the developed strategy for the early diagnosis and/or prognosis of the fatal PDAC disease.

On the stream line of biosensors based on enzyme inhibition effects [10], Worden and coworkers [11] study a novel electrochemical biosensor to detect acetylcholinesterase (AChE) inhibitors that may trigger neurological diseases. The research is based on an integrated approach, combining experimental results within the frame of a theoretical model suitable to be applied to the case of an inhibition-based bi-enzyme (IBE) sensor. Experimentally, AChE and tyrosinase (Tyr) are co-immobilized on the working electrode component of a screen-printed electrode array. Using redox recycling of the electroactive component of the sensor, an amplification mechanism is suitably activated to increase the signal and the sensitivity. The theoretical model is validated by comparison between experimental and calculated results. The model shows its capability to reproduce different trends in the experimental results, ranging from steady-state responses to unsteady-state dynamics of the biosensor, e.g., following the addition of a reactant (phenylacetate) and an ACE inhibitor (PMSF).

In their research article, Kaushik and coworkers [12] present an electrochemical immunosensor for collagen I, chosen as a biomarker for monitoring the regeneration of damaged connective tissue in tendons and ligaments. The proposed immunosensor is fabricated using a self-assembled monolayer (SAM) of a bis-thiol to immobilize gold nanoparticles (AuNPs) which are functionalized with the capture agent, that is a half-reduced monoclonal antibody. Detection is performed by electrochemical impedance spectroscopy and/or SPR, the former technique providing the lower detection limits. Interestingly, the sensor shows improved sensitivity with respect to the commonly used ELISA procedure for the same analysis.

In diagnostics and theranostics, a key issue concerns the capability of detecting cancer biomarkers. Such a role is played by microRNA (miRNA), which are small RNA sequences (18–25 mers), whose expression level is correlated with the onset and development of diseases, including cancer, diabetes and heart disease. In their review article, Amine and coworkers [13] focus on direct miRNA electrochemical biosensors based on redox markers with different designs, such as DNA-intercalating redox systems, redox catalysts as well as free redox indicators. The authors discuss the advantages and drawbacks of these approaches, presenting the state of the art and the challenges still open to improve validation, clinical application and possible commercialization of electrochemical biosensors for the detection of circulating miRNA.

Increasing attention is paid to the development of the biorecognition element able to promote a wider applicability of electrochemical biosensors. In their review, Palchetti and coworkers [14] present the state of the art and prospects on a key point crucial for the future of bioanalytical sensing, which is the development of electrochemical biosensors based on synthetic peptides. The advantages of easily synthetized peptides vs. antibodies are evident in terms of cost effectiveness and high yields. The authors discuss the different roles of peptides in the design of electrochemical biosensors, from their use as antifouling agents to their role in the development of catalytic and affinity electrochemical biosensors. Moreover, the authors discuss and compare the procedures used for the selection and synthesis of peptides as well as the different electrochemical detection strategies based on both label and label-free approaches, together with application for clinical diagnostics.

The drastic effect of viral infections and their transmission at an alarming rate has highlighted the need for advanced and rapid diagnostic techniques, as dramatically demonstrated by the COVID-19 pandemic. In their review, Arduini and coworkers [15] analyze the most recent achievements in the field of the quick detection of SARS-CoV-2 with biosensors. At first, the article presents and discusses the guidelines on COVID-19 for in vitro diagnostic tests and their performance, developed by the European Commission in 2020. Afterwards, the review examines technical and scientific aspects of the different biosensors developed up to the publication of the review, focusing on biosensors designed for the quantitative analysis of SARS-CoV-2 antigens, as tested on real matrices, such as nasopharynx swabs, saliva, serum and droplets. A critical comparison between biosensors able to provide quantitative responses vs. qualitative tests is presented. Finally, the authors discuss the pros and cons of available analytical tools to address a feasible strategy for fabricating an ideal biosensor suitable for the specific detection of SARS-CoV-2, hopefully offering the possibility of a wide range use and commercialization.

Thanking all the authors for their contributions, we hope that the articles presented in this Special Issue can offer a stimulating panorama of some of the open challenges for advancing research in the field of electrochemical and opto-electrochemical biosensors, in particular for the detection of viruses and disease markers. In our opinion, these contributions can constitute a useful starting point for further development in this important field, with a focus on some specific areas. Moreover, they show that when biochemistry, electrochemistry and analytical chemistry meet, it is possible to offer at least a partial answer to the need for real improvements in the quality of life and public health.

Author Contributions: All authors contributed equally to this editorial. All authors have read and agreed to the published version of the manuscript.

Funding: This research received no external funding.

Data Availability Statement: Detailed information is available on request to the corresponding author.

Conflicts of Interest: The authors declare no conflict of interest.

References

1. Turner, A.P.F. Biosensors: Sense and sensibility. *Chem. Soc. Rev.* **2013**, *42*, 3184–3196. [CrossRef] [PubMed]
2. Ugo, P.; Marafini, P.; Meneghello, M. *Bioanalytical Chemistry—From Biomolecular Recognition to Nanobiosensing*; De Gruyter: Berlin, Germany, 2021.
3. Sohrabi, H.; Kordasht, H.K.; Pashazadeh-Panahi, P.; Nezhad-Mokhtari, P.; Hashemzaei, M.; Majidi, M.R.; Mosafer, J.; Oroojalian, F.; Mokhtarzadeh, A.; de la Guardia, M. Recent advances of electrochemical and optical biosensors for detection of C-reactive protein as a major inflammatory biomarker. *Microchem. J.* **2020**, *158*, 105287. [CrossRef]
4. Ugo, P. Editorial overview: Sensors and biosensors: New sense for electrochemical sensors. *Curr. Opin. Electrochem.* **2019**, *16*, A4–A7. [CrossRef]
5. Kumar, D.P.; Amgoth, T.; Annavarapu, C.S.R. Machine learning algorithms for wireless sensor networks: A survey. *Inf. Fusion* **2019**, *49*, 1. [CrossRef]
6. Li, Q.; Dou, X.; Zhang, L.; Zhao, X.; Luo, J.; Yang, M. Oriented assembly of surface plasmon resonance biosensor through staphylococcal protein A for the chlorpyrifos detection. *Anal. Bioanal. Chem.* **2019**, *411*, 6057–6066. [CrossRef] [PubMed]

7. Masson, J.-F. Surface plasmon resonance clinical biosensors for medical diagnostics. *ACS Sens.* **2017**, *2*, 16–30. [CrossRef] [PubMed]
8. Kazmi, S.A.R.; Qureshi, M.Z.; Masson, J.-F. Drug-based gold nanoparticles overgrowth for enhanced SPR biosensing of doxycycline. *Biosensors* **2020**, *10*, 184. [CrossRef] [PubMed]
9. Torrente-Rodríguez, R.M.; Martín, C.M.S.; Gamella, M.; Pedrero, M.; Martínez-Bosch, N.; Navarro, P.G.; de Frutos, P.G.; Pingarrón, J.M.; Campuzano, S. Electrochemical immunosensing of ST2: A checkpoint target in cancer diseases. *Biosensors* **2021**, *11*, 202. [CrossRef] [PubMed]
10. Upadhyay, L.S.B.; Verma, N. Enzyme inhibition based biosensors: A review. *Anal. Lett.* **2012**, *46*, 225–241. [CrossRef]
11. Rafat, N.; Satoh, P.; Worden, R.M. Electrochemical biosensor for markers of neurological esterase inhibition. *Biosensors* **2021**, *11*, 459. [CrossRef] [PubMed]
12. Gwiazda, M.; Bhardwaj, S.K.; Kijeńska-Gawrońska, E.; Swieszkowski, W.; Sivasankaran, U.; Kaushik, A. Impedimetric and plasmonic sensing of collagen I using a half-antibody-supported, Au-modified, self-assembled monolayer system. *Biosensors* **2021**, *11*, 227. [CrossRef] [PubMed]
13. El Aamri, M.; Yammouri, G.; Mohammadi, H.; Amine, A.; Korri-Youssoufi, H. Electrochemical biosensors for detection of microRNA as a cancer biomarker: Pros and cons. *Biosensors* **2020**, *10*, 186. [CrossRef] [PubMed]
14. Sfragano, P.S.; Moro, G.; Polo, F.; Palchetti, I. The role of peptides in the design of electrochemical biosensors for clinical diagnostics. *Biosensors* **2021**, *11*, 246. [CrossRef] [PubMed]
15. Fabiani, L.; Caratelli, V.; Fiore, L.; Scognamiglio, V.; Antonacci, A.; Fillo, S.; De Santis, R.; Monte, A.; Bortone, M.; Moscone, D.; et al. State of the art on the SARS-CoV-2 toolkit for antigen detection: One year later. *Biosensors* **2021**, *11*, 310. [CrossRef] [PubMed]

biosensors

MDPI

Article

Drug-Based Gold Nanoparticles Overgrowth for Enhanced SPR Biosensing of Doxycycline

Syed Akif Raza Kazmi [1,2,*], Muhammad Zahid Qureshi [1] and Jean-Francois Masson [2,*]

1 Department of Chemistry, Government College University Lahore, Lahore 54000, Pakistan; dr.zahidqureshi@gcu.edu.pk
2 Département de Chimie, Québec Centre for Advanced Materials and Regroupement Québécois sur les Matériaux de Pointe, C.P 6128 Succursale Centre-Ville Université de Montréal, Montreal, QC H3C 3J7, Canada
* Correspondence: akifr1@gmail.com (S.A.R.K.); Jf.masson@umontreal.ca (J.-F.M.)

Received: 22 October 2020; Accepted: 18 November 2020; Published: 19 November 2020

Abstract: In clinical chemistry, frequent monitoring of drug levels in patients has gained considerable importance because of the benefits of drug monitoring on human health, such as the avoidance of high risk of over dosage or increased therapeutic efficacy. In this work, we demonstrate that the drug doxycycline can act as an Au nanoparticle (doxy-AuNP) growth and capping agent to enhance the response of a surface plasmon resonance (SPR) biosensor for this drug. SPR analysis revealed the high sensitivity of doxy-AuNPs towards the detection of free doxycycline. More specifically, doxy-AuNPs bound with protease-activated receptor-1 (PAR-1) immobilized on the SPR sensing surface yield the response in SPR, which was enhanced following the addition of free doxy (analyte) to the solution of doxy-AuNPs. This biosensor allowed for doxycycline detection at concentrations as low as 7 pM. The study also examined the role of colloidal stability and growth of doxy-AuNPs in relation to the response-enhancement strategy based on doxy-AuNPs. Thus, the doxy-AuNPs-based SPR biosensor is an excellent platform for the detection of doxycycline and demonstrates a new biosensing scheme where the analyte can provide enhancement.

Keywords: gold nanoparticles; doxycycline; tetracycline; SPR biosensor; signal amplification; clinical diagnosis

1. Introduction

It is important in the analytical community to develop sensors for frequent monitoring of drugs. In particular, clinical diagnosis and therapeutic procedures demand sensors to assess drug levels in patients. There is a need to obtain accurate test results in a short time for a large number of samples to decide on the course of medical treatments [1]. As such, different laboratory-based techniques are often employed to measure the drug concentrations in biofluid of patients, which serves to adjust medication knowing the active concentration of drugs in blood. As such, regular monitoring of drug levels in patients can prevent its toxicity and damage to organs [2,3].

Doxycycline is a wide-spectrum drug belonging to the tetracycline family of antibiotics, which has been a drug of choice for treatment of several types of bacterial infections [4]. Protease-activated receptor-1 (PAR-1) is the member of PARs (protease-activated receptors) family that was identified in 1991 by two independent laboratories during the investigation of thrombin signaling pathway in both hamster and human cells. PAR-1 is expressed in all kinds of blood cells as well as in immune cells epithelium, astrocytes, and neurons [5]. PAR-1 is the receptor protein with which doxycycline binds to inhibit the tumor progression [6].

According to FDA, safe dose of doxycycline is 200 mg on first day of treatment followed by 100 mg per day. In case of prolonged high dose, patient may suffer from gastrointestinal and renal diseases. It is a relatively low-toxicity drug and has been recommended for human use for a long time. However, the long-term use of doxycycline may lead to some side effects. Elzeinová et al. reported the adverse effects of doxycycline on testicular tissue and sperm parameters in CD1 outbred mice [7]. According to them, the treatment of male mice with doxycycline in puberty led to long-lasting effects on reproductive organs and spermatozoa in adult males. They reported that the effect of doxycycline was concentration dependent. In addition, antitumor activities of doxycycline against different types of malignancies have also been reported elsewhere. For example, Sun et al. and Liu et al. have reported cytotoxicity and antimetastatic activity of doxycycline in melanoma and breast carcinomas [8,9]. According to Son et al., doxycycline has potential to show apoptotic activities in pancreatic cancer cells [10]. Duivenvoorden et al. has reported that doxycycline treatment could be effective to reduce the tumor burden in bone metastasis mouse model of human breast cancer [11]. All these studies suggest that this valuable antibiotic also has potential to treat other types of human cancers and thus a candidate anticancer drug of high research value. It is, therefore, important to monitor the concentration of doxycycline (doxy) in blood to optimize the dosage and reducing the side effects.

Currently, methods used for doxycycline detection involve analytical techniques such as high-performance liquid chromatography (HPLC) [12], sequential injection chromatography (SIC) [13], and potentiometry [14]. These techniques provide accuracy and reasonably good detection limits but have disadvantages such as need of complicated sample preparation, trained personnel, and sophisticated instruments and thus cannot provide onsite and fast detection. Therefore, there is a need to develop alternative methods that can provide onsite, fast, and sensitive detection of doxycycline.

Surface plasmon resonance (SPR) biosensor is an optical technique that measures the binding events quantitatively in real time without labeling the interacting molecules [15]. The physical principle of SPR technique involves the measurement of changes in refractive index when the interaction of molecules takes place at the sensor surface [16]. The benefits of the SPR technique include label-free detection, high sensitivity, real-time monitoring, and crude sample analysis [17]. These advantages make this SPR technique a reliable and convenient one to examine the binding specificity and interaction of biomolecules, as first reported in 1982 when Liedberg et al. initially reported the use of a SPR-based biosensor for the detection of biomolecular interaction [18]. Till now, this technique has been primarily used as an effective tool for biomolecular interaction analysis, but more recently, clinical analysis is increasingly reported [19]. SPR sensing proceeds without altering or damaging the composition of original analyte [20] and is increasingly proposed for clinical diagnostics [21,22], drug monitoring [23], environmental monitoring [24,25], food analysis [26,27], and biochemistry [28].

Despite the many advantages of SPR biosensors, the binding of small molecules to the sensor surface typically results in small shifts, which constitutes a limitation of SPR biosensors. Most portable and small SPR instruments are not sensitive enough to assess such small refractive index changes, which make them unfit to use for ultrasensitive detection of small organic drugs [29]. To overcome this limitation, different groups have employed various enhancement strategies in conjugation with SPR, such as enzyme [30], polymerase chain reaction (PCR) [31], and gold nanoparticles (AuNPs) enhancement methods [32]. Among them AuNPs-based enhancement strategies have received considerable attention and played a significant role in response amplification of SPR biosensors [33]. The ease of synthesis, good stability, biocompatibility, low toxicity, and ability of surface functionalization of AuNPs make them an attractive tool for biomedical applications [34]. AuNPs support localized surface plasmon resonances (LSPR), arising from the combined oscillations of electrons present in the conduction band of the metal [35]. The electronic coupling between the LSPR of gold nanostructures and SPR is often applied as a strategy to amplify the response signals of biosensors. For example, this strategy has been designed for the detection of methotrexate [23] and testosterone [36].

AuNPs are extensively applied in SPR biosensors, as such the effect of size of nanoparticles on SPR interactions is increasingly well understood. According to Kelly et al., size and shape of the nanomaterials could be effectively used to control the plasmonic characteristics as well as the electromagnetic field amplification of AuNPs [37]. Comparatively, larger nanostructures give higher sensitivity towards changes in refractive index than the smaller nanostructures. Uludag and Tothill studied the effect of size of AuNPs over the SPR sensor response. According to them, increasing the size of AuNPs resulted in higher sensor response [38]. Springer et al. observed that the size of AuNPs affects the diffusion mass transfer rate as well as the SPR signal and resulted in optical enhancement of SPR biosensor [39]. All these considerations suggested that the size of AuNP is critical and needs more attention while studying the biomolecular interaction via SPR biosensor.

To further build on the use of AuNPs-enhanced SPR for drug detection, we report on the fabrication of a doxy-AuNPs-based SPR biosensor for fast and sensitive detection of doxycycline. The use of the analyte to trigger AuNPs overgrowth is used as a novel sensing principle, where the signal of the SPR sensor is proportional to the concentration of doxycycline, in opposition to the usual competition assays resulting in a reduced response of the SPR sensor with concentration. Synthesized doxy-AuNPs were characterized by UV–VIS, X-ray diffraction (XRD), FT-IR, and transmission electron microscopy (TEM). SPR analysis was performed to demonstrate the detection of doxycycline. Various conditions were optimized to improve the SPR response. In this study, doxy-AuNP containing sodium chloride (NaCl) was employed as reagent providing further increase in the biosensor response. Thus, the doxy-AuNPs-based SPR biosensor is an excellent platform for the ultrasensitive detection of doxycycline.

2. Experimental

2.1. Materials

Gold (III) chloride trihydrate, doxycycline hyclate, N-hydroxysuccinimide (NHS), 16-mercapto-hexadecanoic acid (16-MHA), 11-mercapto-1-undecanol, ethanolamine hydrochloride, and sodium chloride were purchased from Sigma Aldrich (Oakville, Canada). Sodium hydroxide and N-ethyl-N′-(3-dimethylaminopropyl)-carbodiimide (EDC) were purchased from Fluka chemicals. Protease-activated receptor (PAR-1) was purchased from Cedarlane (Burlington, Canada).

2.2. Preparation of the Doxy-AuNPs

To prepare doxy-AuNPs, aqueous solutions of 4 mL gold chloride (0.4 mM) and 2 mL doxycycline (0.8 mM) were added in a conical flask. To the mixture, 3 mL sodium hydroxide (0.01 M) was added. The mixture was continuously stirred for 3 min. After 3 min, a ruby red color was observed (Figure 1). A UV–Vis spectrophotometer (Model Cary 100 Bio, Varian, Palo Alto, USA) was used to monitor the synthesis of doxy-AuNPs in wavelength range of 300–800 nm.

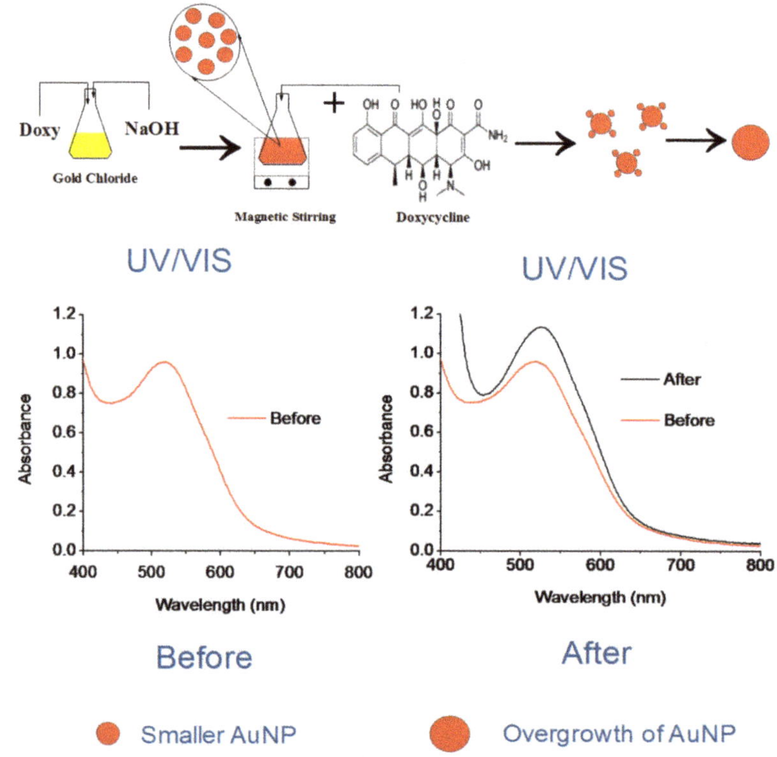

Figure 1. Scheme illustration of doxycycline effect on overgrowth of doxycycline Au nanoparticles (doxy-AuNPs).

2.3. Characterization of the Doxy-AuNPs

The crystalline nature of doxy-AuNPs was confirmed via XRD studies. The solution containing doxy-AuNPs was centrifuged three times at 10,000 rpm for 30 min and washed with deionized water each time. Then, the pellet obtained after centrifugation was left overnight to dry under fume hood. Powder XRD analysis was performed with Bruker D2 Phaser using Cu Kα radiation (1.54 Å λ) in the 2θ region, from 0 to 80°. Transmission electron microscopy (TEM) (FEI Tecnai t12) with voltage 80 kV and final emission 10 μA was used to examine the size and shape of doxy-AuNPs. Moreover, 2k AMT camera was applied to take micrographs of doxy-AuNPs. Sample for TEM was prepared by placing 10 μL of doxy-AuNPs colloidal solution on copper grid coated with carbon and formvar film. The sample was left for 24 h to dry and then analyzed with TEM. The FT-IR is the most widely used technique to study the interaction of biomolecules with the nanomaterials. The appearance of certain spectral changes enables to identify the interaction of certain functional groups with the nanomaterials [40]. The doxy-AuNPs were also characterized with FT-IR. The solution containing doxy-AuNPs was centrifuged three times at 10,000 rpm for 30 min and washed with deionized water each time. Then the pellet obtained after centrifugation was dried under fume hood for 24 h, transferred, and analyzed with FT-IR.

2.4. Fabrication of the SPR Sensor

SPR measurements were performed on a portable SPR instrument (Affinité Instruments, Montréal, QC, Canada) [23]. A dove prism with a gold film (1 nm Cr and 45 nm Au) was immobilized with a self-assembled monolayer (SAM) of 16-mercaptohexadecanoic acid and 11-mercapto-1-undecanol

(Supporting Information, page S2). The SAM has the ability to bind receptor (protease-activated receptor-1) PAR-1 and is capable for resisting nonspecific adsorption on sensing surface for quantification of biomolecule [41]. This modified gold-coated prism with SAM was placed into the chip holder of the SPR setup. Then, a disposable PDMS flow cell was mounted over the prism and tighten with a clamp. The reference and sample solutions were injected at different sensing areas via separate injection ports. In PDMS flow cell, there are two separate flow channels, one for sample solution and other for reference solution. For the sample solution, the flow channel is S-shaped and comprise three different sensing areas, providing analysis of sample in triplicate. The total volume of the channel for sample analysis is 16 μL. For the reference solution, the flow channel covers the fourth sensing area with a volume of 5 μL. The whole SPR system was connected to custom LabView software via a laptop. Data acquired by the SPR system was controlled by software and minimum finding algorithm based on a second-order polynomial fit was used to integrate SPR signal at each time point. The sensorgrams for all four sensing areas were recorded in real time.

2.5. Immobilization of Receptor on Sensor Surface

In all SPR experiments, the SAM-modified gold-coated prism was inserted in the SPR instrument. First, Milli-Q water was added into the flow cell and left for 15–20 min for stabilization. Afterwards, the sensing surface was activated with EDC/NHS and left for 5 min until the resonant wavelength was constant. Then, the sensing surface was rinsed with PBS, followed by the injection of the receptor solution of protease-activated receptor-1 (PAR-1) at 5 μg mL^{-1} and reacted for 15 min. The receptor PAR-1 was covalently attached to the SAM through activated carboxylic acid group from EDC/NHS. Subsequently, nonspecific binding sites on the sensing surfaces were blocked by injecting 1 M ethanolamine hydrochloride (pH 8.0) for 10 min followed by rinsing with PBS to remove noncovalently attached receptor PAR-1. This procedure was repeated for all SPR experiments.

2.6. Electrolytic Stability of Doxy-AuNPs

To examine the electrolytic stability of doxy-AuNPs, different concentrations of NaCl (from 50 to 1000 mM) were added in doxy-AuNPs colloidal solutions and their UV spectra were recorded (Model Cary 100 Bio, Varian, Palo Alto, USA) in the wavelength range of 300–800 nm. To select the suitable electrolytic condition of doxy-AuNPs, which can give larger SPR response, doxy-AuNPs containing varying concentrations of NaCl (from 50 to 1000 mM) were injected in SPR followed by rinsing each time before and after each injection with same concentration of NaCl in water to record the refractive index baseline. A control experiment of doxy-AuNPs without NaCl was also conducted and sensorgrams were recorded in real time.

2.7. Sequential Analysis for Determination of Concentration of Doxycycline

To examine the effect of doxycycline on the growth of synthesized doxy-AuNPs, varying concentrations of doxycycline (from 1 nM to 1 mM) were added in suspensions of doxy-AuNPs and their UV spectra were recorded in the wavelength range of 300–800 nm. Furthermore, to carry out detection of doxycycline with the SPR system, varying concentrations of doxycycline (0.1 nM to 100 μM) were added in the colloidal suspension of doxy-AuNPs and injected sequentially in flow cell at room temperature for 30 min followed by rinsing each time before and after each injection with 100 mM NaCl in water for 5 min to record baseline. Interaction between biological receptor PAR-1 and doxy-AuNPs was measured as binding shift by SPR biosensor in real time. Control experiments were performed by injecting doxy-AuNPs (containing optimized NaCl concentration) without adding free doxycycline in SPR system. Origin software was used to process the data utilizing the minimum wavelength finding algorithm. From the sensorgram, last 50 data points of 100 mM NaCl steps before and after the doxycycline sensing steps were used to calculate the binding shift from sensorgram. The logarithm of doxy concentration was plotted against the binding shift to find the correlation between concentration of doxycycline and binding shift. Triplicate measurements were carried for all conditions. Reproducibility was obtained from the triplicate SPR measurements of 100 nM doxycycline and measured as a coefficient of variation resulting from the ratio of the standard deviation and the mean response, in percentage.

3. Results and Discussion

3.1. Strategy of the Assay

Doxycycline is a broad-spectrum drug with its antimicrobial as well as antitumor activities [4,8,10,11]. PAR-1 is the receptor protein with which doxycycline binds to inhibit the tumor progression [6]. Therefore, SPR analysis for doxycycline detection mainly depends upon the interaction of doxy-AuNPs with PAR-1 immobilized on sensor surface. The interaction of doxy-AuNPs with PAR-1 resulted in change of refractive index, which consequently gives SPR response in the form of wavelength shift. In this work, doxy-AuNPs containing NaCl were employed as an amplification element to enhance the SPR response. Furthermore, addition of free doxycycline in doxy-AuNPs colloidal solution causes overgrowth of doxy-AuNPs, which consequently further enhances the SPR biosensor response. The concentration of doxy was correlated with biosensor response. This concept could be applied to other small molecules that can act as reducing agents for gold ions. It is advantageous of synthesizing the AuNP with the analyte as it provides a simple method for synthesis and functionalization in a single step and allowed for the efficient overgrowth of the AuNP in presence of the analyte.

3.2. Synthesis and Stability of Doxy-AuNPs

A wet chemical reduction method was used to synthesize the doxy-AuNPs [42]. Doxycycline, being a polyphenolic compound, reduces and stabilizes the AuNPs. The polyphenolic groups are oxidized to their respective quinones by $AuCl_4^-$ with H^+ transfer and AuNPs formation. Recently, He et al. has reported the similar phenomena [43]. The b-agonists that possess monophenolic group or aniline showed the capability of reducing $HAuCl_4$ into AuNPs at elevated temperature, which means the reducing capability of such compounds are weaker than the one of the polyphenolic compounds, such as doxycycline. Immediately after addition of doxycycline and sodium hydroxide in gold chloride solution, AuNPs were synthesized in 3 min with characteristic ruby red color, similar to another synthesis previously reported for L-methionine [44]. Synthesis of doxy-AuNPs was confirmed using UV–Vis spectrophotometry. A sharp surface plasmon resonance was observed at 520 nm, which is a characteristic LSPR (localized surface plasmon resonance) in spherical gold nanoparticles [45], thus confirming the synthesis of doxy-AuNPs (Figure 2a). TEM images were then acquired for further supporting the synthesis of doxy-AuNPs. Homogenously distributed spherical gold nanoparticles were obtained with this method (Figure 2b). Average particle size of doxy-AuNPs calculated was 4.7 ± 0.7 nm ($n = 169$, histogram in Supporting Information, Figure S1). The crystalline nature of doxy-AuNPs was examined through XRD analysis. XRD pattern of doxy-AuNPs showed strong diffraction peaks at 38.5°, 46.1°, 64.5°, and 78.6° corresponding to {111}, {200}, {220}, and {311}, respectively, which reflects the crystalline nature of doxy-AuNPs (Figure 2c) [46].

To examine the electrolytic stability of synthesized doxy-AuNPs, different concentrations of NaCl (from 50 to 1000 mM) were added in doxy-AuNPs colloidal solutions and their UV spectra were recorded. Doxy-AuNPs showed good electrolytic stability with slight red shift (from 520 to 530 nm) and small decrease in intensity up to 100 mM NaCl, whereas in case of higher concentrations from 250 to 1000 mM NaCl, LSPR band of doxy-AuNPs further red shifted from 530 to 540 nm with significant broadening and decrease in intensity (Figure 2d). It was likely due to the refractive index shift of high salt solution and screening of surface charge on the AuNP. Srivastava and Gupta have also reported this phenomenon. According to them, resonance wavelength increases with higher salt content due to interaction of the salts with the metal film [47]. The effect of salt has been previously shown to have an impact on the Debye length and the interaction of ligand-modified AuNP for a methotrexate SPR sensor [48]. As such, the stability of the doxy-AuNP was essential to carry the SPR measurements reported in this paper.

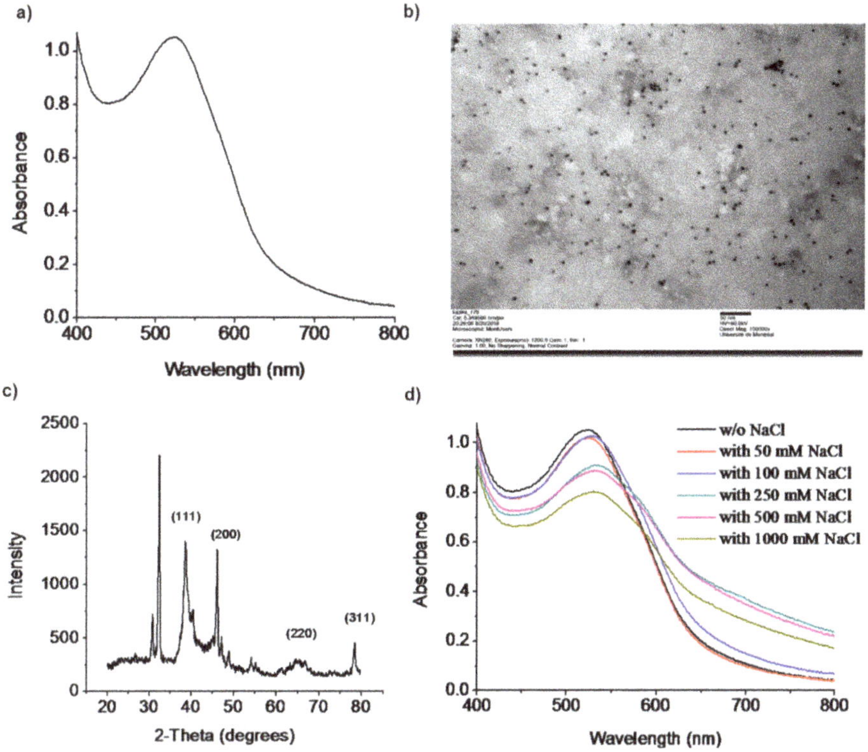

Figure 2. (**a**) UV–Vis spectrum of doxy-AuNPs. (**b**) TEM image of doxy-AuNPs, acquired at 80 kV, with exposure of 1200 ms and magnification of 150,000X. The scale bar represents 50 nm. (**c**) XRD spectra of doxy-AuNPs. (**d**) UV–Vis spectra showing the electrolytic stability of doxy-AuNPs in the presence of different concentrations of NaCl.

The interaction of doxycycline in synthesis of AuNPs was studied through FT-IR (Figure 3). In case of pure doxycycline, the absorption band was observed in the range of 3400–3200 cm^{-1} for O-H and N-H bonds but this band completely disappeared in case of doxy-AuNPs. This observation hints about the involvement of these moieties in the modification process. Likewise, the absorption bands in the range of 1700–1500 cm^{-1} were attributed to α,β-unsaturated carbonyl of amide and ketone functionalities of doxycycline. These signals moved to higher values in case of doxy-AuNPs, although the intensity of signals is low. The shifting to higher values justified the involvement of hydroxyl group resulting into disappearance of C=C conjugation.

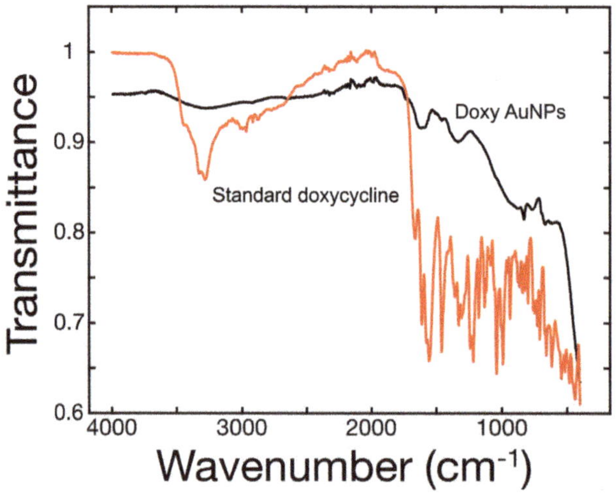

Figure 3. FT-IR spectra of doxycycline (red) and doxycycline-modified gold nanoparticles (black).

3.3. SPR Analysis for Detection of Doxycycline

3.3.1. Optimization of Electrolytic Conditions of Doxy-AuNPs

A shorter Debye length and, as a consequence, decreased colloidal stability are required for the molecular interaction of target analyte to occur on a surface-bound receptor. The presence of NaCl causes the electrostatic screening of surface charges by dissolved ions and reduces the Debye length, and resulted in the higher SPR response reported previously for a methotrexate assay [48]. To select the suitable electrolytic condition of doxy-AuNPs, which can give higher SPR response, doxy-AuNPs without NaCl and with varied concentrations of NaCl (from 50 to 1000 mM) were injected in SPR system. In the absence of NaCl, very low and undetectable SPR response was observed for doxy-AuNPs, whereas significantly higher SPR response was observed for doxy-AuNPs in the presence of NaCl (Figure 4 and Figures S2 and S3 in Supporting Information page S3). Very low SPR response of doxy-AuNPs is mainly attributed to the small size (4.7 nm) and larger Debye length of doxy-AuNPs in absence of salt, which makes them unfit to enter deep in the binding pocket of receptors bound to the sensor surface [49,50]. On the contrary, addition of NaCl to doxy-AuNPs causes the electrostatic screening of surface charges by dissolved ions and reduces the Debye length, and thus resulted in the largest SPR response [48]. The control with the same NaCl concentration before injection of the doxy-AuNP led to changes in SPR shifts much smaller (i.e., 1 nm) than with the doxy-AuNP. Doxy-AuNP with 50 mM NaCl led to a SPR shift of 9.5 nm, whereas the doxy-AuNP with 100 mM NaCl provided a 25 nm SPR shift. Since the doxy-AuNPs containing 100 mM NaCl generated maximum SPR response signal (Figure 4), these conditions were selected for all further SPR bioassays for detection of doxycycline.

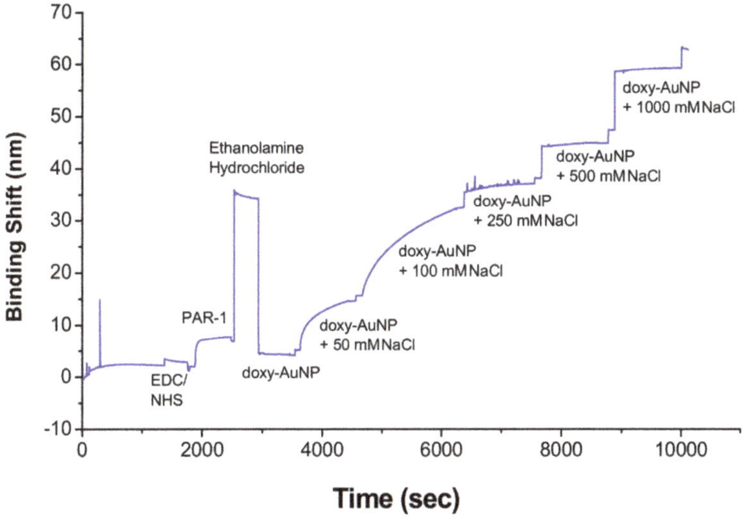

Figure 4. Effect of sodium chloride (NaCl) concentration on the surface plasmon resonance (SPR) response of doxy-AuNPs. The SPR response was measured in the Kretschmann configuration, and the binding shift refers to the propagating plasmon of the gold film.

3.3.2. SPR Bioassay for Doxycycline Detection

Sequential SPR analysis was performed for the detection of doxycycline (analyte). As the Au salt and doxycycline were reacted in equimolar conditions, it is hypothesized that the reaction is incomplete and thus, leaves unreacted Au ions in solution in addition to the AuNPs. Different concentrations of doxycycline (0.1 nM to 10 μM) were added in the colloidal solution of doxy-AuNPs (containing 100 mM NaCl) and injected sequentially into the flow cell of SPR system. In comparison, a control sample was run in which doxy-AuNPs (containing 100 mM NaCl) were injected in flow cell of SPR system. For the control sample, a 25 nm binding shift was observed with doxy-AuNPs (Figure 5a, red trace) without the addition of doxycycline in solution while an increase in binding shift was observed with successive addition of increasing concentrations of free doxycycline in the doxy-AuNPs colloidal solutions (Figure 5a, black trace). This enhancement of SPR response on successive addition of free doxycycline is mainly because increased concentration of doxycycline resulted in rapid growth of doxy-AuNPs, similar to reported elsewhere for other tetracyclines [50], which consequently give higher SPR response.

We conclude that the growth was likely due to the already present doxy-AuNPs in colloidal solution working as nuclei for the gold atoms remaining from the AuNP synthesis and doxycycline (analyte). This caused the rapid growth of seeds of doxy-AuNPs (Figure 1), which consequently resulted in higher SPR response. Our UV–Vis results showing the effect of doxycycline addition in doxy-AuNPs colloidal solution also supports this overgrowth. On addition of varying concentrations of doxycycline (from 1 nM to 1 mM) in doxy-AuNPs colloidal solution, the LSPR of doxy-AuNPs showed slight red shift with increase in intensity (Figure 5b), a typical feature of nanoparticle growth. Shen et al. has also reported the similar phenomena for effect of tetracycline addition to the *in situ* growth mechanism of AuNPs. According to them, AuNPs seeds (citrate stabilized) present in the solution work as nuclei for the conjugation and growth of gold atoms produced as result of reaction between tetracycline and $HAuCl_4$ [50]. Furthermore, a similar effect of size of AuNPs on SPR response was reported by Bukar et al. According to them, gold nanoparticles with large size and smaller Debye length on the SPR sensor surface prevail over interaction with surface-bound receptors and lead to a higher SPR response [48].

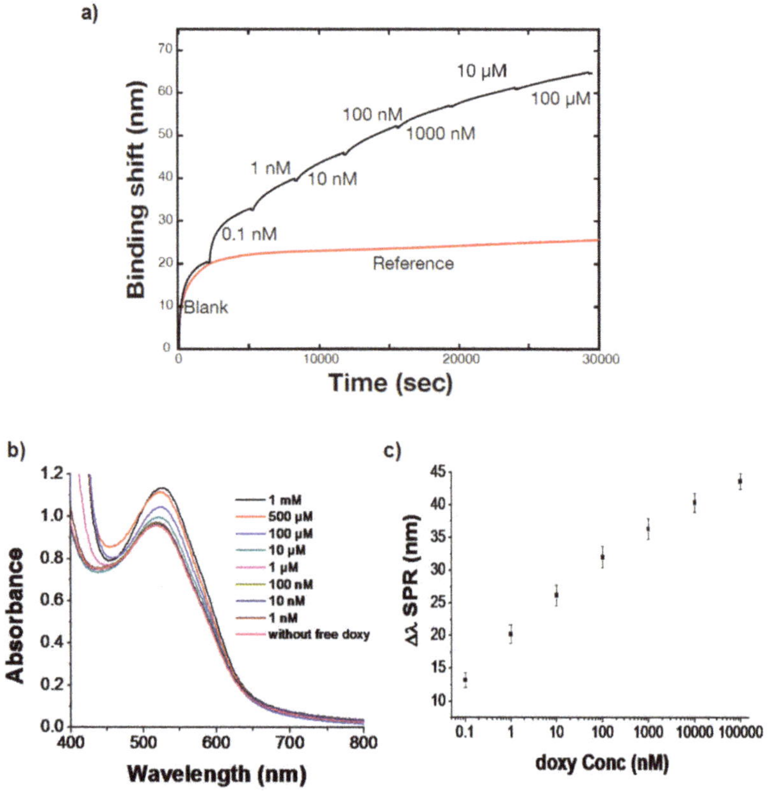

Figure 5. (**a**) Propagating SPR response of doxy-AuNPs (control, red trace) and of doxy-AuNPs with varying concentrations of doxy (analyte, black trace). (**b**) UV–Vis spectra indicating the effect of addition of doxycycline on growth of doxy-AuNPs. (**c**) Sequential binding curve presenting a correlation between log of doxy concentration and SPR response. Error bars indicate standard deviation of triplicate measurements.

Calibration of this SPR sensor shows linearity over several orders of magnitude and detection of doxycycline from nanomolar to micromolar (Figure 5c), which is in the clinical range, demonstrating the applicability of the sensor for doxycycline. The blood serum levels of doxycycline reach 1–10 mg/mL within about 2 h after administration of a dose, which corresponds to approximately 2–22 µM [51]. The sensor also showed high reproducibility with a coefficient of variation around 5% and a limit of detection of 7 pM (established from the sensitivity and noise level of the sensor). This low limit of detection compared favorably to the other analytical techniques developed earlier for doxycycline detection (Table 1) and therefore highlights the advantages of the SPR sensor for doxycycline. In addition to the excellent analytical performance, the SPR sensor is relatively simple to use on a portable instrument that would be conducive for point-of-care measurements.

Table 1. Comparison with other analytical techniques developed for doxycycline detection.

Ref.	Method	Linearity Range	Limit of Detection (LOD)	
			As Reported in Paper	Value in mol/L
Jeyabaskaran et al., 2014 [52]	RP-HPLC	25–150 μg/mL	0.02 μg/mL	3.7×10^{-8} mol/L
Adrian et al., 2012 [53]	ELISA	0.25–6.7 μg/mL	0.1 μg/L	1.95×10^{-10} mol/L
Kogawa et al., 2012 [54]	HPLC–UV	50–100 μg/mL	2.83 μg/mL	5.2×10^{-6} mol/L
Selvadurai et al., 2010 [55]	Liquid chromatography–mass spectrometric (LC-MS)	0.5–5 μg/mL	50 ng/mL	9.2×10^{-8} mol/L
Ramesh et al., 2010 [56]	RP-HPLC	30–300 μg/mL	0.02 μg/mL	3.7×10^{-8} mol/L
This work	Surface plasmon resonance biosensor	0.1 nM–100 μM	7 pM	7×10^{-12} mol/L

4. Conclusions

An ultrasensitive SPR biosensor based on doxy-AuNPs has been successfully developed for the detection of doxycycline. Variation in size and growth of doxy-AuNPs affected the biosensor response. To overcome the limitation of low molecular weight of analyte, doxy-AuNPs (containing 100 mM NaCl) have been applied as an amplification element to obtain significantly enhanced SPR response. The reported biosensor allowed for the detection of doxycycline as low as 7 pM. The high sensitivity, low limit of detection, excellent signal response time (less than half an hour), good stability, and reproducibility make this SPR biosensor an excellent alternative to the conventional methods for the detection of doxycycline. In future, the present biosensor can be applied in different fields of medical diagnostics and environmental monitoring for the detection of doxycycline.

Supplementary Materials: The following are available online at http://www.mdpi.com/2079-6374/10/11/184/s1, Figure S1: Histogram of doxy-AuNPs, Figure S2: SPR sensorgram indicating the response of doxy-AuNP (without NaCl) towards the doxycycline determination, Figure S3: SPR sensorgram indicating the response of doxy-AuNP (with and without NaCl) towards the doxycycline determination and additional information on the fabrication of SPR sensor using 16-mercaptohexadecanoic acid (16-MHA) and 11-mercapto-1-undecanol, on Protease activated receptor 1 (PAR-1) and on the role of NaCl in SPR sensing of doxycycline

Author Contributions: S.A.R.K. designed and performed the experiments, interpreted the data, and wrote the article. M.Z.Q. supervised the research. J.-F.M. designed the study, interpreted the data, wrote the article and supervised the research. All authors have read and agreed to the published version of the manuscript.

Funding: This work was funded by the Higher Education Commission of Pakistan (HEC-Pakistan grant to S.A.R.K.), the Canadian Foundation for Innovation (CFI; grant 12910 to J.-F.M.), and the Natural Science and Engineering Research Council of Canada (NSERC; grant RGPIN-2016-03864 to J.-F.M.).

Conflicts of Interest: J.-F.M. has financial interest in Affinité Instruments commercializing the SPR instrument used in this study.

References

1. Ronkainen, N.J.; Halsall, H.B.; Heineman, W.R. Electrochemical biosensors. *Chem. Soc. Rev.* **2010**, *39*, 1747–1763. [CrossRef] [PubMed]
2. Cohen, M.R. Why error reporting systems should be voluntary. *Br. Med. J.* **2000**, *320*, 728–729. [CrossRef] [PubMed]
3. Booth, M.A.; Gowers, S.A.N.; Leong, C.L.; Rogers, M.L.; Samper, I.C.; Wickham, A.P.; Boutelle, M.G. Chemical Monitoring in Clinical Settings: Recent Developments toward Real-Time Chemical Monitoring of Patients. *Anal. Chem.* **2018**, *90*, 2–18. [CrossRef]
4. Haddada, M.B.; Jeannot, K.; Spadavecchia, J. Novel Synthesis and Characterization of Doxycycline-Loaded Gold Nanoparticles: The Golden Doxycycline for Antibacterial Applications. *Part. Part. Syst. Charact.* **2019**, *36*, 1800395. [CrossRef]
5. Liu, X.; Yu, J.; Song, S.; Yue, X.; Li, Q. Protease-activated receptor-1 (PAR-1): A promising molecular target for cancer. *Oncotarget* **2017**, *8*, 107334–107345. [CrossRef]
6. Zhong, W.; Chen, S.; Zhang, Q.; Xiao, T.; Qin, Y.; Gu, J.; Sun, B.; Liu, Y.; Jing, X.; Hu, X.; et al. Doxycycline directly targets PAR1 to suppress tumor progression. *Oncotarget* **2017**, *8*, 16829–16842. [CrossRef]

7. Elzeinová, F.; Pěknicová, J.; Děd, L.; Kubátová, A.; Margaryan, H.; Dorosh, A.; Makovický, P.; Rajmon, R. Adverse effect of tetracycline and doxycycline on testicular tissue and sperm parameters in CD1 outbred mice. *Exp. Toxicol. Pathol.* **2013**, *65*, 911–917. [CrossRef]
8. Sun, T.; Zhao, N.; Ni, C.S.; Zhao, X.L.; Zhang, W.Z.; Su, X.; Zhang, D.F.; Gu, Q.; Sun, B.C. Doxycycline inhibits the adhesion and migration of melanoma cells by inhibiting the expression and phosphorylation of focal adhesion kinase (FAK). *Cancer Lett.* **2009**, *285*, 141–150. [CrossRef]
9. Liu, S.; Liu, X.; Wang, H.; Zhou, Q.; Liang, Y.; Sui, A.; Yao, R.; Zhao, B.; Sun, M. Lentiviral vector-mediated doxycycline-inducible USP39 shRNA or cDNA expression in triple-negative breast cancer cells. *Oncol. Rep.* **2015**, *33*, 2477–2483. [CrossRef] [PubMed]
10. Son, K.; Fujioka, S.; Iida, T.; Furukawa, K.; Fujita, T.; Yamada, H.; Chiao, P.J.; Yanaga, K. Doxycycline induces apoptosis in PANC-1 pancreatic cancer cells. *Anticancer Res.* **2009**, *29*, 3995–4003. [PubMed]
11. Duivenvoorden, W.C.M.; Popović, S.V.; Lhotük, Š.; Seidlitz, E.; Hirte, H.W.; Tozer, R.G.; Singh, G. Doxycycline decreases tumor burden in a bone metastasis model of human breast cancer. *Cancer Res.* **2002**, *62*, 1588–1591. [PubMed]
12. Hadad, G.M.; El-Gindy, A.; Mahmoud, W.M.M. HPLC and chemometrics-assisted UV-spectroscopy methods for the simultaneous determination of ambroxol and doxycycline in capsule. *Spectrochim. Acta Part A Mol. Biomol. Spectrosc.* **2008**, *70*, 655–663. [CrossRef] [PubMed]
13. Šatínský, D.; Dos Santos, L.M.L.; Sklenářová, H.; Solich, P.; Montenegro, M.C.B.S.M.; Araújo, A.N. Sequential injection chromatographic determination of ambroxol hydrochloride and doxycycline in pharmaceutical preparations. *Talanta* **2005**, *68*, 214–218. [CrossRef] [PubMed]
14. Sun, X.X.; Aboul-Enein, H.Y. Internal solid contact sensor for the determination of doxycycline hydrochloride in pharmaceutical formulation. *Talanta* **2002**, *58*, 387–396. [CrossRef]
15. Abadian, P.N.; Kelley, C.P.; Goluch, E.D. Cellular analysis and detection using surface plasmon resonance techniques. *Anal. Chem.* **2014**, *86*, 2799–2812. [CrossRef] [PubMed]
16. Špringer, T.; Homola, J. Biofunctionalized gold nanoparticles for SPR-biosensor-based detection of CEA in blood plasma. *Anal. Bioanal. Chem.* **2012**, *404*, 2869–2875. [CrossRef] [PubMed]
17. Li, Q.; Dou, X.; Zhang, L.; Zhao, X.; Luo, J.; Yang, M. Oriented assembly of surface plasmon resonance biosensor through staphylococcal protein A for the chlorpyrifos detection. *Anal. Bioanal. Chem.* **2019**, *411*, 6057–6066. [CrossRef]
18. Liedberg, B.; Nylander, C.; Lunström, I. Surface plasmon resonance for gas detection and biosensing. *Sens. Actuators* **1983**, *4*, 299–304. [CrossRef]
19. Masson, J.F. Surface Plasmon Resonance Clinical Biosensors for Medical Diagnostics. *ACS Sens.* **2017**, *2*, 16–30. [CrossRef]
20. Yuan, H.; Ji, W.; Chu, S.; Qian, S.; Wang, F.; Masson, J.F.; Han, X.; Peng, W. Fiber-optic surface plasmon resonance glucose sensor enhanced with phenylboronic acid modified Au nanoparticles. *Biosens. Bioelectron.* **2018**, *117*, 637–643. [CrossRef]
21. Mariani, S.; Minunni, M. Surface plasmon resonance applications in clinical analysis. *Anal. Bioanal. Chem.* **2014**, *406*, 2303–2323. [CrossRef] [PubMed]
22. Bocková, M.; Chadtová Song, X.; Gedeonová, E.; Levová, K.; Kalousová, M.; Zima, T.; Homola, J. Surface plasmon resonance biosensor for detection of pregnancy associated plasma protein A2 in clinical samples. *Anal. Bioanal. Chem.* **2016**, *408*, 7265–7269. [CrossRef] [PubMed]
23. Zhao, S.S.; Bukar, N.; Toulouse, J.L.; Pelechacz, D.; Robitaille, R.; Pelletier, J.N.; Masson, J.F. Miniature multi-channel SPR instrument for methotrexate monitoring in clinical samples. *Biosens. Bioelectron.* **2015**, *64*, 664–670. [CrossRef]
24. Brulé, T.; Granger, G.; Bukar, N.; Deschênes-Rancourt, C.; Havard, T.; Schmitzer, A.R.; Martel, R.; Masson, J.F. A field-deployed surface plasmon resonance (SPR) sensor for RDX quantification in environmental waters. *Analyst* **2017**, *142*, 2161–2168. [CrossRef] [PubMed]
25. Herranz, S.; Bocková, M.; Marazuela, M.D.; Homola, J.; Moreno-Bondi, M.C. An SPR biosensor for the detection of microcystins in drinking water. *Anal. Bioanal. Chem.* **2010**, *398*, 2625–2634. [CrossRef] [PubMed]
26. Pilolli, R.; Visconti, A.; Monaci, L. Rapid and label-free detection of egg allergen traces in wines by surface plasmon resonance biosensor. *Anal. Bioanal. Chem.* **2015**, *407*, 3787–3797. [CrossRef] [PubMed]
27. McGrath, T.F.; Elliott, C.T.; Fodey, T.L. Biosensors for the analysis of microbiological and chemical contaminants in food. *Anal. Bioanal. Chem.* **2012**, *403*, 75–92. [CrossRef] [PubMed]

28. Graybill, R.M.; Bailey, R.C. Emerging Biosensing Approaches for microRNA Analysis. *Anal. Chem.* **2016**, *88*, 431–450. [CrossRef] [PubMed]
29. Chang, Y.F.; Wang, W.H.; Hong, Y.W.; Yuan, R.Y.; Chen, K.H.; Huang, Y.W.; Lu, P.L.; Chen, Y.H.; Chen, Y.M.A.; Su, L.C.; et al. Simple Strategy for Rapid and Sensitive Detection of Avian Influenza A H7N9 Virus Based on Intensity-Modulated SPR Biosensor and New Generated Antibody. *Anal. Chem.* **2018**, *90*, 1861–1869. [CrossRef]
30. Jabbari, S.; Dabirmanesh, B.; Arab, S.S.; Amanlou, M.; Daneshjou, S.; Gholami, S.; Khajeh, K. A novel enzyme based SPR-biosensor to detect bromocriptine as an ergoline derivative drug. *Sens. Actuators B Chem.* **2017**, *240*, 519–527. [CrossRef]
31. Carrascosa, L.G.; Calle, A.; Lechuga, L.M. Label-free detection of DNA mutations by SPR: Application to the early detection of inherited breast cancer. *Anal. Bioanal. Chem.* **2009**, *393*, 1173–1182. [CrossRef] [PubMed]
32. Xue, C.S.; Erika, G.; Jiří, H. Surface plasmon resonance biosensor for the ultrasensitive detection of bisphenol A. *Anal. Bioanal. Chem.* **2019**, *411*, 5655–5658. [CrossRef] [PubMed]
33. Wang, J.; Zhou, H.S. Aptamer-based Au nanoparticles-enhanced surface plasmon resonance detection of small molecules. *Anal. Chem.* **2008**, *80*, 7174–7178. [CrossRef] [PubMed]
34. Kazmi, S.A.R.; Qureshi, M.Z.; Ali, S.; Masson, J.F. In Vitro Drug Release and Biocatalysis from pH-Responsive Gold Nanoparticles Synthesized Using Doxycycline. *Langmuir* **2019**, *35*, 16266–16274. [CrossRef]
35. Frederix, F.; Friedt, J.M.; Choi, K.H.; Laureyn, W.; Campitelli, A.; Mondelaers, D.; Maes, G.; Borghst, G. Biosensing Based on Light Absorption of Nanoscaled Gold and Silver Particles. *Anal. Chem.* **2003**, *75*, 6894–6900. [CrossRef]
36. Yockell-Lelièvre, H.; Bukar, N.; McKeating, K.S.; Arnaud, M.; Cosin, P.; Guo, Y.; Dupret-Carruel, J.; Mougin, B.; Masson, J.F. Plasmonic sensors for the competitive detection of testosterone. *Analyst* **2015**, *140*, 5105–5111. [CrossRef]
37. Kelly, K.L.; Coronado, E.; Zhao, L.L.; Schatz, G.C. The optical properties of metal nanoparticles: The influence of size, shape, and dielectric environment. *J. Phys. Chem. B* **2003**, *107*, 668–677. [CrossRef]
38. Uludag, Y.; Tothill, I.E. Cancer biomarker detection in serum samples using surface plasmon resonance and quartz crystal microbalance sensors with nanoparticle signal amplification. *Anal. Chem.* **2012**, *84*, 5898–5904. [CrossRef]
39. Špringer, T.; Ermini, M.L.; Špačková, B.; Jabloňků, J.; Homola, J. Enhancing sensitivity of surface plasmon resonance biosensors by functionalized gold nanoparticles: Size matters. *Anal. Chem.* **2014**, *86*, 10350–10356. [CrossRef]
40. Sapsford, K.E.; Tyner, K.M.; Dair, B.J.; Deschamps, J.R.; Medintz, I.L. Analyzing nanomaterial bioconjugates: A review of current and emerging purification and characterization techniques. *Anal. Chem.* **2011**, *83*, 4453–4488. [CrossRef]
41. Bolduc, O.R.; Lambert-Lanteigne, P.; Colin, D.Y.; Zhao, S.S.; Proulx, C.; Boeglin, D.; Lubell, W.D.; Pelletier, J.N.; Féthière, J.; Ong, H.; et al. Modified peptide monolayer binding His-tagged biomolecules for small ligand screening with SPR biosensors. *Analyst* **2011**, *136*, 3142–3148. [CrossRef] [PubMed]
42. Herizchi, R.; Abbasi, E.; Milani, M.; Akbarzadeh, A. Current methods for synthesis of gold nanoparticles. *Artif. Cells Nanomed. Biotechnol.* **2016**, *44*, 596–602. [CrossRef] [PubMed]
43. He, P.; Shen, L.; Liu, R.; Luo, Z.; Li, Z. Direct detection of β-agonists by use of gold nanoparticle-based colorimetric assays. *Anal. Chem.* **2011**, *83*, 6988–6995. [CrossRef] [PubMed]
44. Raza, A.; Javed, S.; Qureshi, M.Z.; Khan, M.U.; Khan, M.S. Synthesis and study of catalytic application of l-methionine protected gold nanoparticles. *Appl. Nanosci.* **2017**, *7*, 429–437. [CrossRef]
45. Zhang, J.J.; Gu, M.M.; Zheng, T.T.; Zhu, J.J. Synthesis of gelatin-stabilized gold nanoparticles and assembly of carboxylic single-walled carbon nanotubes/Au composites for cytosensing and drug uptake. *Anal. Chem.* **2009**, *81*, 6641–6648. [CrossRef] [PubMed]
46. Divakaran, D.; Lakkakula, J.R.; Thakur, M.; Kumawat, M.K.; Srivastava, R. Dragon fruit extract capped gold nanoparticles: Synthesis and their differential cytotoxicity effect on breast cancer cells. *Mater. Lett.* **2019**, *236*, 498–502. [CrossRef]
47. Srivastava, S.K.; Gupta, B.D. Influence of ions on the surface plasmon resonance spectrum of a fiber optic refractive index sensor. *Sens. Actuators B Chem.* **2011**, *156*, 559–562. [CrossRef]

48. Bukar, N.; Zhao, S.S.; Charbonneau, D.M.; Pelletier, J.N.; Masson, J.F. Influence of the Debye length on the interaction of a small molecule-modified Au nanoparticle with a surface-bound bioreceptor. *Chem. Commun.* **2014**, *50*, 4947–4950. [CrossRef]
49. Mitchell, J.S.; Wu, Y.; Cook, C.J.; Main, L. Sensitivity enhancement of surface plasmon resonance biosensing of small molecules. *Anal. Biochem.* **2005**, *343*, 125–135. [CrossRef]
50. Shen, L.; Chen, J.; Li, N.; He, P.; Li, Z. Rapid colorimetric sensing of tetracycline antibiotics with in situ growth of gold nanoparticles. *Anal. Chim. Acta* **2014**, *839*, 83–90. [CrossRef]
51. Agwuh, K.N.; MacGowan, A. Pharmacokinetics and pharmacodynamics of the tetracyclines including glycylcyclines. *J. Antimicrob. Chemother.* **2006**, *58*, 256–265. [CrossRef] [PubMed]
52. Jeyabaskaran, M.; Rambabu, C.; Sree Janardhanan, V.; Rajinikanth, V.; Pranitha, T.; Dhanalakshmi, B. RP-HPLC method development and validation of doxycycline in bulk and tablet formulation. *Int. J. Pharm. Anal. Res.* **2014**, *3*, 397–404.
53. Adrian, J.; Fernández, F.; Sánchez-Baeza, F.; Marco, M.P. Preparation of antibodies and development of an enzyme-linked immunosorbent assay (ELISA) for the determination of doxycycline antibiotic in milk samples. *J. Agric. Food Chem.* **2012**, *60*, 3837–3846. [CrossRef] [PubMed]
54. Kogawa, A.C.; Salgado, H.R.N. Quantification of doxycycline hyclate in tablets by HPLC-UV method. *J. Chromatogr. Sci.* **2013**, *51*, 919–925. [CrossRef]
55. Selvadurai, M.; Meyyanathan, S.N. Determination of Doxycycline in Human Plasma by Liquid Chromatography-Mass Spectrometry after Liquid-Liquid Extraction and its Application in Human Pharmacokinetics Studies. *J. Bioequiv. Availab.* **2010**, *02*, 93–97. [CrossRef]
56. Ramesh, P.; Basavaiah, K.; Tharpa, K.; Basavaiah, K.; Revanasiddappa, H.D. Development and validation of RP-HPLC method for the determination of doxycycline hyclate in spiked human urine and pharmaceuticals. *J. Preclin. Clin. Res.* **2010**, *4*, 101–107.

biosensors

MDPI

Article

Electrochemical Immunosensing of ST2: A Checkpoint Target in Cancer Diseases

Rebeca M. Torrente-Rodríguez [1], Cristina Muñoz-San Martín [1], Maria Gamella [1], María Pedrero [1,*], Neus Martínez-Bosch [2], Pilar Navarro [2,3,4], Pablo García de Frutos [3,4], José M. Pingarrón [1] and Susana Campuzano [1,*]

1 Departamento de Química Analítica, Facultad de CC. Químicas, Universidad Complutense de Madrid, 28040 Madrid, Spain; rebecamt@ucm.es (R.M.T.-R.); cmunoz04@ucm.es (C.M.-S.M.); mariagam@quim.ucm.es (M.G.); pingarro@quim.ucm.es (J.M.P.)
2 Cancer Research Program, Hospital del Mar Medical Research Institute (IMIM), Unidad Asociada IIBB-CSIC, 08003 Barcelona, Spain; nmartinez@imim.es (N.M.-B.); PNavarro@imim.es (P.N.)
3 Departamento de Muerte y Proliferación Celular, Instituto de Investigaciones Biomédicas de Barcelona–Centro Superior de Investigaciones Científicas (IIBB-CSIC), 08036 Barcelona, Spain; pablo.garcia@iibb.csic.es
4 Institut d'Investigacions Biomédiques August Pi i Sunyer (IDIBAPS), 08036 Barcelona, Spain
* Correspondence: mpedrero@quim.ucm.es (M.P.); susanacr@quim.ucm.es (S.C.); Tel.: +34-913-945159 (M.P.); +34-913-944219 (S.C.)

Abstract: A magnetic beads (MB)-involved amperometric immunosensor for the determination of ST2, a member of the IL1 receptor family, is reported in this work. The method utilizes a sandwich immunoassay and disposable screen-printed carbon electrodes (SPCEs). Magnetic immunoconjugates built on the surface of carboxylic acid-microsized magnetic particles (HOOC-MBs) were used to selectively capture ST2. A biotinylated secondary antibody further conjugated with a streptavidin peroxidase conjugate (Strep-HRP) was used to accomplish the sandwiching of the target protein. The immune platform exhibits great selectivity and a low limit of detection (39.6 pg mL^{-1}) for ST2, allowing the determination of soluble ST2 (sST2) in plasma samples from healthy individuals and patients diagnosed with pancreatic ductal adenocarcinoma (PDAC) in only 45 min once the immunoconjugates have been prepared. The good correlation of the obtained results with those provided by an ELISA kit performed using the same immunoreagents demonstrates the potential of the developed strategy for early diagnosis and/or prognosis of the fatal PDAC disease.

Keywords: electrochemical immune platform; human ST2; plasma; pancreatic cancer

Citation: Torrente-Rodríguez, R.M.; Martín, C.M.-S.; Gamella, M.; Pedrero, M.; Martínez-Bosch, N.; Navarro, P.; García de Frutos, P.; Pingarrón, J.M.; Campuzano, S. Electrochemical Immunosensing of ST2: A Checkpoint Target in Cancer Diseases. *Biosensors* **2021**, *11*, 202. https://doi.org/10.3390/bios11060202

Received: 29 May 2021
Accepted: 16 June 2021
Published: 21 June 2021

1. Introduction

IL1RL1/IL33R encodes a member of the interleukin 1 receptor family known as ST2 (or IL-33R), which consists of a transmembrane receptor (ST2L) and truncates soluble (sST2) isoforms. ST2 has well-known relations with inflammatory diseases; elevated circulating levels of sST2 are found in the serum of patients suffering from several disorders such as systemic lupus erythematosus pulmonary fibrosis, rheumatoid arthritis, collagen vascular and asthma, as well as in inflammatory conditions including septic shock or trauma [1–6].

In addition, serum sST2 has been reported as a promising prognostic biomarker to manage cardiovascular diseases [5,7–9] but, as is the case with other biomarkers, sST2 is not only related to cardiovascular diseases. Recent studies have shown that sST2 can be used as a biomarker of hepatic cystic echinococcosis (CE) activity; it has been reported that it can differentially work at the cut-off value of 1246 pg mL^{-1} [10]. Moreover, the survey carried out within the Oulu Project Elucidating Risk of Atherosclerosis (OPERA) dedicated to explore the connections among cardio metabolic risk factors, different diseases, and total mortality, showed higher sST2 levels among subjects suffering from cardiovascular disease, cancer, mild cognitive decline, and diabetes, while elevated sST2 concentrations indicated a worse prognosis and could provide prognostic information on an individual mortality before any particular diagnostic [11]. In addition, it was reported that patients suffering from severity of metabolic syndrome (MetS), which comprises a group of metabolic abnormalities including central obesity, hypertension, diabetes mellitus (DM) or hyperglycaemia, high triglyceride (TG) levels, and low levels of high-density lipoprotein cholesterol (HDL-C), showed high serum sST2 levels, regardless of sex and age [12]. Additionally, the role of sST2 in pathogenesis and prognosis of different types of cancer, such as glioblastoma [13], breast cancer [14], pancreatic cancer [15], and leukaemia [16] has been described. ST2 is considered as a key molecule regulating cell proliferation [6] and exerting a pro-tumorigenic effect on diverse types of cancer, including breast, colon, liver, lung, and pancreatic cancers, among others [17]. Moreover, high ST2 expression has been associated with poor survival and it is considered as a potential target for colorectal cancer immunotherapy [18]. A study with chemotherapy-treated advanced pancreatic ductal adenocarcinoma (PDAC) patients showed that sST2-plasma levels lower than 13,064 pg mL^{-1} were related to higher overall survival (16 months) than those over the median (4 months) [19]. Increased levels of sST2 correlating with severity have also been reported in plasma samples from patients with pancreatitis [20], a risk factor for PDAC initiation.

The evaluation of sST2 levels is generally undertaken using enzyme-linked immunosorbent assays (ELISA), sometimes limited by their low sensitivity and poor precision [5]. However, the ELISA assay reported in 2009 by Dieplinger et al. [3], known as Presage® ST2, has been suggested as the only one to be used clinically [5], due to its high precision, sensitivity, and in vitro stability, with a limit of detection (LOD) <2 ng mL^{-1} [21]. Only two more methods for the determination of ST2 have been reported. One consisted of the production of molecularly imprinted polymer nanoparticles (nanoMIPs) used as synthetic antibodies for ST2 and using surface plasmon resonance (SPR), providing a LOD of 8.79 ng mL^{-1} [22]. The second method was an impedimetric immunosensor using a fullerene C60-modified disposable graphite paper electrode allowing a low LOD of 0.124 fg mL^{-1}. However, the impedimetric immunosensor needed more than 14 h for preparation, followed by 30 min for antigen incubation before measurement [23].

In this paper, we describe a simple, sensitive, specific, precise, and fast electrochemical immunoassay for the determination of ST2. The method was successfully applied to the analysis of sST2 in human plasma from healthy individuals and from patients diagnosed with PDAC. The target analyte in the plasma samples was specifically captured with immunoconjugates prepared on the surface of MBs, sandwiched with a biotinylated detector antibody (btn-DAb), and labelled with a Strep-HRP conjugate. SPCEs were used as amperometric transductors to detect the activity of the enzyme magnetically captured at the surface of the working electrode in the presence of H_2O_2 and hydroquinone (HQ).

2. Materials and Methods

2.1. *Apparatus and Electrodes*

A CHI812B potentiostat (CH Instruments, Inc., Austin, TX, USA) operated by the software CHI812B was used for the electrochemical measurements. Screen-printed carbon electrodes (SPCEs, DRP-110) and the mandatory cable connector (DRP-CAC) were purchased from Methrom Hispania, S.I., (Madrid, Spain). A magnetic concentrator (DynaMag™-2, 123.21D, Invitrogen Dynal AS, Carlsbad, CA, USA) was used to efficiently separate and handle MBs. Other instruments employed include: a constant temperature incubator shaker (Optic Ivymen® System, Comecta S.A, Scharlab, Madrid, Spain), a magnetic stirrer (Inbea S.L.), a Vortex Bunsen AGT-9, a Basic pH-meter (Basic 20+, Crison, Barcelona, Spain), and a homemade polymethacrylate (PMMA) casing with a neodymium magnet (AIMAN GZ) embedded. ELISA flat-bottom plates and a Magellan V 7.1 (TECAN) ELISA plate reader were used to compare the results obtained with the developed electrochemical immune platform.

2.2. Materials and Reagents

MBs functionalized with carboxylic acid groups (HOOC-MBs, 2.7 μm Ø 10 mg mL^{-1}, Dynabeads® M-270 carboxylic acid, Cat. No: 14305D) were acquired from Invitrogen-Thermo Fisher. Furthermore, 2-(N-morpholino) ethanesulfonic acid (MES), sodium chloride, potassium chloride, sodium dihydrogen phosphate, di-sodium hydrogen phosphate, and Tris-hydroxymethyl-aminomethane-HCl (Tris-HCl) from Scharlab were used. N-(3-dimethyl-aminopropyl)-N′-ethylcabodiimide (EDC), N-hydroxysulfosuccinimide (Sulfo-NHS), ethanolamine, Tween® 20, hydroquinone (HQ), and hydrogen peroxide (H_2O_2, 30% w/v) were purchased from Sigma-Aldrich. Blocker casein solution (BB) (consisting of a 1% w/v purified casein PBS solution, pH 7.4) from Thermo Scientific was used. Anti-ST2 murine monoclonal capture antibody (anti-ST2-CAb), recombinant human ST2 standard, and goat anti-human ST2 detector antibody modified with biotin (btn-DAb) were used; all of which were included in the Human ST2/IL-33R DuoSet® ELISA (Cat. No: DY523B-05, R&D Systems, Inc.). Human hemoglobin (Hb), human serum albumin, (HSA) and IgG from human serum were purchased from Sigma-Aldrich. Streptavidin peroxidase conjugate (Strep-HRP) from Roche Diagnostics GmbH was used.

Next, 0.05 M of pH 6.0 phosphate buffer, 0.1 M of pH 8.0 phosphate buffer, pH 7.4 phosphate-buffered saline (PBS), 0.025 M of pH 5.0 MES buffer, and 0.1 M of pH 7.2 Tris−HCl buffer solutions were prepared with deionized water from a Millipore Milli-Q purification system (18.2 MΩ cm).

2.3. Preparation of the Magnetic Immunoconjugates and Electrochemical Readout

The protocol for the biofunctionalization of the MBs was carried out under continuous stirring (950 rpm) at 25 °C. A 3 μL-aliquot of the commercial HOOC-MBs solution was deposited into a 1.5 mL centrifuge tube and, after the two washing steps with 50 μL of MES buffer for 10 min, the surface carboxylic groups of the MBs were activated with 25 μL of a 50 mg mL^{-1} mixture solution of EDC/Sulfo-NHS prepared in MES buffer for 35 min. Once activated, the beads were washed twice with 50 μL MES buffer and incubated with 25 μL of a 10 μg mL^{-1} anti-ST2-CAb solution in MES buffer for 15 min. Thereafter, the blocking of the activated free remaining MBs sites was made with 25 μL of 1 M ethanolamine solution prepared in 0.1 M of phosphate buffer at a pH of 8.0, for 60 min. The modified beads were then washed twice with 50 μL of 0.1 M Tris-HCl buffer at a pH of 7.2, and once more with 50 μL of BB. Subsequently, they were incubated in a 25 μL-aliquot of human ST2 standard (or the properly diluted plasma sample to be analyzed) in BB for 15 min. Thereafter, the modified beads were washed twice with 50 μL of BB and incubation with 25 μL of a mixture solution containing 1.0 μg mL^{-1} btn-DAb and 1:1000 diluted Strep-HRP conjugate, prepared in BB, and accomplished for 30 min to form the sandwich immunocomplexes. Two latter additional washings with 50 μL BB were finally made.

The as-modified MBs were re-suspended in 0.05 M of pH 6.0 sodium phosphate buffer (50 μL) and magnetically concentrated by drop-casting onto the WE surface of the SPCE previously placed into the PMMA casing. The embedded magnet was positioned just below the carbon working electrode of the SPCE to ensure the reproducible capture of the modified MBs onto the working electrode surface. The ensemble SPCE/magnet holding block was connected to the electrochemical station through the cable connector and immersed into an electrochemical cell containing 10mL of the same buffer solution and 1.0 mM of freshly prepared HQ. Amperometric readings in stirred solutions were recorded at−0.20 V (vs. Ag pseudo-reference electrode) upon the addition of 50 μL of a fresh 0.1 M H_2O_2 solution. The provided signals correspond to the difference between the steady-state and the background currents, the error bars having been estimated as the triple of the standard deviation of three replicates (confidence intervals calculated for $\alpha = 0.05$).

2.4. Analysis of sST2 in Plasma

The developed immunosensor was used to determine the sST2 concentration in plasma samples, both from healthy individuals and PDAC-diagnosed patients. These samples were provided by the Hospital del Mar Medical Research Institute (IMIM) and approved by the corresponding ethical permission (IMIM 2020/9067/I). Signed informed consent from all the involved subjects, were obtained.

Due to the demonstrated absence of the matrix effect, quantification was performed by simple interpolation of the amperometric responses provided by the immunosensor for plasma samples diluted 25-fold or 50-fold for healthy subjects or PDAC patients, respectively, into the calibration plot constructed with ST2 standards.

In addition, the same samples were analyzed by applying the ELISA method which used the same immunoreagents according to the previously reported protocol [24] with minor modifications (1.0 $\mu g\,mL^{-1}$ anti-ST2-CAb solution, prepared in PBS; 200 $ng\,mL^{-1}$ btn-DAb solution (in Reagent Diluent solution), and Strep-HRP prepared by diluting 40 times with Reagent Diluent solution the solution provided in the commercial kit). The absorbance values obtained for plasma samples that were 25-times diluted from healthy individuals and 100-times diluted from PDAC patients were interpolated into the calibration graph constructed with ST2 standards.

3. Results

Figure 1a schematically shows the developed platform involving magnetic immunocarriers prepared by the covalent immobilization of a specific capture antibody (anti-ST2-CAb) onto HOOC-MBs, which selectively capture ST2. This protein was subsequently recognized with a specific biotinylated detector antibody (btn-DAb) which was enzymatically labeled with a (Strep-HRP) polymer. Amperometric detection at –0.20 V (*vs.* Ag pseudo-reference electrode) was performed onto SPCEs where the MBs bearing the sandwich immunocomplexes were magnetically located using a magnet-holding block. The bioaffinity reactions taking place on the surface of the immunocarriers were evaluated in the presence of HQ as a redox mediator, using H_2O_2 as an enzymatic substrate (Figure 1b). The recorded cathodic current was proportional to the target protein level (Figure 1c).

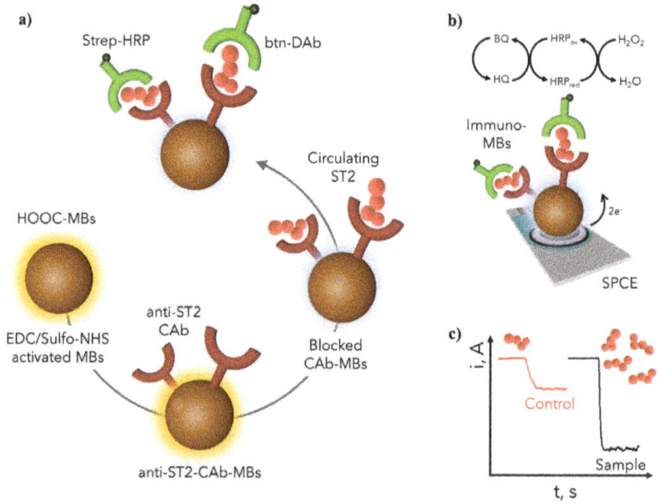

Figure 1. Preparation of the MB-based immunosensor for the determination of ST2. (**a**) Steps involved in the sandwich immunoassay; (**b**) Electrochemical transducer and reactions involved in the amperometric readout; (**c**) Example of amperometric traces recorded for control and high ST2 content samples.

3.1. Optimization of Experimental Variables

The fundamentals of the proposed immune platform were verified by comparing the amperometric responses measured using both unmodified MBs and anti-ST2-CAb-MBs in the presence of 0.0 (B) and 1000 pg mL^{-1} (S) ST2 standards, as well as the corresponding S/B ratio values. To ensure that the variation in the S/B ratio values was related only to the presence and concentration of ST2, the same buffer solution (BB) was used to perform both S and B measurements. Figure 2a confirmed negligible non-specific adsorptions of ST2, Strep-HRP and btn-DAb when no specific anti-ST2-CAb was attached onto the HOOC-MBs, confirming the rationale of the proposed sandwich-based immunoassay.

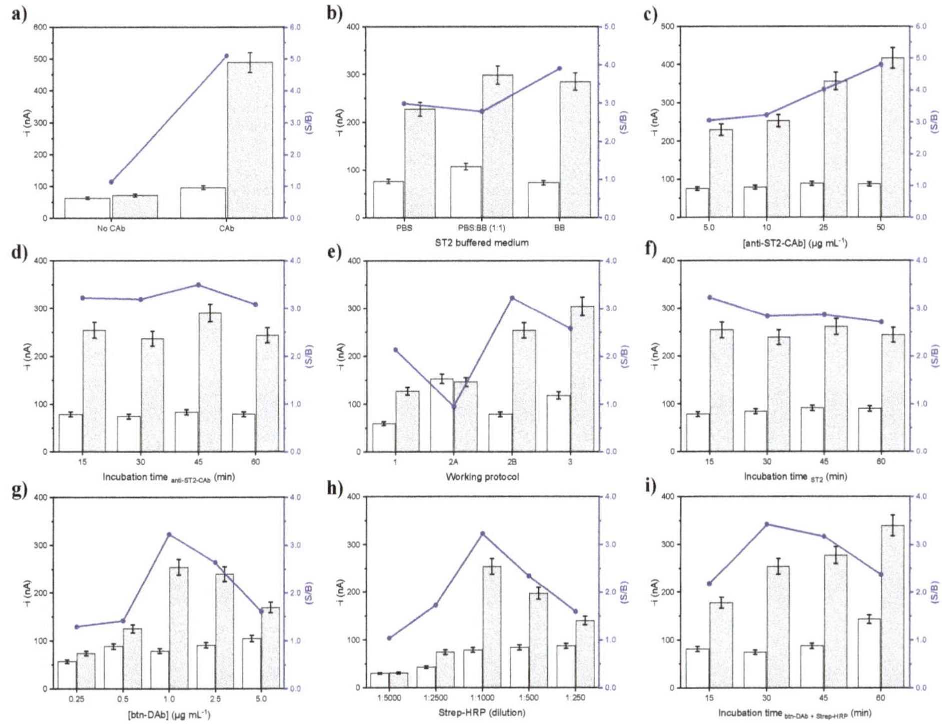

Figure 2. Feasibility of the immunosensor design (**a**), and effect of the working variables on the amperometric response provided by the developed immune platform (**b–i**): (**b**) different buffered medium for the preparation of ST2 standard solutions; (**c**) concentration and (**d**) incubation time of anti-ST2-CAb; (**e**) steps involved in the working protocol; (**f**) incubation time with ST2; (**g**) concentration of btn-DAb; (**h**) Strep-HRP dilution; and (**i**) incubation time of the mixture containing btn-DAb and Strep-HRP. Amperometric responses measured in the presence of 0.0 (white bars) and 1000 (**a**) or 500 (**b–i**) (grey bars) pg mL^{-1} ST2 and the resulting signal-to-blank ratios ((S/B), blue dots and lines).

The main experimental variables involved in the preparation and performance of the immune platform were optimized. The comparison of the amperometric measurements (–0.20 V vs. the Ag pseudo-reference electrode) in the absence (B) and in the presence of 500 pg mL^{-1} (S) ST2, according to the S/B ratio, was taken as the selection criterion. The amount of magnetic micro-carriers and the variables involved in the amperometric detection, including the detection potential, the pH, and composition of the supporting electrolyte and the concentrations of H_2O_2 and HQ, were the same as those optimized in previous works [25,26]. The selected pH value of 6.0 [26] agrees with the optimum pH range (6.0–6.5) reported for HRP [27]. The study of the applied potential influence on the amperometric detection at SPCEs using the HRP/H_2O_2/HQ system in 0.05 M of pH 6.0 sodium phosphate buffer led to the selection of a potential value of −0.20 V as appropriate to achieve good sensitivity and precision [25,26].

The tested ranges for each variable as well as the selected values are summarized in Table 1, while the obtained results are displayed in Figure 2b–i.

Table 1. Assessed experimental variables optimized for the ST2 immunosensor development.

Variable	Tested Range	Selected Value
ST2 standard buffered medium	PBS; PBS:BB; BB	BB
[anti-ST2-CAb] (μg mL^{-1})	0.0–50	10
Incubation time $_{\text{anti-ST2 CAb}}$ (min)	15–60	15
Number of steps for the assay	1–3	2
Incubation time $_{\text{ST2}}$ (min)	15–60	15
[btn-DAb] (μg mL^{-1})	0.25–5.0	1.0
Strep-HRP dilution	1:250–1:5000	1:1000
Incubation time $_{\text{btn-DAb + Strep-HRP}}$ (min)	15–60	30

Figure 2b shows the effect of the buffer solution composition on the ST2 recognition and non-specific adsorptions. BB, PBS, and a (1:1) PBS:BB mixture were tested, with a larger S/B ratio observed when using BB, which was selected as a buffer medium to carry out the assay.

The amperometric responses in the presence of ST2 increased with the concentration of the specific anti-ST2-CAb solution to be immobilized onto the surface of the MBs, while there was no significant variation in the B response (Figure 2c). Nevertheless, a concentration of 10 μg mL^{-1} anti-ST2-CAb was chosen for further work because of the sufficiently large S/B ratio achieved and to improve the assay affordability. It is clear that if higher sensitivity for ST2 determination was required, 50 μg mL^{-1} anti-ST2-CAb can be used. As it is observed in Figure 2d, an incubation time of 15 min was enough for the immobilization of the anti-ST2-CAb onto the activated MBs.

The number of steps involved in the assay was optimized by checking different working protocols, requiring different stages of incubation in solutions of different composition, all of these started from the prepared anti-ST2-CAb-MBs: (1) a protocol involving three successive incubation steps with the ST2 standard (30 min), btn-DAb (30 min), and Strep-HRP (15 min) solutions; (2A) a protocol involving two successive steps involving incubations in a mixture solution containing ST2 standard and btn-DAb (30 min), and in a Strep-HRP solution (30 min); (2B) a protocol involving two successive steps consisting of incubation with the ST2 standard solution (30 min) followed by another incubation in a btn-DAb/Strep-HRP mixture solution (30 min); and (3) a protocol involving a single incubation in a mixture solution containing the ST2 standard, btn-DAb, and Strep-HRP (30 min). Figure 2e shows that larger S/B ratios were reached for protocols 2B and 3, probably due to an improved efficiency in biorecognition events when the reagents are in homogeneous solution. As evidenced, a better S/B ratio was reached when ST2 was first captured on the anti-ST2-CAb-MBs, and subsequently incubated in a btn-DAb and Strep-HRP mixture solution (Figure 2e, bars 2B). From this result we can deduce that when target ST2 is firstly captured by the detector antibody, the effect of steric hindrance of the ST2-btn-DAb complex is more apparent in hampering the efficient recognition by the anti-ST2-CAb modified MBs. Therefore, this two-step working protocol (protocol 2B) was selected for further work. According to this optimized protocol, the time required for the complete modification of the MBs, and therefore for the preparation of the biosensor and the determination, is 175 min. However, it should be noted that the biosensor can be prepared, or the determination performed in as little as 45 min if starting from anti-ST2-

CAb-MBs, which, according to the results discussed in Section 3.2, are stable for at least 22 days.

Figure 2g,h display the effect of btn-DAb and Strep-HRP concentration on the immunosensor response, respectively. The S/B ratio increased with btn-DAb concentration up to 1.0 μg mL^{-1} and progressively decreased for larger concentrations due to the slight increase in the blank signal (B) and the decrease in the specific response in the presence of ST2 (S), which can be explained because of a hindered molecular recognition in the presence of large btn-DAb amounts. As expected, smaller S/B ratio values were obtained when low Strep-HRP tracer was loaded onto the modified MBs (Figure 2h). According to Figures 2f and 2i, incubation times of 15 and 30 min, were selected for capturing ST2 and for its simultaneous recognition and labeling through the HRP-Strep-btn-DAb mixture, respectively.

3.2. Calibration Curves and Analytical Characteristics of the Immune Platform

Calibration graphs for ST2 constructed with immune platforms were prepared with either a 10 or 50 μg mL^{-1} capture antibody and loaded onto the magnetic microcarriers (Figure 3a,b).

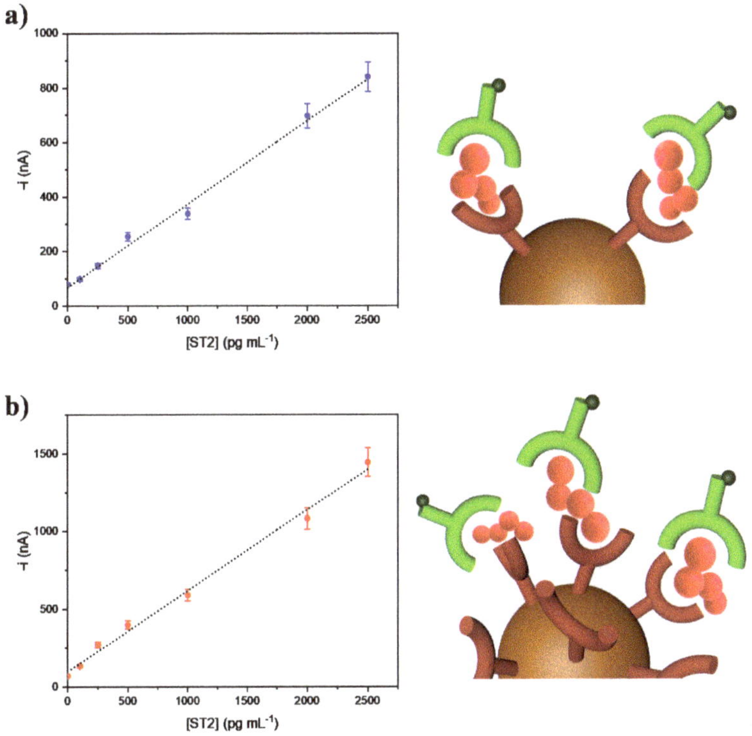

Figure 3. Calibration curves constructed for the amperometric determination of ST2 with immune platforms prepared from MBs modified with (**a**) 10 μg mL^{-1} or (**b**) 50 μg mL^{-1} anti-ST2-CAb solutions. Comparative fictitious pictures of the anti-ST2-CAb loading onto the magnetic immunoconjugates are also shown.

The amperometric responses increased with the ST2 concentration over the 141 to 2500 pg mL^{-1} and 76 to 2500 pg mL^{-1} ranges for the immunosensors prepared using 10 or 50 μg mL^{-1} anti-ST2-CAb solutions, respectively. According to the $3 \times s_b/m$ criterion, where

s_b is the standard deviation for 10 amperometric measurements in the absence of ST2, and m is the slope of the corresponding linear calibration plot, LODs of 39.6 and 26.7 pg mL^{-1}, respectively, were calculated. Besides, as expected, an increase in the sensitivity (0.52 nA mL pg^{-1} *vs.* 0.30 nA mL pg^{-1}) was apparent when using the larger loading of anti-ST2-CAb on the MBs. Importantly, both LODs values were significantly lower than the reference intervals reported for sST2 in human plasma and serum from males (11–45 ng mL^{-1} and 8.6–49.3 ng mL^{-1}) and females (9–35 ng mL^{-1} and 7.32–33.5 ng mL^{-1}) [28,29].

Compared with the only two (bio)sensors reported to date for ST2 determination, an extremely low LOD was claimed for the impedimetric immunosensor (0.124 fg mL^{-1}). However, the method, involving disposable graphite paper electrodes coated with fullerene C60, took more than 14 h, and was applied to the analysis of spiked serum samples from healthy individuals [23]. The proof of concept SPR sensor using affinity MIP nanoparticles achieved a LOD value of 8.79 ng mL^{-1} and was just applied to the analysis of spiked fetal bovine serum [22].

The developed immune platform can be prepared in 3 h without tedious synthesis procedures, and has an acceptable reproducibility (RSD value of 6.4% for the measurements of 500 pg mL^{-1} ST2 carried out with five biosensors prepared in the same manner and tested the same day), and great stability (no significant differences in terms of S/B ratio values were observed for amperometric measurements of 0.0 and 1000 pg mL^{-1} ST2 with immune platforms prepared from anti-ST2-CAb-MBs immunoconjugates which were stored in filtered PBS at 4 °C for at least 22 days, as seen in Figure 4).

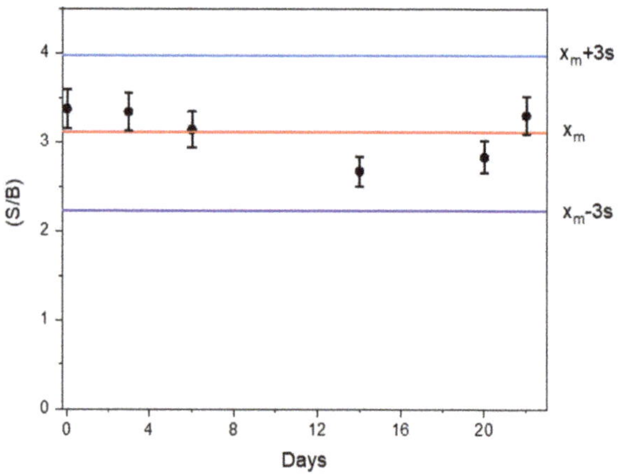

Figure 4. Stability of anti-ST2-CAb-MBs immunoconjugates stored in filtered PBS at 4 °C after their preparation. S/B ratio values were obtained for 0.0 and 1000 pg mL^{-1} ST2 standards with immune platforms prepared from the stored immunoconjugates each control day. Control limits (blue lines) were set as ±3 s of the mean value obtained the first day of the study (n = 3).

ASPECT-PLUS ST2 test, a commercially available cassette (Critical Diagnostics), allows the performance of a point-of-care test (POCT) for the determination of sST2 in human plasma within a concentration range from 12.5 to 250 ng mL^{-1} [30]. This fast (less than 35 min), quantitative lateral flow immunoassay makes use of murine mouse monoclonal antibodies against human ST2, and goat polyclonal antibodies against murine IgG performing fluorescence detection. Moreover, Dieplinger et al. performed a clinical comparison of the ASPECT-PLUS ST2 test, MBL and PRESAGE ST2 ELISAs. These authors concluded that, despite ASPECT-PLUS meeting the analytical requirements for POCT and providing comparable results to those obtained with the PRESAGE ST2 ELISA kit, there were large variation coefficients, close to 17%, and a considerable high LOD (about 12 ng mL^{-1}), and thus that ASPECT-PLUS is probably not suitable for risk stratification of healthy and/or population-based cohorts with endogenous sST2 levels below this concentration [31]. PRESAGE ST2 and MBL ST2 sandwich-based ELISA kits provided LODs of 1.3 ng mL^{-1} and 32 pg mL^{-1}, respectively, which are comparable to that achieved with the developed amperometric immune platform. However, ELISAs have important comparative limitations in terms of multiplexing ability and portability.

3.3. Selectivity of the ST2 Immune Platform

The responses of the developed immunosensor were checked in the presence of some potential interfering proteins usually found in serum. Amperometric responses were measured for 0.0 (B) and 1000 pg mL^{-1} ST2 (S) in the absence and in the presence of 5 mg mL^{-1} HSA, 1.0 and 0.1 mg mL^{-1} human IgG, and 5 mg mL^{-1} Hb. Figure 5 shows that 1.0 mg mL^{-1} human IgG and HSA significantly affected the immunosensor response. As it is well known, the presence of human anti-mouse antibodies (HAMAs) leads to significant errors in sandwich assay configurations using murine monoclonal antibodies, due to the possible cross-link between them and as they both capture and label detector antibodies in the absence of a target analyte [32]. The interference in the presence of HSA was also observed in an electrochemical aptasensor for the determination of MUC1 [33], as well as between HSA and monoclonal immunoglobulins [34]. It appears that the degree of interference of HSA in immunoassays may be conditioned by its degree of purification, which depends on the presence of IgGs with a wide range of specificities that may perturb the assay.

Moreover, according to specifications of the DY523B-05 DuoSet® ELISA, IL-1α, IL-1β, IL-1rα, IL-1RAcP/Fc chimera, IL-1 RI, IL-1 RII and recombinant mouse ST2/Fc chimera do not exhibit cross-reactivity with the antibodies involved in the immunosensor at a concentration level of 50 ng mL^{-1}, and the recombinant human IL-33 only interferes at concentrations above 97.7 pg mL^{-1}.

It is important to note that, as it is shown in the next section, the interferences observed for high human IgG and HSA did not hinder the reliable determination of sST2 in plasma.

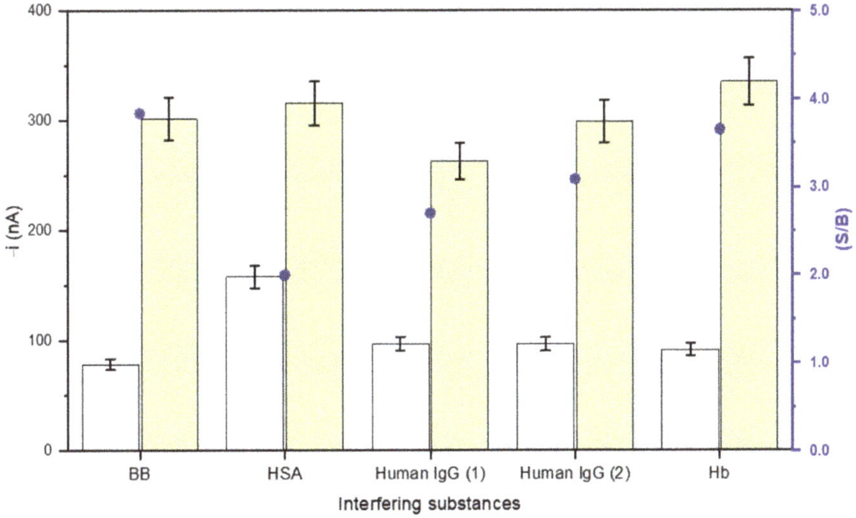

Figure 5. Amperometric measurements carried out with the developed immunosensor in the presence of different serum proteins: 0.0 (white bars) and 1000 pg mL^{-1} (green bars) ST2 standards (and the corresponding S/B ratio, blue dots) prepared in the absence or in the presence of 5.0 mg mL^{-1} HSA, 1.0 and 0.1 mg mL^{-1} human IgG (human IgG (1) and (2), respectively) and 5.0 mg mL^{-1} Hb.

3.4. sST2 determination in Plasma

The determination of sST2 was carried out in plasma from healthy individuals and patients diagnosed with PDAC. The possible matrix effect was assessed by comparing the slope values of the calibration plots prepared with ST2 buffered standard solutions (0.30 ± 0.01 nA mL pg^{-1}) using 10 μg mL^{-1} anti-ST2-CAb, and by adding ST2 standards to a 25-times diluted plasma sample from a healthy individual (0.31 ± 0.06 nA mL pg^{-1}) (Figure 6a). The values calculated using the Student's t-test ($t_{exp} = 0.335 < t_{tab} = 2.571$) showed no significant differences between the slope values for both calibration curves, which means that there were no matrix effects in the diluted sample.

In this regard, the analysis was done by interpolating the amperometric readings for 25 (healthy individuals) or 50 (PDAC patients) times diluted plasma samples into the calibration constructed with standards. Different dilutions were applied to the samples due to the significantly higher concentration of sST2 in those from oncology patients with the aim of obtaining amperometric signals around the midpoint of the linear calibration plot constructed with ST2 standards to minimize the error in the concentration quantification by interpolation. The obtained results are summarized in Table 2, which also includes the results provided by the ELISA methodology for the same samples according to the protocol described in Section 2.4.

Figure 6b shows the results obtained with the immune platform by patient pool. Figure 6c displays representative amperograms from plasma samples of healthy individuals and PDAC patients. In addition, the correlation plot of the results provided by both methodologies are shown in Figure 6d.

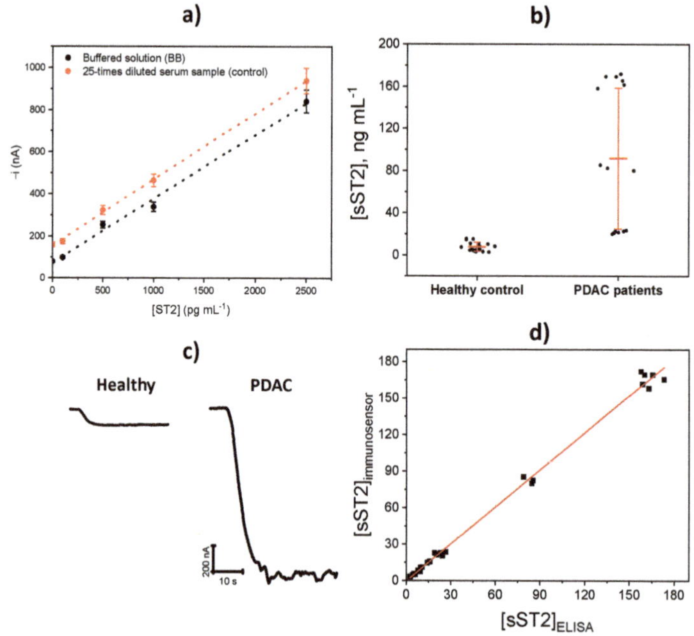

Figure 6. (**a**) Comparison of the calibration plots constructed with ST2 buffered standard solutions and by adding ST2 standards to a 25-times diluted plasma sample from a healthy individual. (**b**) Concentration of sST2 (in ng mL^{-1}) obtained with the developed immune platform in plasma samples grouped into pools. (**c**) Examples of the real amperometric traces recorded with the immune platform for diluted plasma samples (25-times for healthy individuals and 50-times for PDAC patients) for samples 6 (healthy individual) and 9 (PDAC patient) of Table 2. (**d**) Correlation plot for the sST2 concentration values provided by the developed immune platform and the ELISA method (individual replicates performed for the determinations in the 11 plasma samples are included in the plot).

Table 2. Concentration of sST2 (in ng mL^{-1}) obtained from the measurements carried out with the immune platform and the ELISA method in plasma samples.

Subjects	Sample	Immune Platform		ELISA		t_{exp}	t_{tab}
		[sST2] [1]	**$RSD_{n=3}$, %**	**[sST2]** [1]	**$RSD_{n=3}$, %**		
Healthy individuals	1	(5.5 ± 0.8)	6.1	(5 ± 1)	9.3	0.009	2.776
	2	(4.7 ± 0.2)	1.3	(4.4 ± 0.7)	6.8	1.519	
	3	(15 ± 1)	3.6	(15 ± 2)	6.3	0.016	
	4	(3.1 ± 0.6)	7.7	(2.6 ± 0.5)	7.9	2.518	
	5	(10.8 ± 0.7)	2.5	(10 ± 2)	6.6	1.752	
	6	(8 ± 1)	6.0	(8 ± 4)	9.8	0.680	
PDAC patients	7	(168 ± 6)	1.3	(166 ± 28)	3.9	0.468	
	8	(22 ± 2)	3.6	(20 ± 4)	4.5	2.515	
	9	(164 ± 18)	4.4	(160 ± 12)	1.7	0.933	
	10	(83 ± 6)	3.2	(83 ± 15)	4.3	0.098	
	11	(22 ± 4)	8.1	(25 ± 7)	6.9	1.767	

[1] (mean value $\pm t \times s/\sqrt{n}$, n = 3).

As expected, larger average sST2 concentrations were found for PDAC patients. Remarkably, two patients with larger sST2 concentrations (samples 7 and 10 in Table 2) suffered from high-grade metastatic tumors (stage 4) and showed worse prognosis (4.06 and 0.63 months, respectively). These results agree well with data reported by Kieler et al. [19], indicating a significant negative association of sST2 levels in plasma with the median overall survival rates (mOS).

In addition, the statistical comparison shown in Table 2 ($t_{exp} < t_{tab} = 2.776$) and the correlation parameters (slope (1.02 ± 0.02); intercept (0 ± 1) ng mL^{-1}; R^2 =0.996) confirmed the absence of significant differences between the results provided by the developed immune platform and the ELISA method, which is incompatible with decentralized and multiplexed determinations.

4. Conclusions

This work reports a novel immune platform, involving the use of MBs and disposable carbon electrodes, for the simple and rapid (45 min) determination of ST2. Sandwich immunocomplexes labeled with HRP were prepared on the MBs surface and amperometric transduction was performed, upon MBs magnetic capture on the surface of SPCEs. The immune platform exhibits a high sensitivity (LOD value in the low pg mL^{-1} level) and a selectivity compatible with the clinical application. In fact, the immune platform was successfully applied to the analysis of plasma samples from patients diagnosed with PDAC upon a simple dilution and without matrix effect. The obtained results clearly confirmed the usefulness of the developed immune platform and the good agreement with those provided by the ELISA method, thus allowing for the minimally invasive diagnosis of PDAC.

Importantly, considering the reported data on the sST2 expression in several cancers, it is tempting to speculate that the immune platform can also be useful for the diagnosis of other tumors where this protein is overexpressed [17]. Large-scale clinical trials are needed to further evaluate the performance of this method before it can be used for definitive clinical diagnosis and/or prognosis. Nevertheless, the exhibited attributes in terms of versatility, affordable cost, and the ability to perform multiplexed determinations in an endpoint manner at POCT settings, allow envisioning the immune platform translation to the clinic to assist in the identification and/or follow-up of patients with high-prevalence and mortal cancer diseases.

Author Contributions: Conceptualization, R.M.T.-R., M.G., M.P., J.M.P., S.C.; methodology, R.M.T.-R., C.M.-S.M.; investigation, R.M.T.-R., C.M.-S.M.; resources, N.M.-B., P.N., P.G.d.F.; writing—original draft preparation, R.M.T.-R., M.G., M.P., S.C.; writing—review and editing, N.M.-B., P.N., P.G.d.F., J.M.P.; supervision, M.G., M.P., S.C.; funding acquisition, P.N., P.G.d.F., S.C. All authors have read and agreed to the published version of the manuscript.

Funding: This research was funded by Spanish Ministerio de Ciencia e Innovación. PID2019-103899RB-I00, Spanish Ministerio de Ciencia, Innovación y Universidades, RTI2018-095672-B-I00, Comunidad de Madrid, S2018/NMT-4349, and AES-ISCIII/FEDER, PI20/00625.

Institutional Review Board Statement: The study was conducted according to the guidelines of the Declaration of Helsinki and approved by the Institutional Review Board of Hospital del Mar Medical Research Institute (protocol IMIM 2020/9067/I).

Informed Consent Statement: Informed consent was obtained from all subjects involved in the study.

Data Availability Statement: The data that support the findings of this study are available from the corresponding authors upon reasonable request.

Acknowledgments: The financial support of PID2019-103899RB-I00 to S.C. (Spanish Ministerio de Ciencia e Innovación), RTI2018-095672-B-I00 to P.G-F (Spanish Ministerio de Ciencia, Innovación y Universidades) S2018/NMT-4349 to S.C. (Comunidad de Madrid) and PI20/00625 to P.N. (AES-ISCIII/FEDER) Research projects are gratefully acknowledged. C. Muñoz-San Martín acknowledges a predoctoral contract from Complutense University of Madrid. R.M. Torrente-Rodríguez acknowledges Talento-Contract from Comunidad de Madrid (2019-T2/IND-15965).

Conflicts of Interest: The authors declare no conflict of interest.

References

1. Iwahana, H.; Yanagisawa, K.; Ito-Kosaka, A.; Kuroiwa, K.; Tago, K.; Komatsu, N.; Katashima, R.; Itakura, M.; Tominaga, S.-I. Different promoter usage and multiple transcription initiation sites of the interleukin-1 receptor-related human ST2 gene in ut-7 and tm12 cells. *Eur. J. Biochem.* **1999**, *264*, 397–406. [CrossRef]
2. Rehman, S.U.; Mueller, T.; Januzzi, J.L. Characteristics of the novel Interleukin family biomarker ST2 in patients with acute heart failure. *J. Am. Coll. Cardiol.* **2008**, *52*, 1458–6145. [CrossRef] [PubMed]
3. Dieplinger, B.; Januzzi, J.L., Jr.; Steinmair, M.; Gabriel, C.; Poelz, W.; Haltmayer, M.; Mueller, T. Analytical and clinical evaluation of a novel high-sensitivity assay for measurement of soluble ST2 in human plasma—The Presage™ ST2 assay. *Clin. Chim. Acta* **2009**, *409*, 33–40. [CrossRef] [PubMed]
4. Konukoglu, D. Is soluble ST2 a new marker in heart failure? *Int. J. Med. Biochem.* **2018**, *1*, 44–51. [CrossRef]
5. McCarthy, C.P.; Januzzi, J.L., Jr. Soluble ST2 in heart failure. *Heart Fail. Clin.* **2018**, *14*, 41–48. [CrossRef] [PubMed]
6. Kikuchi, M.; Takase, K.; Hayakawa, M.; Hayakawa, H.; Tominaga, S.; Ohmori, T. Altered behavior in mice overexpressing soluble ST2. *Mol. Brain* **2020**, *13*, 74. [CrossRef]
7. Gül, İ.; Yücel, O.; Zararsız, A.; Demirpençe, Ö.; Yücel, H.; Zorlu, A.; Yılmaz, M.B. Prognostic role of soluble suppression of tumorigenicity-2 on cardiovascular mortality in outpatients with heart failure. *Anatol. J. Cardiol.* **2017**, *18*, 200–205. [CrossRef]
8. Bahuleyan, C.G.; Alummoottil, G.K.; Abdullakutty, J.; Lorsdson, A.J.; Babu, S.; Krishnakumar, V.V.; Pillai, A.M.; Abraham, G.; Dilipb, M.N. Prognostic value of soluble ST2 biomarker in heart failure patients with reduced ejection fraction—A multicenter study. *Indian Heart J.* **2018**, *70S*, S79–S84. [CrossRef]
9. Bai, J.; Han, L.; Liu, H. Combined use of high-sensitivity ST2 and NT-proBNP for predicting major adverse cardiovascular events in coronary heart failure. *Ann. Palliat. Med.* **2020**, *9*, 1976–1989. [CrossRef] [PubMed]
10. An, M.; Zhu, Y.; Xu, C.; Li, Y.; Pang, N.; Zhao, X.; Li, Z.; Wang, H.; Zhang, F.; Ding, J. Soluble ST2 (sST2) as potential marker for hepatic cystic echinococcosis activity. *J. Infect.* **2020**, *80*, 462–468. [CrossRef]
11. Filali, Y.; Kesäniemi, Y.A.; Ukkola, O. Soluble ST2, a biomarker of fibrosis, is associated with multiple risk factors, chronic diseases and total mortality in the OPERA study. *Scand. J. Clin. Lab. Investig.* **2021**, *1–8*. [CrossRef]
12. Zong, X.; Fan, Q.; Zhang, H.; Yang, Q.; Xie, H.; Chen, Q.; Zhang, R.; Tao, R. Soluble ST2 levels for predicting the presence and severity of metabolic syndrome. *Endocr. Connect.* **2021**, *10*, 336–344. [CrossRef]
13. Zhang, Y.; Davis, C.; Shah, S.; Hughes, D.; Ryan, J.C.; Altomare, D.; Pena, M.M. IL-33 promotes growth and liver metastasis of colorectal cancer in mice by remodeling the tumor microenvironment and inducing angiogenesis. *Mol. Carcinog.* **2017**, *56*, 272–287. [CrossRef] [PubMed]
14. Jovanovic, I.; Radosavljevic, G.; Mitrovic, M.; Juranic, V.L.; McKenzie, A.N.; Arsenijevic, N.; Jonjic, S.; Lukic, M.L. ST2 deletion enhances innate and acquired immunity to murine mammary carcinoma. *Eur. J. Immunol.* **2011**, *41*, 1902–1912. [CrossRef]
15. Fang, M.; Li, Y.; Huang, K.; Qi, S.; Zhang, J.; Zgodzinski, W.; Majewski, M.; Wallner, G.; Gozdz, S.; Macek, P.; et al. IL33 Promotes colon cancer cell stemness via JNK activation and macrophage recruitment. *Cancer Res.* **2017**, *77*, 2735–2745. [CrossRef] [PubMed]

16. Yoshida, K.; Arai, T.; Yokota, T.; Komatsu, N.; Miura, Y.; Yanagisawa, K.; Tetsuka, T.; Tominaga, S. Studies on natural ST2 gene products in the human leukemic cell line UT-7 using monoclonal antihuman ST2 antibodies. *Hybridoma* **1995**, *14*, 419–427. [CrossRef]
17. Larsen, K.M.; Minaya, M.K.; Vaish, V.; Peña, M.M.O. The role of IL-33/ST2 pathway in tumorigenesis. *Int. J. Mol. Sci.* **2018**, *19*, 2676. [CrossRef] [PubMed]
18. Van der Jeught, K.; Sun, Y.; Fang, Y.; Zhou, Z.; Jiang, H.; Yu, T.; Yang, J.; Kamocka, M.M.; So, K.M.; Li, Y.; et al. ST2 as checkpoint target for colorectal cancer immunotherapy. *JCI Insight* **2020**, *5*, e136073. [CrossRef]
19. Kieler, M.; Unseld, M.; Wojta, J.; Kaider, A.; Bianconi, D.; Demyanets, S.; Prager, G.W. Plasma levels of interleukin-33 and soluble suppression of tumorigenicity 2 in patients with advanced pancreatic ductal adenocarcinoma undergoing systemic chemotherapy. *Med. Oncol.* **2019**, *36*, 1. [CrossRef]
20. Ouziel, R.; Gustot, T.; Moreno, C.; Arvanitakis, M.; Degré, D.; Trépo, E.; Quertinmont, E.; Vercruysse, V.; Demetter, P.; Le Moine, O.; et al. The ST2 pathway is involved in acute pancreatitis. A translational study in humans and mice. *Am. J. Pathol.* **2012**, *180*, 2330–2339. [CrossRef]
21. Mueller, T.; Jaffe, A.S. Soluble ST2-analytical considerations. *Am. J. Cardiol.* **2015**, *115*, 8B–21B. [CrossRef]
22. Crapnell, R.D.; Canfarotta, F.; Czulak, J.; Johnson, R.; Betlem, K.; Mecozzi, F.; Down, M.P.; Eersels, K.; van Grinsven, B.; Cleij, T.J.; et al. Thermal detection of cardiac biomarkers heart-fatty acid binding protein and ST2 using a molecularly imprinted nanoparticle-based multiplex sensor platform. *ACS Sens.* **2019**, *4*, 2838–2845. [CrossRef] [PubMed]
23. Demirbakan, B.; Sezgintürk, M.K. An impedimetric biosensor system based on disposable graphite paper electrodes: Detection of ST2 as a potential biomarker for cardiovascular disease in human serum. *Anal. Chim. Acta* **2021**, *1144*, 43–52. [CrossRef] [PubMed]
24. Munoz-San Martin, C.; Gamella, M.; Pedrero, M.; Montero-Calle, A.; Barderas, R.; Campuzano, S.; Pingarrón, J.M. Magnetic beads-based electrochemical immunosensing of HIF-1α, a biomarker of tumoral hypoxia. *Sens. Actuators B* **2020**, *307*, 127623. [CrossRef]
25. Eguílaz, M.; Moreno-Guzmán, M.; Campuzano, S.; González-Cortés, A.; Yáñez-Sedeño, P.; Pingarrón, J.M. An electrochemical immunosensor for testosterone using functionalized magnetic beads and screen-printed carbon electrodes. *Biosens. Bioelectron.* **2010**, *26*, 517–522. [CrossRef]
26. Conzuelo, F.; Gamella, M.; Campuzano, S.; Pinacho, D.G.; Reviejo, A.J.; Marco, M.P.; Pingarrón, J.M. Disposable and integrated amperometric immunosensor for direct determination of sulfonamide antibiotics in milk. *Biosens. Bioelectron.* **2012**, *36*, 81–88. [CrossRef]
27. Schomberg, D.; Salzmann, M.; Stephan, D. *Enzyme Handbook*; Springer: Berlin/Heidelberg, Germany, 1993; Volume 7, pp. 1–6.
28. Lu, J.; Snider, J.V.; Grenache, D.G. Establishment of reference intervals for soluble ST2 from a United States population. *Clin. Chim. Acta* **2010**, *411*, 1825–1826. [CrossRef] [PubMed]
29. Coglianese, E.E.; Larson, M.G.; Vasan, R.S.; Ho, J.E.; Ghorbani, A.; McCabe, E.L.; Cheng, S.; Fradley, M.G.; Kretschman, D.; Gao, W.; et al. Distribution and clinical correlates of the interleukin receptor family member soluble ST2 in the Framingham heart study. *Clin. Chem.* **2012**, *58*, 1673–1681. [CrossRef]
30. Hartopo, A.B.; Sukmasari, I.; Puspitawati, I. The utility of point of care test for soluble ST2 in predicting adverse cardiac events during acute care of ST-segment elevation myocardial infarction. *Cardiol. Res. Pract.* **2018**, *2018*, 3048941. [CrossRef]
31. Dieplinger, B.; Egger, M.; Gegenhuber, A.; Haltmayer, M.; Mueller, T. Analytical and clinical evaluation of a rapid quantitative lateral flow immunoassay for measurement of soluble ST2 in human plasma. *Clin. Chim. Acta* **2015**, *451*, 310–315. [CrossRef]
32. Melanson, S.E.F.; Tanasijevic, M.J.; Jarolim, P. Cardiac troponin assays: A view from the clinical chemistry laboratory. *Circulation* **2007**, *116*, e501–e504. [CrossRef] [PubMed]
33. Zhao, R.N.; Feng, Z.; Zhao, Y.N.; Jia, L.P.; Ma, R.-N.; Zhang, W.; Shan, L.; Xue, Q.W.; Wang, H.-S. A sensitive electrochemical aptasensor for Mucin 1 detection based on catalytic hairpin assembly coupled with PtPdNPs peroxidase-like activity. *Talanta* **2019**, *200*, 503–510. [CrossRef] [PubMed]
34. Padelli, M.; Labouret, T.; Labarre, M.; Le Reun, E.; Rouillé, A.; Kerspern, H.; Capaldo, C.; Chauvet, J.; Plée-Gautier, E.; Carré, J.L.; et al. Systematic overestimation of human serum albumin by capillary zone electrophoresis method due to monoclonal immunoglobulin interferences. *Clin. Chim. Acta* **2019**, *491*, 74–80. [CrossRef] [PubMed]

biosensors

MDPI

Article

Impedimetric and Plasmonic Sensing of Collagen I Using a Half-Antibody-Supported, Au-Modified, Self-Assembled Monolayer System

Marcin Gwiazda [1,2,3], Sheetal K. Bhardwaj [3,4,*], Ewa Kijeńska-Gawrońska [1,5], Wojciech Swieszkowski [1], Unni Sivasankaran [3] and Ajeet Kaushik [6,*]

1 Faculty of Materials Science and Engineering, Warsaw University of Technology, 141 Woloska Str., 02-507 Warsaw, Poland; marcin.gwiazda@postgrad.manchester.ac.uk (M.G.); ewa.kijenska@pw.edu.pl (E.K.-G.); wojciech.swieszkowski@pw.edu.pl (W.S.)
2 Department of Chemistry, The University of Manchester, Manchester M13 9PL, UK
3 Institute of Animal Reproduction and Food Research, Polish Academy of Sciences, Tuwima 10, 10-748 Olsztyn, Poland; unni.siva.info@gmail.com
4 Van't Hoff Institute for Molecular Sciences, University of Amsterdam Science Park 904, 1098 XH Amsterdam, The Netherlands
5 Centre for Advanced Materials and Technologies CEZAMAT, Poleczki 19, 02-822 Warsaw, Poland
6 NanoBioTech Laboratory, Department of Natural Sciences, Florida Polytechnic University, Lakeland, FL 33805, USA
* Correspondence: sheeturo@gmail.com or s.k.bhardwaj@uva.nl (S.K.B.); ajeet.npl@gmail.com or akaushik@floridapoly.edu (A.K.)

Citation: Gwiazda, M.; Bhardwaj, S.K.; Kijeńska-Gawrońska, E.; Swieszkowski, W.; Sivasankaran, U.; Kaushik, A. Impedimetric and Plasmonic Sensing of Collagen I Using a Half-Antibody-Supported, Au-Modified, Self-Assembled Monolayer System. *Biosensors* **2021**, *11*, 227. https://doi.org/10.3390/bios11070227

Received: 18 May 2021
Accepted: 5 July 2021
Published: 8 July 2021

Abstract: This research presents an electrochemical immunosensor for collagen I detection using a self-assembled monolayer (SAM) of gold nanoparticles (AuNPs) and covalently immobilized half-reduced monoclonal antibody as a receptor; this allowed for the validation of the collagen I concentration through two different independent methods: electrochemically by Electrochemical Impedance Spectroscopy (EIS), and optically by Surface Plasmon Resonance (SPR). The high unique advantage of the proposed sensor is based on the performance of the stable covalent immobilization of the AuNPs and enzymatically reduced half-IgG collagen I antibodies, which ensured their appropriate orientation onto the sensor's surface, good stability, and sensitivity properties. The detection of collagen type I was performed in a concentration range from 1 to 5 pg/mL. Moreover, SPR was utilized to confirm the immobilization of the monoclonal half-antibodies and sensing of collagen I versus time. Furthermore, EIS experiments revealed a limit of detection (LOD) of 0.38 pg/mL. The selectivity of the performed immunosensor was confirmed by negligible responses for BSA. The performed approach of the immunosensor is a novel, innovative attempt that enables the detection of collagen I with very high sensitivity in the range of pg/mL, which is significantly lower than the commonly used enzyme-linked immunosorbent assay (ELISA).

Keywords: collagen type I; 4,4′-thiobisbenzenethiol; nanogold; electrochemical impedance spectroscopy; surface plasmon resonance; half antibody; medical diagnostic devices

1. Introduction

Currently, significant medical developments require the use of modern technologies to continuously monitor a patient's state. Accordingly, it is highly demanded to construct and apply wearable sensors or in situ biomarkers, which are capable of detecting targets through real-time sensing [1–3]. One such crucial biomarker is collagen. This protein is distributed in different human tissues, such as bone, cartilage, tendons, ligaments and the cornea, and plays an important role in the regeneration of damaged connective tissue in tendons and ligaments [4–6]. Moreover, collagen is contained in the composition of the extracellular matrix (ECM) and ensures the high mechanical properties required for connective tissue [7]. Collagen type I triple helix consists of two identical α1(I)-chains and one α2(I)-chain. Thus, it provides relatively good biomechanical properties, including load-bearing, tensile strength and torsional stiffness [4,8]. Collagen fibrils are directly responsible for the mechanism of tendon regeneration [9]. Additionally, the determination of collagen type I protein has an important function in the case of tendon inflammation [8–10]. Tendons and ligaments exhibit high tensile strength [11] because they are mostly composed of connective tissue, proteoglycans, elastin and collagen type I and III fibrils with spindle-shaped tenocytes. [12,13] Nevertheless, this structure contributes to the low vascularization of those tissues and reduce their capability for efficient regeneration. [14] To improve and accelerate the regeneration mechanism, it is demanded to initially very precisely evaluate the presence of collagen type I [15], which indicates the occurrence of a mechanism for the synthesis of the collagenous fibrils and thus starting the self-healing process. [10] This directly determines the appropriate selection of applied therapies [16] or invasive surgical reconstruction. [15] The currently performed techniques are based on a biopsy of the damaged tendon or ligament tissue and usually allow to determine the collagen content with the maximum accuracy of ng/mL. [17] Accordingly, the application of in situ, direct biomarkers to evaluate the content of the collagen type I [18] with a highly sensitive level in the picomolar range can significantly improve the diagnosis of the occurrence of the potential healing process and allow for the appropriate treatment sooner using either percutaneous injection of collagen and hyaluronic acid or the implementation of invasive surgery [16]. The presence of even a very small amount of collagen type I, in the picogram range, can induce and accelerate the selection of the appropriate treatment earlier, to apply, for example, different doses of hyaluronic acid or collagen type I/III injection, aiming to avoid the implementation of highly invasive surgery. [10,15,16] To increase the retreatment process, it is significantly relevant to indicate the concentration of collagen type I that directly enhances the regeneration of damaged tendon tissue. For this reason, it is required to implement sensitive systems suitable for detecting collagen type I with an accurate level of selectivity.

The development of chemical, physical, histochemical and immunochemical methods allowed for the detection of collagen in the micromolar concentration range at the end of the last century [19,20]. Afterward, the application of the enzyme-linked immunosorbent assay (ELISA) based on hydroxyproline allowed for the verification of collagen proteins in the range of μg/mL [21,22]. Currently, electrochemical sensing platforms [23,24] that incorporate specific antibodies responsible for selective antigen detection are at the centre of research interest. These kinds of sensors are highly effective tools to recognise the target analyte, with significant sensitivity and selectivity [1,2,25,26]. However, a major challenge is related to the successful immobilization of biomolecules (enzyme/antibodies/DNA) on the surface of the applied transducer [25–30]. For this purpose, it is fundamental to modify the surface of the working electrode to enhance the connection with the antibody receptor. Common methods are based on 'lock and key' approaches, such as G and A proteins, which enable immobilization of the receptor antibody on the surface of the transducer [31–35]. The application of G and A proteins is highly efficient for non-covalently binding antibodies, also providing to orientate them on-tail [36]. Hence, those intermediate proteins have five and two specific domains, which allow them to appropriately terminate with the crystallizable region (Fc) and also support the orientation of the on-tail antibodies [37]; this ensures obtaining a uniform arrangement of the receptor of their antigen-binding fragment (Fab) against the complementary antigen, consequently increasing their sensitivity properties. [38] Nevertheless, the high molecular weights of the intermediate proteins and their insulating electric properties [39] between the redox marker and transducer substrate have a negative influence on the electrochemical sensor's performance, revealing higher electron transfer resistance through Electrochemical Impedance Spectroscopy (EIS).

Alternative solutions are sensors based on redox-active platforms, which are responsible for the immobilization of antibodies as well as for the transduction of analytical signals. Their main advantage is the ability to work without applying redox markers in the sample [40–43]. Furthermore, there have been different attempts to allow for biosensing that excluded additional redox species [44], such as label-free, impedance-derived redox capacitance for Flavivirus dengue detection [45]. Another appropriate approach is related to the immobilization of antibodies directly on the surface of the transducer through metal nanoparticles [46–50]. These surface forms have high electrical conductivity and compatibility towards protein receptor molecules [51–54]. In addition, the preformed surface with its noble metal nanoparticles [55] is a capable environment for maintaining the physiological activity of immobilized proteins. Metal nanoparticle monolayers are suitable for the immobilization of whole molecules of antibodies via electrostatic interactions [52,53], as well as for covalent immobilization of the Fab part of antibodies via Au–S covalent bonds [51,54]. The main benefit of using the F_{ab} parts of antibodies is the immobilization of the stable sensing elements, ensuring their appropriate orientation [52,55,56].

Moreover, the application of the 4,4′-thiobisbenzenethiol (TBBT) AuNPs SAM [56,57] offers a significant advantage compared to the commonly used 1,6-hexanedithiol (HDT) AuNPs SAM because of its relatively lower electron transfer resistivity [51,58–60]. Furthermore, the efficiency of the sensitivity properties could be related to the physical features of the used nanomaterial, which directly depends on the size of the nanoparticles and their electrical conductivity. Application of the SAM gold nanoparticles reveals high electrical conductivity and low resistivity (2.44×10^{-6} Ω·cm) [61,62], which consequently improved the analytical parameters of the immunosensors and sensitivity properties. Application of system-based, orientated, half-reduced antibodies allows obtaining a highly specific immunosensor to the target protein. The recognition of the analyte contributes to the decreasing of the accessibility of the redox-active marker registered through the Electrochemical Impedance Spectroscopy (EIS). Analogically, the highly sensitive orientation of a half-antibody contributes to the efficiency of the interaction with complementary antigens, inducing the mechanism of plasmonic resonance and allowing to detect the shift SPR angle. Consequently, it is not required to use any additional amplification mechanism to verify the changes in the optical or electrochemical signals towards various concentrations of the analyte.

In this work, we construct a biosensor composed of 4,4′-thiobisbenzenethiol (TBBT) SAM, enabled to covalently bound gold nanoparticles (AuNPs). It has been applied for immobilization of half-antibody fragments via metal nanoparticles using disulphide-bridge covalent bonds. The half IgG was derived by the process of the enzymatic digestion using tris(2-carboxyethyl) phosphine hydrochloride (TECP) [63]. In this approach, the further separation process of the reaction mixture was not necessary because the other fractions of the half-Fc and Fab with half-Fab antibody fragments contribute to the mechanism of efficiently blocking empty spaces onto the receptor layer. Additionally, the mechanism of the covalently bonded, reduced IgG half-antibody is stable over the wide range of pH. This is an important advantage in comparison to the electrostatic immobilization, where the various pH ranges have an impact on the isoelectric point of the whole IgG antibody, and it determines the specific value of pH that allows for the stable, controlled attachment of the receptor onto the transducer substrate.

The main aim of the present research is to fabricate an immunosensor that can verify the collagen I concentration under conditions of a low limit of detection, and to be compatible for detection using two different electrochemical and optical methods. This universal system can allow to quickly verify the collagen I content, with the miniaturized portable electrochemical device based on an evaluation of the accessibility of the redox marker to the sensor surface through the EIS measurement of the electron transfer resistance corresponding to the appropriate value of the analyte concentration. Implementation of Electrochemical Spectroscopy Impedance as a quantifying method enables to record very precisely the electrochemical signal of the electron transfer resistance with high sensitivity. [64] The adapted parameters of EIS, such as bias potential and frequency, ensure not having any negative impact on the stability of the receptor layer, in comparison to cyclic voltammetry (CV), which requires a wide range of applied potential. [65] Impedance spectroscopy plays an important role to evaluate the electrochemical condition, stability of the sensor electrode and to detect the rate of charge transfer, absorption of the proteins, ion exchange and interaction between the antibody–antigen recognition. [66] All of those factors have as a fundamental aspect the utilization of the EIS technique to obtain a highly sensitive and specific biosensor, where the determined values of the electron transfer resistance are correlated with the accessibility of the used redox marker to the electrode interface, allowing to very accurately verify the concentration of the analyte. [67] Subsequently, Electrochemical Impedance Spectroscopy was selected as one of the methods used in the collagen I-sensing platform. Moreover, the same biosensing system using an independent optical technique was applied, where the interaction between the specific half-reduced antibody and antigen is generated through excitation of the plasmonic effect shift of the recorded SPR angle. This duality of the verification of the collagen I content supports applying it as a multipurpose system and gives the opportunity to translate it into other biosensing platforms. Furthermore, this extraordinary approach consisted of the application of stable covalent immobilization of AuNPs through the thiol groups and half-reduced monoclonal antibodies. Additionally, the Au layer of the AuNPs ensured an increased surface area of the working electrode and consequently immobilized more half-reduced antibody receptors in comparison to the plain surface [68–70]. AuNPs have also been used for the enhancement of the SPR signal response, which leads to enhance the sensitivity and specificity for biomolecule detection. AuNPs favour biosensing amplification due to their plasmonic properties and large dielectric constant. The conducted experiments have value for the construction of novel immunosensors based on the half-IgG reduced antibody for collagen I detection, to obtain high stability, sensitivity and selectivity properties.

2. Materials and Methods

2.1. Reagents and Materials

Gold colloidal solution (AuNPs, 0.01% concentration of nanoparticles with a 20 nm diameter), monoclonal antibody Anti-Collagen Type I (IgG1 isotype) produced in mouse, bovine collagen solution Type I, tris(2-carboxyethyl) phosphine hydrochloride (TECP), ferro- and ferricyanides and bovine serum albumin (BSA) was procured from Sigma-Aldrich (Poland). Methanol, potassium hydroxide, ethanol and sulfuric acid were supplied by POCh (Poland). Alumina polishing suspensions of 0.30 μm and 0.05 μm were obtained from Buehler (USA). Milli-Q water with a resistivity of 18.2 $M\Omega \cdot cm^{-1}$ was purchased from Millipore, Germany. The 4,4′-thiobisbenzenethiol (TBBT) compound was received from Leuven University [51]. All the utilized chemical reagents and solvents were used without any further specific purification because they were of analytical quality. All the experiments of this research were conducted at room temperature.

2.2. Preparation of the Half-Antibody Fragment

In order to obtain a half-antibody fragment, the procedure described by Sharma et al. [63] (Figure 1) was applied. Initially, a 5 mM TECP solution was prepared in 10 mM PBS buffer. Then, 2 μL of 5 mM TECP was mixed with 200 μL of 10 μg/mL monoclonal collagen type I antibody in PBS buffer. Afterward, the solutions of TECP and monoclonal collagen type I were mixed at room temperature for 1 h. TECP ('bond breaker') reduced the disulphide bridges from both the F_c and F_{ab} parts of the antibody. Consequently, the suspension contained a mixture of half-antibody chains of the F_c and F_{ab} regions. The separation of the half-IgG and F_{ab} parts from the reaction mixture was not necessary [63].

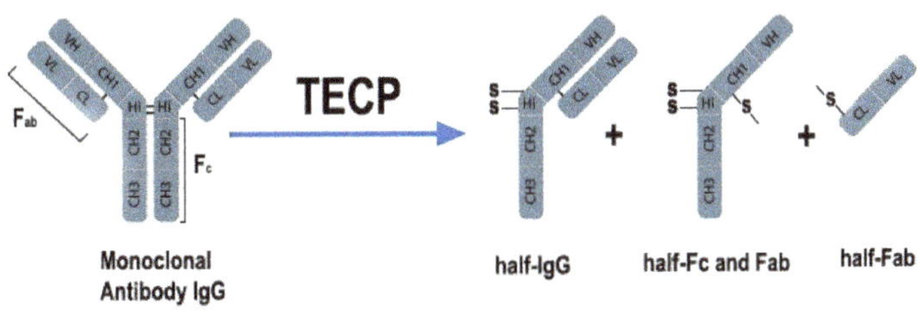

Figure 1. Llustration of the enzymatic reduction of the monoclonal antibody IgG by the disulphide-bridge-bond-breaker TECP (tris (2-carboxyethyl) phosphine hydrochloride) [63].

2.3. Fabrication of the Immunosensor to Estimate Collagen I

The electrodes were polished using alumina slurries (0.30 μm) for 15 min followed by gentle washing with methanol and Milli-Q water. Then, this procedure was conducted again, but using 0.05 μm of alumina slurries, to obtain a smooth gold surface following the rinsing of the electrodes with methanol and Milli-Q water. Afterwards, electrochemical cleaning of the Au electrodes was performed by cyclic voltammetry (CV) using an AutoLab potentiostat/galvanostat. CV cycles (n = 100) were performed by immersing the working electrode in a 0.5 M KOH solution with an applied potential from 0.4 V to −1.2 V using a 0.1 V/s scan rate. Thereafter, the Au electrode was again electrochemically cleaned using a 0.5 M H_2SO_4 solution. Eventually, the Au surface of the working electrode was pre-treated by the activation through the application of 10 CV cycles in a 0.5 M KOH solution. This stage ensured removing any residual impurities absorbed on the gold electrode surface. Thereafter, the working electrode was cleaned by the rising of the Milli-Q water and ethanol. Subsequently, the Au electrode was immersed in a solution of 1.0 mM 4,4′-thiobisbenzenethiol (TBBT) in ethanol for 0.5 h. Then, the electrode was rinsed with ethanol and Milli-Q water.

Once the SAM layer of TBBT was created on the Au/TBBT substrate, the electrode was flipped to spot the top with 10 μL droplets of the Au colloid solution of AuNPs (Au/TBBT/AuNPs) for 2 h. In the following step, 10 μL droplets of the 10 μg/mL half-antibody fragment solution were used, immobilized for 2 h directly on the surface of Au/TBBT/AuNPs, to obtain the Au/TBBT/AuNPs/half-IgG electrode, and which was further rinsed with PBS buffer. In total, 10 μL droplets of a 1% solution of bovine serum albumin (BSA), dissolved in 0.1 M PBS, pH 7.4, were placed on each electrode (Au/TBBT/AuNPs/half-IgG/BSA) for 0.5 h to block unspecific binding. The overall scheme of the electrode modification steps is represented in Figure 2. Eventually, the modified electrodes were rinsed using a solution of 0.1 M PBS.

Once the process of the modification was completed, the electrodes were immersed in 0.1 M PBS, and after that, they were incubated in a refrigerator at +4 °C overnight. Electrochemical measurements (CV and EIS) were carried out after each stage of the modification to confirm the successful fabrication of the sensor.

2.4. Collagen I Detection Using Au/TBBT/AuNPs/half-IgG

After fabrication, the electrodes (n = 6) were exposed to various concentrations of collagen I (range of concentration: 1, 2, 3, 4 and 5 pg/mL). For the interaction of antigen (collagen I) with half-IgG, 10 μL drops of collagen I, diluted in 0.1 M PBS buffer, were deposited on the modified electrode surfaces. Then, the electrodes were prevented from air contamination and evaporation of the solutions by covering them with black Eppendorf tubes. The incubation time was 30 min at room temperature. After that, the remaining unbound antigens were removed from the electrode surfaces by rinsing with 1 mL of a 0.1 M PBS buffer (pH 7.4).

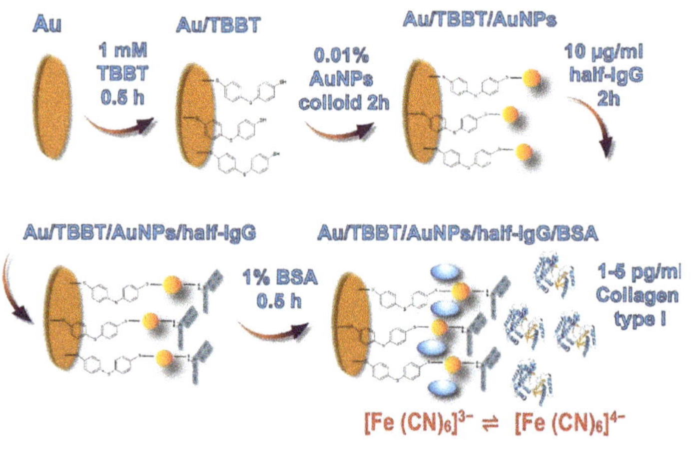

Figure 2. Illustration of the enzymatic reduction of the monoclonal antibody IgG by the disulphide-bridge-bond-breaker TECP (tris(2-carboxyethyl) phosphine hydrochloride) [63].

2.5. Electrochemical Measurements

The applied electrochemical system was based on the AutoLab potentiostat/galvanostat (Eco Chemie, Netherlands) with three combined electrodes. The working electrode was represented by the circular electrode with a 2 mm diameter made from polycrystalline Au, the Ag/AgCl as the reference electrode and the platinum wire as a counter electrode. Electrochemical experiments were performed in the electrolyte composed of 0.1 M PBS (aqueous salts solution with 2.7 mM KCl, 137 mM NaCl, 1.8 mM Na_2HPO_4, 10 mM KH_2PO_4 and pH 7.4) with the addition of 0.5 mM ferro- and ferricyanides ($K_3[Fe (CN)_6]/K_4[Fe (CN)_6]$; (1:1)) as a redox-active probe. The cyclic voltammetry (CV) measurements were recorded in the potential range from 0.6 V to −0.2 V at a 0.1 V/s scan rate. Electrochemical Impedance Spectroscopy (EIS) was conducted to determine the value of the electron transfer resistance (R_{et}) in a frequency from 0.01 Hz to 100 kHz at 0.17 V of the bias potential for 10 mV of the ac amplitude. The concentration of collagen I was determined by EIS measurements. EIS spectra were fitted using a specific equivalent circuit supported by AutoLab Metrohm NOVA software to determine the value of the electron transfer resistance (R_i). The response of the immunosensor toward collagen I is represented as $(R_i - R_0)/R_0 \times 100\%$, where R_0 is the electron transfer resistance for the electrodes after all the steps of the modifications before the detection of any analyte; and R_i is related to the electron transfer resistance of the completely modified electrodes after the application of a particular concentration of the analyte.

2.6. Atomic Force Microscopy Analyses

Atomic Force Microscopy (AFM) was performed using a Universal SPM Quesant (Agoura Hills, CA, USA), on mica plates coated with thin films of Au (111) of 200 nm thickness. Before the analysis, the Au surfaces were annealed with a hydrogen flame followed by cleaning in an ozone/UV chamber. The intermittent-contact mode was used with a NSC16 tip (CW2, Si_3N_4) as a cantilever. A bare Au surface, TBBT-modified Au surface and AuNPs attached to the TBBT-modified Au surfaces were analysed immediately after preparation. The average roughness (R_a) and thickness from each modification stage were measured. A significant statistical difference (at $p < 0.005$) was evaluated by one-way ANOVA with a post-hoc Tukey test.

2.7. Surface Plasmon Resonance Measurements

Surface Plasmon Resonance (SPR) analyses were performed in an Autolab Springle SPR system (Eco Chemie, Netherlands) coupled with a thermostatic water bath at a wavelength of 670 nm and constant temperature of 25 °C. The sensing surface (Au/TBBT/AuNPs/half-IgG/BSA) was placed inside the cuvette, and the sample solution (collagen I) was injected on the active surface at a flow rate of 20 µL/s. After each measurement, the surface was washed with phosphate buffer by switching the flow back to the buffer. The total volume of each sample injection was kept at 100 µL. All the measurements were repeated three times.

3. Results

3.1. Characterization of Nano-Enabled SAM Using Atomic Force Microscopy

AFM analyses were conducted to study the surface topography of the modified electrodes. These studies were made on bare and modified (with TBBT SAM and TBBT SAM together with AuNPs) Au substrates. For comparison, a 2 µm × 2 µm area scanning was performed and is represented in Figure 3. The average roughness parameter from five different scans was calculated to study the porosity/topography of the obtained surfaces. Bare Au showed terraces on the surface over the scanned area of 0.1 by 0.1 µm (Figure S1). The summary comparison with the measured values for the average roughness (R_a) and thickness are presented in Figure S2, with the marked presence of the statistically significant differences. The average roughness parameter for the bare Au surface was found to be 21.3 ± 0.7 nm (Figure 3A). The obtained roughness (19.4 ± 3.6 nm) and thickness (21.1 ± 6.3 nm) after the immobilization of TBBT on the Au surface (Figure 3B) was not significantly changed and it was in the same range in relation to the plain gold surface. After the incorporation of Au nanoparticles, the topography of the TBBT-modified surface again changed, and the attached particles became visible in the corresponding AFM images. The roughness of the modified surfaces changed to 22.6 ± 3.8 nm and the measured thickness significantly increased to 27.6 ± 4.3 nm in comparison to the Au/TBBT sample for AuNPs (Figure 3C), which correspond to similar research performed by Park et al. [71] for a SAM AuNP layer. The value of the average roughness was increased in comparison to the previous stage of the functionalization of the electrode surface using the TBBT compound. The condition of the bare Au surface and occurrence of the scratches provided for the relatively high roughness of the base modification substrate. The diameter of the used gold nanoparticles is commonly determined for a colloid solution by the dynamic light scattering (DLS) technique [72]. Consequently, the appearance of the surrounded ions onto the surface of AuNPs led to obtaining a higher hydrodynamic diameter in the range of approximately 20 nm, although the average dimension of the particles usually has quite a wide distribution [73]. In our study, the performance of the AFM measurements was important to validate the mechanism of the formation of the self-assembled monolayer of AuNPs after modification of the Au substrate by the TBBT compound. The heights of the particles obtained from the analysis of the AFM images (at lower area) confirm the presence of nano-sized materials on the modified surfaces. The size of the particles was achieved from AFM 2D images. The corresponding 2D images of the 3D images in Figure 3C are given in Figure S3. The average length and breadth of the particles for the AuNP-modified Au surface were 411.5 ± 35.6 nm and 168.6 ± 38.7 nm, respectively. These results indicate the formation of a larger aggregated cluster of the combined gold nanoparticles, which are arranged in a highly packed density on the surface of the electrode.

It was observed that the magnitude of the length and breadth showed the aggregation of particles on the surface, contributing to the increase in surface roughness and surface area of the previously plain smooth Au substrate. Therefore, the higher surface area and roughness of the formed Au self-assembled monolayer had a significant impact by binding more half-antibody receptors on the transducer surface, consequently amplifying the received signal and obtaining a much higher sensitivity towards to collagen type I.

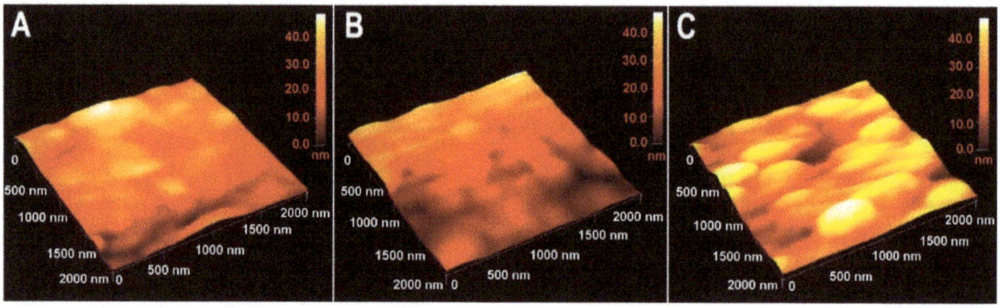

Figure 3. AFM 3D images (2 μm × 2 μm) of (**A**) the mica substrate coated with a thin film of Au (111), (**B**) the TBBT monolayer, and (**C**) the AuNP-modified Au surface.

3.2. *SPR-Assisted Confirmation of Half-Antibody Fragment Collagen I Immobilization*

SPR is a direct, label-free, real-time measurement of binding kinetics and affinity. It is an optical detection method that utilises the conjugation of prisms that permit biomolecular interactions in real time. The interaction between biomolecules is analysed by determining the change in the refractive index in real time. This change in refractive index is obtained from the interaction between the immobilized biomolecule and the analyte. It is the most convenient tool to study the interfacial interaction between the analyte (antigen) and the immobilized biomolecules (antibody) in real time [74–77]. Therefore, we have applied this technique to confirm the immobilization of half-IgG collagen I antibodies on the transducer surface [78–81]. Upon deposition of the reaction mixture obtained after antibody digestion using TECP [63], an increase in the SPR angle was observed. Real-time, label-free biomolecular interactions between half-IgG and collagen I were recorded using an Auto lab Springle SPR system (Eco Chemie, Netherlands). A 50 nm-thick, gold-coated glass disc was supplied along with the instrument. It is an open cuvette-based dual channel system, where channel-1 was used to measure the interactions between half-IgG and collagen I and channel-2 was used to monitor the signals due to changes in the refractive index of the buffers, and also acted as a reference. Different reagents, samples and buffers were injected in the desired amounts into two cuvettes (assembled over the gold disc). This SPR technique is used to characterize the binding interactions between half-IgG and collagen I without any labelling requirements.

The SPR angle increased from 10° to 155° after the immobilization of the antibody on the surface of Au. After the deposition of AuNPs on the Au surface, the angle shifted from 10° to 100°, and later, after immobilization of the half-IgG antibodies (Au/TBBT/AuNPs/half-IgG), the angle shifted to 155°, as shown in Figure S4. After the immobilization of half-IgG, steady-state conditions were obtained, and the surface was washed using PBS buffer to remove any unbounded species. The obtained results validated the successful half-IgG antibody immobilization on the Au/TBBT/AuNPs surface within approximately 1 h and 20 min (Figure S4). The shift in angle at each step is shown in Figure S4A and described in the Supplementary Materials. In the next step, the time of interfacial interaction between half-IgG and collagen I was checked using SPR. The golden disc support, modified with TBBT/AuNPs/half-IgG/BSA, was placed into an SPR chamber filled with 100 μL PBS buffer. For the specific interaction, the SPR response of the TBBT/AuNPs/half-IgG/BSA sensing platform at various concentrations of collagen type I was recorded in PBS buffer. While the Au/TBBT/AuNPs/half-IgG/BSA surface was exposed to various concentrations of collagen I, the obtained sensogram revealed three phases for each concentration: (i) baseline (1st phase); (ii) association of collagen I with the Au/TBBT/AuNPs/half-IgG/BSA surface (2nd phase); and (iii) dissociation of collagen I (3rd phase). With the inoculation of 1 pg/mL of collagen I, an increase in angle shift is observed from 10° to 40° during the association phase. The SPR response signal increases consistently upon the exposure of collagen I up to 5 pg/mL; after that, the response signal decreases, as shown in Figure 4A. The decreasing value of the SPR angle shift could be caused by the adherence and interaction of the target collagen protein with the binding part of the antibody on the receptor layer. Accordingly, the detection of the analyte in the higher concertation range was impeded. Figure 4B depicts the calibration curve of the SPR signal attained as a function of the collagen I concentrations and signifies linearity between 1 pg/mL and 5 pg/mL. After the association phase, the residual analyte is discarded by using a flushing buffer to clean the surface. The antigen–antibody interaction was measured by injecting collagen I for 6 to 20–25 min followed by a rinsing period of 10 min with pure running buffer. Each experiment was repeated thrice.

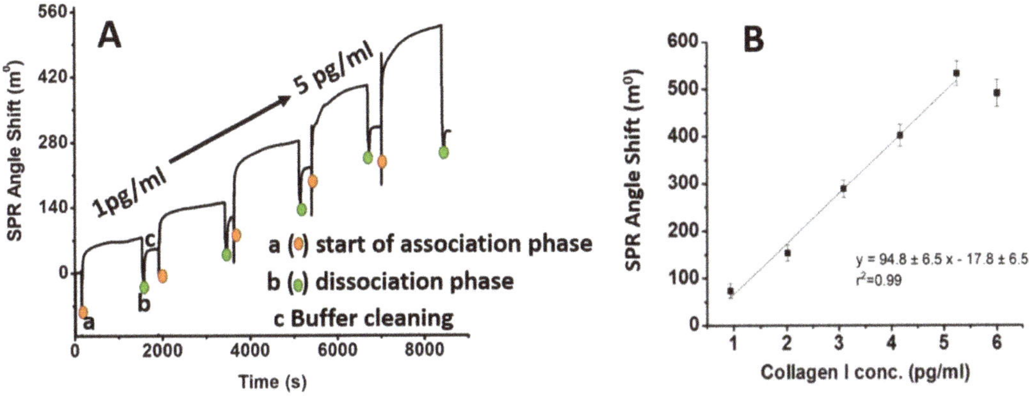

Figure 4. (**A**) SPR response, and (**B**) calibration curve of Au/TBBT/AuNPs/half-IgG/BSA towards collagen I in the concentration range from 1–5 pg/mL in PBS buffer.

The Au/TBBT/AuNPs/half-IgG/BSA immunosensor shows a linear range between 1 and 5 pg/mL; beyond this, it shows a decrease in the SPR angle shift. This decrease in angle after 5 pg/mL shows that the device cannot detect collagen I beyond 5 pg/mL. In our approach, we used the SPR technique to determine the actual dynamic range of the performed collagen immunosensor and consequently validated it through impedance spectroscopy. Therefore, we have decided to conduct the experiment with a range of collagen concentration from 1 to 5 pg/mL. Based on these results, the concentration range of collagen I from 1 pg/mL to 5 pg/mL was selected for the electrochemical sensing, with a time of 30 min for the half IgG–collagen I interaction. The lowest concentration detected by the SPR technique was 1 pg/mL. The same surface was reused several times for the measurements (Au/TBBT/AuNPs). The fabricated Au/TBBT/AuNPs/half-IgG/BSA immunosensor is highly sensitive. Most of the extant research report on a full-antibody-immobilized immunosensor, which leads to random antibody immobilization on the transducer surface [82–84]. However, in the present work, an Au/TBBT/AuNPs/half-IgG/BSA immunosensor, thiol (−SH) group of the antibody is conjugated onto the Au surface. The half-IgG antibody immobilization can precisely bind the F_c part of the antibody to accomplish an oriented antibody immobilization, as shown in Figure 2. The oriented intact antibody shows higher sensitivity as compared to full-antibody immobilization. It is reported that the half antibody shows a 3–8 times higher sensitivity than the full antibody [85].

3.3. Electrochemical Characterization of the Immunosensor Fabrication

The crucial parts of the immunosensors are the specific antibodies responsible for selective recognition of the antigens, as well as the transducer layers, which are mainly responsible for sensor sensitivity. The focus of this work was to verify the optimized stage of the electrode modification and detection of collagen I. Application of the 4,4′-

thiobisbenzenethiol (TBBT) compound contained two SH groups that played an important role in the covalent deposition on the Au substrate, as well as covalent immobilization of the AuNPs.

The parameters characterizing TBBT SAM are superior when compared to 1,6-hexanedithiol SAM, widely applied in immunosensor fabrications [51,58–60,62]. It was confirmed that TBBT SAM has a charged transfer resistance of approximately 500 kΩ. This value is three times lower than the charged transfer resistance of 1,6-hexanedithiol dithiol [51,52]. Accordingly, it enables receiving a higher electrical signal, detecting the analyte across a wider concentration range and reduced the potential negative effect of electrode blocking. In addition, the foundation of the TBBT SAM on the Au electrode platform is more reproducible and it amplifies the intensity of the recorded signal, because of higher electrical conductivity in comparison to the 1,6-hexanedithiol dithiol SAM. Therefore, TBBT SAM was applied in the present research.

Another important point of immunosensors is the stable immobilization of specific antibodies to maintain their right orientation and physiological activity at the same time [59,60]. The AuNPs SAM has a minus charge due to the citrate anions used for nanoparticle stabilization, which creates an environment suitable for the electrostatic immobilization of antibodies. For these approaches, the selection of the pH conditions preserves the plus charges on the F_c part of the antibodies and allows for the right immobilization of whole antibodies with F_{ab} parts, which are responsible for antigen recognition, exposed in the sample solution [53,54,64].

The AuNPs SAM is also very suitable for covalent immobilization of the F_{ab} parts in which the disulphide groups are incorporated [51,54]. To apply this method, the enzymatic digestion of whole antibodies is necessary. Here, we applied the procedure published by Sharma et al. [63], incorporating the tris(2-carboxyethyl) phosphine hydrochloride (TECP) compound for whole antibodies, cleaving the disulphide bridges. After reducing the antibodies, the half region of F_c with the half region of F_{ab} (heavy constant CH and variable VH chains) and the half region of F_{ab} (light constant CL and variable VL chains) were obtained (Figure 1). In this approach, the separation of products from the reaction mixture is not required. The immunosensor fabrication consists of the following steps (Figure 2): (i) TBBT SAM deposition on the Au electrode; (ii) covalent deposition of AuNPs; (iii) covalent deposition of the half-antibody fragment; and (iv) filling of empty free spaces and eliminating of unspecific binding by BSA. Each step of the modifications of the working Au electrode was evaluated by both the performed electrochemical techniques: CV and EIS in the presence of $K_3[Fe(CN)_6]/K_4[Fe(CN)_6]$ (1:1) as a redox marker, with a 0.5 mM concentration, and using 0.1 M PBS as an electrolyte at a stable pH of 7.4. The CV and EIS curves recorded after each step of the modification are presented in Figure 5. The potential separation (ΔE_p) between the oxidation and reduction peaks equal to 86 ± 9 mV recorded for the pure Au electrode confirmed the good reversibility of the redox marker process and cleanness of the surface. This conclusion was also confirmed by the EIS recorded for the bare electrode (Figure 5C and Table 1). The straight line is related to the diffusion-controlled electrochemical process.

However, after the TBBT SAM deposition, the surface of the working electrode was blocked. This caused a decrease in the accessibility of the ferro- and ferricyanides $[Fe(CN)_6]^{3-/4-}$ redox marker to the interface with the working electrode surface. Consequently, the oxidation and reduction peaks separation increased to 386 ± 44 mV and the electron transfer resistance (R_{et}), estimated with EIS, was 560 ± 58 kΩ. Both parameters confirmed the successful deposition of TBBT SAM. After the immobilization of the AuNPs, the difference between the oxidation and reduction peak potential decreased to the value 168 ± 18 mV (Figure 5A). Correspondingly, the charge transfer resistance was reduced to 120 ± 11 kΩ (Figure 5B and Table 1). This result indicated the presence of the quasi-reversible electron transfer mechanism between the transducer and redox marker [86], and subsequently enhanced to form a higher electric conductivity interface similar to the bare gold electrode.

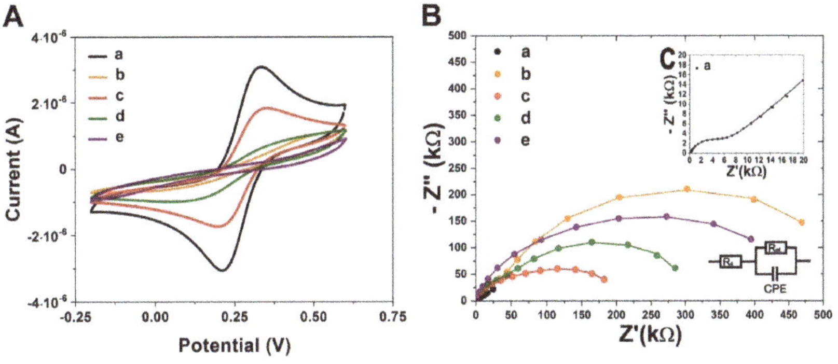

Figure 5. (**A**) Cyclic voltammetry (CV) curves, and (**B**,**C**) electrochemical impedance spectra (EIS) recorded after each step of the Au electrode modifications: (a) bare Au electrode; (b) TBBT SAM deposition; (c) immobilization of the metal nanoparticle colloids AuNPs; (d) immobilization of half-IgG; (e) deposition of BSA. Measuring conditions of EIS: applied frequencies from 0.01 Hz —100 kHz with the bias potential at 0.17 V in 10 mV of ac amplitude. The EIS spectra were fitted to the Nyquist plots for an electrical circuit model, which included R_s—solution resistance; R_{et}—electron transfer resistance; and CPE—constant phase element. Composition of used electrolyte: 0.1 M PBS, pH 7.4 with 0.5 mM $K_3[Fe(CN)_6]/K_4[Fe(CN)_6]$ (1:1).

Table 1. Summary of the fitting results from the EIS plots through the Randles electrical circuit.

Samples	R_{et} (Ω)	R_s (Ω)	CPE (F)
Au/TBBT	560×10^3	13	1.07×10^{-4}
Au/TBBT/AuNPs	120×10^3	7.4	2.46×10^{-4}
Au/TBBT/AuNPs/half-IgG	256×10^3	9.7	1.28×10^{-4}
Au/TBBT/AuNPs/half-IgG/BSA	563×10^3	16	1.71×10^{-4}

The immobilization of the half-IgG caused a substantial decrease in electrode reversibility. The CV peaks separation increased to 358 ± 76 mV for AuNPs. CV data were also confirmed by EIS. After immobilization of half-IgG, the charge transfer resistance increased to 256 ± 35 kΩ in the case of AuNPs. These parameters confirmed the successful deposition of half-IgG on the nanoparticles. The filling of empty space and blocking unspecific binding with BSA caused the additional reversibility to decrease. The final value charge transfer resistance of the immunosensor based on AuNPs was 563 ± 76 kΩ. However, the peaks of the oxidation and reduction process were not clearly distinguishable ($\Delta Ep = 404 \pm 35$ mV). This result confirmed the complete modification of the sensing platform, which, after that, was ready for the detection of the collagen I analyte.

3.4. EIS-Based Collagen Type I Immunosensing

The sensing of collagen I using the prepared immunosensors was carried out with Electrochemical Impedance Spectroscopy (EIS). The cyclic voltammetry (CV) technique was not suitable because of its high irreversibility. The measurements of the sensitivity of the performed immunosensors were conducted with concentrations of 1, 2, 3, 4 and 5 pg/mL of collagen type I in PBS, pH 7.4. The interactions between half-IgG and collagen I impeded the accessibility of the ferro- and ferricyanides to the surface of the transducer and, consequently, increased the electron transfer resistance (Ri). These values were obtained by fitting the EIS spectra using the circuit model presented in Figure 6.

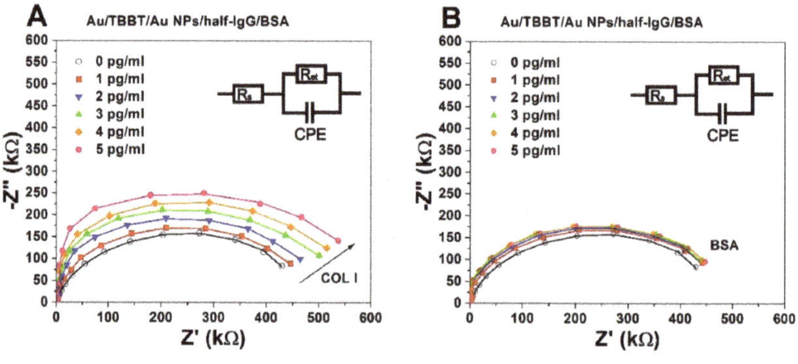

Figure 6. Electrochemical impedance spectra: (**A**) Au/TBBT/AuNPs/half-IgG/BSA in the presence of collagen I, (**B**) Au/TBBT/AuNPs/half-IgG/BSA in the presence of BSA. Concentration range of collagen I analyte: (○) 0, (■) 1, (▼) 2, (▲) 3, (♦) 4, (•) 5 pg/mL. Measuring conditions of the EIS: applied frequencies from 0.01–100 kHz with the bias potential at 0.17 V in 10 mV of ac amplitude. The EIS spectra were fitted to the Nyquist plots for an electrical circuit model, which included R_s—solution resistance, R_{et}—electron transfer resistance, and CPE—constant phase element. Composition of the used electrolyte: 0.1 M PBS, pH 7.4 with 0.5 mM $K_3[Fe(CN)_6]/K_4[Fe(CN)_6]$ (1:1).

To obtain the appropriate calibration curves, the relative changes in electron transfer resistance (ΔR) were expressed using the following equation [51]:

$$\Delta R = \frac{R_i - R_0}{R_0} \times 100\% \quad (1)$$

where R_0 represents the value of the electron transfer resistance of the sensing system recovered in the 0.1 M PBS buffer without application of the analyte. The values of the relative changes in electron transfer resistance increased proportionally with higher concentrations of collagen I for the studied system (Figure 7). The slope of the calibration curve and the range of standard deviations determined the precision sensing of collagen I.

The limit of detection (LOD) was determined by using the following formula [87]:

$$LOD = \frac{3.3\sigma}{S} \quad (2)$$

where σ is the value of the standard deviation for the y-intercept and S represents a slope of the regression line. The determined value of LOD for the collagen immunosensor was 0.38 pg/mL. A selectivity study was performed using bovine serum albumin (BSA), with a concentration range from 1 to 5 pg/mL as a control. These compounds revealed negligible responses towards the presented sensing platform, and the accurate selectivity properties were also confirmed. According to the obtained results, the performance of the collagen immunosensor was validated in the dynamic range from 1 to 5 pg/mL, which was evaluated previously by the SPR measurements. The calculated LOD is only a theoretical value, indicating the minimum concentration of the collagen type that is possible to detect using the performed system.

However, the SPR angle shift for the higher concentration above the dynamic range was not accurate for the further determination of the collagen type I protein. Therefore, this sensor has an important application in the detection of a very low range of collagen content, which is required for future samples taken from patients to confirm the presence of the initial stage of collagen synthesis. The verification of the collagen type I concentration in the picomolar range has a significant impact on the initial and rapid diagnosis of the regeneration mechanism of tendons and ligaments [13,15,17,18]. Accordingly, it allows selecting the appropriate treatment, while also revealing the potential capability of supporting the healing of patients by injection with collagen type I/III and hyaluronic acid, or by applying invasive surgery [10,16].

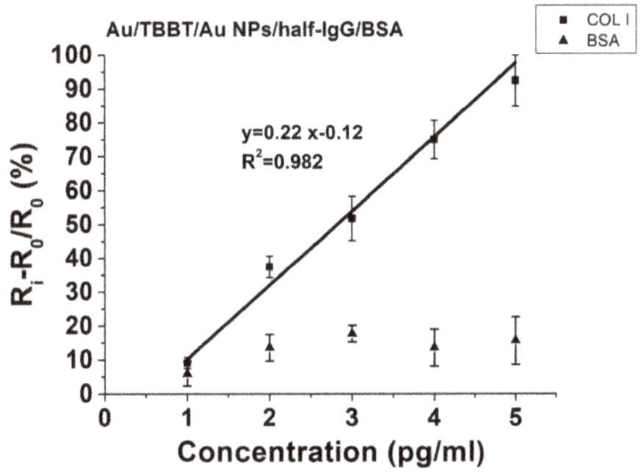

Figure 7. The correlation between $(R_i - R_0)/R_0$ (%) and the applied range of collagen I (COL I) concentrations (pg/mL) and the negative control of bovine serum albumin (BSA), as measured for the Au/TBBT/AuNPs/half-IgG/BSA immunosensor system. R_0 represents the value of the electron transfer resistance of a completely functionalised working electrode without any addition of the collagen I analyte (COL I), and R_i is the electron transfer resistance after all steps of the electrode functionalisation, which were measured in 0.1 M PBS solution for the range of concentrations from 1–5 pg/mL (n = 5) of collagen I (COL I).

4. Discussion

According to the obtained results, the limit of detection demonstrated that the performed immunosensor based on the nano-Au particles had a remarkable high sensitivity range for collagen I detection, which was caused by many factors, such as the high electrical conductivity of the AuNPs with directly immobilized, complementary half-IgG antibodies. Additionally, the application of the AuNPs increased the surface area of the transducer [46–49]. This directly allowed for combining higher amounts of the half-IgG antibody receptors [51,54], which had a crucial role in the sensitivity of the immunosensor. Therefore, these kinds of modifications based on covalent bonding from each side between Au and S can definitely guarantee a better and more stable SAM layer compared to the other immobilization systems based on the G or A proteins [31–35], which have relatively higher resistivity and, consequently, lower electrical signals towards the covalent immobilization of receptors through metal nanoparticles. Moreover, there are various methods for the determination of the collagen content, as summarised in Table 2. One of the most common techniques is ELISA; however, this enables obtaining a minimum detection limit in the range of approximately 1 ng/mL. Subsequently, the application of electrochemical immunosensors based on both techniques, Electrochemical Spectroscopy Impedance, and Surface Plasmon Resonance, allows for achieving significantly higher sensitivity, in the range of picograms per millilitre, against the previous commonly used techniques, such as ELISA.

Table 2. Comparison of the different techniques for the determination of the collagen content.

Method of Measurement	Type of Collagen	Type of Sample	Detection Limit	Range of Detection	References
ELISA	collagen I	synthetic C peptide fragments of type I collagen (α−1)	10 ng/mL	10–1000 ng/mL	[88]
Fluorescence Assays	collagen triple helix GPO	synthetic collagen triple helix GPO	30 nM	100–1000 nM	[89]
Surface Plasmon Resonance Imaging (SPRI)	collagen IV	human blood plasma	2.4 ng/mL	10–1000 ng/mL	[90]
ELISA	collagen I	human serum	0.83 ng/mL	0.83–500 ng/mL	[91]
ELISA	collagen III	human serum	0.6 ng/mL	0.9–200 ng/mL	[92]
Localized Surface Plasmon Resonance (LSPR)	collagen IV	extracted collagen IV from human placenta	10 ng/mL	10–1000 ng/mL	[19]
ELISA	collagen I	human blood plasma	5.3 pg/mL	40–2500 pg/mL	[93]
Electric Field-Induced Accumulation	collagen I	extracted collagen I from human placenta Bornstein and Traub type I	3.0 pg/mL	3–60 pg/mL	[94]
Cyclic Voltammetry (CV)	collagen I	solution of synthetic collagen I	0.5 pg/mL	0.5 pg/mL–0.5 ng/mL	[95]
EIS (AuNPs transducer)	collagen I	bovine collagen solution I	0.38 pg/mL	1.0–5.0 pg/mL	Present work

Additionally, the fabrication of immunosensors presented in this research is rather simple. The important advantage of this platform ensures high and strong stability of the antibody immobilization using covalent bonds against to the weaker electrostatic interactions. Additionally, an independent examination through Surface Plasmon Resonance confirmed this efficiency in collagen detection in the significantly low pg/mL concentration range by the presented immunosensor. However, the electrochemical sensing analyser [96,97] costs much less in comparison to spectroscopic devices [94].

Furthermore, relatively low sample consumption at the µL level enhances the attractiveness of the presented immunosensors. Finally, the portable electrochemical device can be a potential solution to directly use for the medical diagnostic system without specific and expensive ELISA kit assays.

5. Conclusions

The results obtained proved the suitability of the 4,4′-thiobisbenzenethiol SAM formed on the Au electrode for the efficient covalent immobilization of AuNPs. The determined value of the limit of detection was 0.38 pg/mL, which is a remarkably low value in comparison to the current collagen sensors. In the presence of the control compound (BSA), very moderate responses were generated, and this proved the selectivity properties of the presented immunosensor.

The proposed construction of the immunosensor with a nano-Au SAM layer has several significant advantages, such as the high stability of the receptor layer, using covalent bonds through the enzymatically reduced half-IgG antibody, and additionally increasing the surface area of the electrode, which directly supported to immobilize more antibodies. Therefore, the presented immunosensors have improved on the currently used methods by being able to validate the presence of a low concentration of collagen type I, without requiring a large volume of the analysed sample. Overall, the presented immunosensors have the potential to make a great impact on future applications in medical laboratory diagnosis, based on the pg/mL level of sensitivity, good selectivity, very small sample consumption and simple fabrication method at a reasonable cost.

Supplementary Materials: The following are available online at https://www.mdpi.com/article/10.3390/bios11070227/s1, Figure S1. AFM 3D image (0.1 μm × 0.1 μm) of the mica substrate coated with a thin film of Au (111); Figure S2. Results of the average roughness (Ra) and thickness for the bare gold electrode surface (Au), after modification of TBBT (Au/TBBT) and after immobilization of the gold nanoparticles (Au/TBBT/AuNPs). The calculation of the significant differences ($p < 0.05$) was performed by one-way ANOVA and post-hoc Tukey tests, and it was marked by the bars with a star (*). Figure S3. AFM 2D image of a AuNP-modified gold surface (mica substrate coated with thin film of Au (111)). Representative images of (A) length and (B) breadth measurements of one particle.; Figure S4. (A) Plot of the reflectivity vs. angle shift of the surfaces with the change in reflectivity percentage for the (i) Au, (ii) Au/TBBT, (iii) Au/TBBT/AuNPs and (iv) Au/TBBT/AuNPs/half-IgG surface in buffer; and (B) SPR confirmation of half-IgG immobilization on the surface of Au/TBBT/AuNPs in PBS buffer at pH 7.

Author Contributions: Conceptualization, M.G., S.K.B., E.K.-G., W.S. and A.K., methodology, M.G., S.K.B., U.S.; software, M.G., S.K.B.; validation, S.K.B., A.K. formal analysis, M.G., S.K.B., A.K.; investigation, M.G., S.K.B., A.K.; resources, W.S., A.K.; data curation, M.G., S.K.B.; writing—original draft preparation, M.G., S.K.B., E.K.-G., W.S.; writing—review and editing, M.G., S.K.B., A.K.; visualization, M.G., S.K.B.; supervision, W.S., A.K.; project administration, E.K.-G.; funding acquisition, W.S., S.K.B. All authors have read and agreed to the published version of the manuscript.

Funding: This research was funded by THE NATIONAL CENTRE FOR RESEARCH AND DEVELOPMENT (NCBiR, Warsaw, Poland), grant number STRATEGMED1/233224/10/NCBR/2014, and additionally through the statutory funds from the Institute of Animal Reproduction and Food Research of the Polish Academy of Sciences in Olsztyn, Poland.

Institutional Review Board Statement: Not applicable.

Informed Consent Statement: Not applicable.

Data Availability Statement: All presented data from this research are available on request to the corresponding authors.

Acknowledgments: This research was financed by the National Centre for Research and Development (NCBiR, Warsaw, Poland) grant no. STRATEGMED1/233224/10/NCBR/2014, and additionally through the statutory funds from the Institute of Animal Reproduction and Food Research of the Polish Academy of Sciences in Olsztyn, Poland. Additionally, we would like to acknowledge and thank Hanna Radecka and Jerzy Radecki for their support and contribution to this research.

Conflicts of Interest: Authors declare no conflict of interest.

References

1. Gao, W.; Emaminejad, S.; Nyein, H.Y.Y.; Challa, S.; Chen, K.; Peck, A.; Fahad, H.M.; Ota, H.; Shiraki, H.; Kiriya, D.; et al. Fully integrated wearable sensor arrays for multiplexed in situ perspiration analysis. *Nature* **2016**, *529*, 509–514. [CrossRef] [PubMed]
2. Ray, T.R.; Choi, J.; Bandodkar, A.J.; Krishnan, S.; Gutruf, P.; Tian, L.; Ghaffari, R.; Rogers, J.A. Bio-integrated wearable systems: A comprehensive review. *Chem. Rev.* **2019**, 5461–5533. [CrossRef] [PubMed]
3. Mujawar, M.A.; Gohel, H.; Bhardwaj, S.K.; Srinivasan, S.; Hickman, N.; Kaushik, A. Nano-enabled biosensing systems for intelligent healthcare: Towards COVID-19 management. *Mater. Today Chem.* **2020**, *17*, 100306. [CrossRef] [PubMed]
4. Gelse, K.; Po, E.; Aigner, T. Collagens—Structure, function, and biosynthesis. *Adv. Drug Deliv. Rev.* **2003**, *55*, 1531–1546. [CrossRef] [PubMed]
5. Gwiazda, M.; Kumar, S.; Świeszkowski, W.; Ivanovski, S.; Vaquette, C. The effect of melt electrospun writing fiber orientation onto cellular organization and mechanical properties for application in Anterior Cruciate Ligament tissue engineering. *J. Mech. Behav. Biomed. Mater.* **2020**, *104*, 103631. [CrossRef]
6. Miller, E.J. Collagen types: Structure, distribution, and functions. In *Collagen: Volume I: Biochemistry*; Marcel, E.N., Ed.; CRC Press: Boca Raton, FL, USA, 2018; pp. 139–156.

7. Kew, S.J.; Gwynne, J.H.; Enea, D.; Abu-rub, M.; Pandit, A.; Zeugolis, D.; Brooks, R.A.; Rushton, N.; Best, S.M.; Cameron, R.E. Acta Biomaterialia Regeneration and repair of tendon and ligament tissue using collagen fibre biomaterials. *Acta Biomater.* **2011**, *7*, 3237–3247. [CrossRef] [PubMed]
8. Prabhakaran, M.P.; Swieszkowski, W.; Kurzydlowski, K.J. Electrospun bio-composite P (LLA-CL)/collagen I/collagen III scaffolds for nerve tissue engineering. *J. Biomed. Mater. Res. Part B Appl. Biomater.* **2012**, *100*, 1093–1102. [CrossRef]
9. Rinoldi, C.; Costantini, M.; Kijen, E.; Heljak, M.; Monika, C.; Buda, R.; Baldi, J.; Cannata, S.; Guzowski, J.; Gargioli, C.; et al. Tendon Tissue Engineering: Effects of Mechanical and Biochemical Stimulation on Stem Cell Alignment on Cell-Laden Hydrogel Yarns. *Adv. Healthc. Mater.* **2019**, *1801218*, 1–10. [CrossRef]
10. Maffulli, N.; Longo, U.G.; Kadakia, A.; Spiezia, F. Achilles tendinopathy. *Foot Ankle Surg.* **2020**, *26*, 240–249. [CrossRef]
11. O'Brien, T.D.; Reeves, N.D.; Baltzopoulos, V.; Jones, D.A.; Maganaris, C.N. Mechanical properties of the patellar tendon in adults and children. *J. Biomech.* **2010**, *43*, 1190–1195. [CrossRef]
12. Rein, S.; Hagert, E.; Schneiders, W.; Fieguth, A.; Zwipp, H. Histological analysis of the structural composition of ankle ligaments. *Foot Ankle Int.* **2015**, *36*, 211–224. [CrossRef]
13. Thorpe, C.T.; Screen, H.R.C. Tendon structure and composition. *Adv. Exp. Med. Biol.* **2016**, *3–10*. [CrossRef]
14. Theobald, P.; Benjamin, M.; Nokes, L.; Pugh, N. Review of the vascularisation of the human Achilles tendon. *Injury* **2005**, *36*, 1267–1272. [CrossRef] [PubMed]
15. Olesen, J.L.; Langberg, H.; Heinemeier, K.M.; Flyvbjerg, A.; Kjær, M. Determination of markers for collagen type I turnover in peritendinous human tissue by microdialysis: Effect of catheter types and insertion trauma. *Scand. J. Rheumatol.* **2006**, *35*, 312–317. [CrossRef]
16. Lipman, K.; Wang, C.; Ting, K.; Soo, C.; Zheng, Z. Tendinopathy: Injury, repair, and current exploration. *Drug Des. Devel. Ther.* **2018**, *12*, 591. [CrossRef]
17. Buckley, M.R.; Evans, E.B.; Matuszewski, P.E.; Chen, Y.L.; Satchel, L.N.; Elliott, D.M.; Soslowsky, L.J.; Dodge, G.R. Distributions of types I, II and III collagen by region in the human supraspinatus tendon. *Connect. Tissue Res.* **2013**, *54*, 374–379. [CrossRef] [PubMed]
18. Williams, I.F.; McCullagh, K.G.; Silver, I.A. The distribution of types I and III collagen and fibronectin in the healing equine tendon. *Connect. Tissue Res.* **1984**, *12*, 211–227. [CrossRef]
19. Kaushik, B.K.; Singh, L.; Singh, R.; Zhu, G.; Zhang, B.; Wang, Q.; Kumar, S. Detection of Collagen-IV Using Highly Reflective Metal Nanoparticles-Immobilized Photosensitive Optical Fiber-Based MZI Structure. *IEEE Trans. Nanobioscience* **2020**, *19*, 477–484. [CrossRef]
20. Etherington, D.J.; Sims, T.J. Detection and estimation of collagen. *J. Sci. Food Agric.* **1981**, *32*, 539–546. [CrossRef]
21. Cissell, D.D.; Link, J.M.; Hu, J.C.; Athanasiou, K.A. A Modified Hydroxyproline Assay Based on Hydrochloric Acid in Ehrlich's Solution Accurately Measures Tissue Collagen Content. *Tissue Eng. Part C Methods* **2017**, *23*, 243–250. [CrossRef]
22. Yasmin, H.; Kabashima, T.; Rahman, M.S.; Shibata, T.; Kai, M. Amplified and selective assay of collagens by enzymatic and fluorescent reactions. *Sci. Rep.* **2014**, *4*, 1–8. [CrossRef]
23. Goodarzi, Z.; Maghrebi, M.; Zavareh, A.F.; Mokhtari-Hosseini, Z.-B.; Ebrahimi-hoseinzadeh, B.; Zarmi, A.H.; Barshan-tashnizi, M. Evaluation of nicotine sensor based on copper nanoparticles and carbon nanotubes. *J. Nanostructure Chem.* **2015**, 237–242. [CrossRef]
24. Shown, I.; Ganguly, A. Non-covalent functionalization of CVD-grown graphene with Au nanoparticles for electrochemical sensing application. *J. Nanostructure Chem.* **2016**, *6*, 281–288. [CrossRef]
25. Bhardwaj, S.K.; Yadav, P.; Ghosh, S.; Basu, T.; Mahapatro, A.K. Biosensing Test-Bed Using Electrochemically Deposited Reduced Graphene Oxide. *ACS Appl. Mater. Interfaces* **2016**, *8*, 24350–24360. [CrossRef]
26. Bhardwaj, S.K.; Chauhan, R.; Yadav, P.; Ghosh, S.; Mahapatro, A.K.; Singh, J.; Basu, T. Bi-enzyme functionalized electro-chemically reduced transparent graphene oxide platform for triglyceride detection. *Biomater. Sci.* **2019**, *7*, 1598–1606. [CrossRef]
27. Bhardwaj, S.K.; Basu, T.; Mahapatro, A.K. Triglyceride detection using reduced graphene oxide on ITO surface. *Integr. Ferroelectr.* **2017**, *184*, 92–98. [CrossRef]
28. Fuletra, I.; Gupta, C.; Nisar, S.; Bharadwaj, R.; Saluja, P.; Bhardwaj, S.K.; Asokan, K.; Basu, T. Self-assembled gold nano islands for precise electrochemical sensing of trace level of arsenic in water. *Groundw. Sustain. Dev.* **2020**, *12*, 100528. [CrossRef]
29. Bhardwaj, S.K.; Mahapatro, A.K.; Basu, T. Benzymatic triglyceride biosensor based on electrochemically reduced graphene oxide. *Int. J. ChemTech Res.* **2015**, *7*, 858–866.
30. Paliwal, P.; Sargolzaei, S.; Bhardwaj, S.K.; Bhardwaj, V.; Dixit, C.; Kaushik, A. Grand Challenges in Bio-Nanotechnology to Manage the COVID-19 Pandemic. *Front. Nanotechnol.* **2020**, *2*, 3389. [CrossRef]
31. Jeong, M.L.; Hyun, K.P.; Jung, Y.; Jin, K.K.; Sun, O.J.; Bong, H.C. Direct immobilization of protein G variants with various numbers of cysteine residues on a gold surface. *Anal. Chem.* **2007**, *79*, 2680–2687.
32. Neumann, L.; Wohland, T.; Whelan, R.J.; Zare, R.N.; Kobilka, B.K. Functional immobilization of a ligand-activated G-protein-coupled receptor. *ChemBioChem* **2002**, *3*, 993–998. [CrossRef]
33. Chammem, H.; Hafaid, I.; Bohli, N.; Garcia, A.; Meilhac, O.; Abdelghani, A.; Mora, L. A disposable electrochemical sensor based on protein G for High-Density Lipoprotein (HDL) detection. *Talanta* **2015**, *144*, 466–473. [CrossRef] [PubMed]
34. Rosenbaum, D.M.; Rasmussen, S.G.F.; Kobilka, B.K. The structure and function of G-protein-coupled receptors. *Nature* **2009**, *459*, 356–363. [CrossRef]

35. Jarocka, U.; Sawicka, R.; Góra-Sochacka, A.; Sirko, A.; Zagórski-Ostoja, W.; Radecki, J.; Radecka, H. Electrochemical immunosensor for detection of antibodies against influenza A virus H5N1 in hen serum. *Biosens. Bioelectron.* **2014**, *55*, 301–306. [CrossRef]
36. Trilling, A.K.; Beekwilder, J.; Zuilhof, H. Antibody orientation on biosensor surfaces: A minireview. *Analyst* **2013**, *138*, 1619–1627. [CrossRef] [PubMed]
37. Choe, W.; Durgannavar, T.A.; Chung, S.J. Fc-binding ligands of immunoglobulin G: An overview of high affinity proteins and peptides. *Materials* **2016**, *9*, 994. [CrossRef]
38. Tajima, N.; Takai, M.; Ishihara, K. Significance of antibody orientation unraveled: Well-oriented antibodies recorded high binding affinity. *Anal. Chem.* **2011**, *83*, 1969–1976. [CrossRef]
39. Zhang, B.; Song, W.; Pang, P.; Lai, H.; Chen, Q.; Zhang, P.; Lindsay, S. Role of contacts in long-range protein conductance. *Proc. Natl. Acad. Sci. USA* **2019**, *116*, 5886–5891. [CrossRef]
40. Jarocka, U.; Sawicka, R.; Stachyra, A.; Góra-Sochacka, A.; Sirko, A.; Zagórski-Ostoja, W.; Saczyńska, V.; Porebska, A.; Dehaen, W.; Radecki, J.; et al. A biosensor based on electroactive dipyrromethene-Cu(II) layer deposited onto gold electrodes for the detection of antibodies against avian influenza virus type H5N1 in hen sera. *Anal. Bioanal. Chem.* **2017**, *407*, 7807–7814. [CrossRef] [PubMed]
41. Radecki, J.; Radecka, H. Mechanisms of Analytical Signals Generated by Electrochemical Genosensors: Review. *J. Mex. Chem. Soc.* **2015**, *59*, 276–281.
42. Malecka, K.; Stachyra, A.; Góra-Sochacka, A.; Sirko, A.; Zagórski-Ostoja, W.; Dehaen, W.; Radecka, H.; Radecki, J. New redox-active layer create via epoxy-amine reaction—The base of genosensor for the detection of specific DNA and RNA sequences of avian influenza virus H5N1. *Biosens. Bioelectron.* **2015**, *65*, 427–434. [CrossRef]
43. Piro, B.; Reisberg, S. Recent advances in electrochemical immunosensors. *Sensors* **2017**, *17*, 794. [CrossRef]
44. Ben Aissa, S.; Mars, A.; Catanante, G.; Marty, J.L.; Raouafi, N. Design of a redox-active surface for ultrasensitive redox capacitive aptasensing of aflatoxin M1 in milk. *Talanta* **2019**, *195*, 525–532. [CrossRef]
45. Santos, A.; Bueno, P.R.; Davis, J.J. A dual marker label free electrochemical assay for Flavivirus dengue diagnosis. *Biosens. Bioelectron.* **2018**, *100*, 519–525. [CrossRef]
46. Lu, J.; Liu, S.; Ge, S.; Yan, M.; Yu, J.; Hu, X. Ultrasensitive electrochemical immunosensor based on Au nanoparticles dotted carbon nanotube-graphene composite and functionalized mesoporous materials. *Biosens. Bioelectron.* **2012**, *33*, 29–35. [CrossRef] [PubMed]
47. Chen, A.; Chatterjee, S. Nanomaterials based electrochemical sensors for biomedical applications. *Chem. Soc. Rev.* **2013**, *42*, 5425–5438. [CrossRef] [PubMed]
48. Liu, G.; Qi, M.; Zhang, Y.; Cao, C.; Goldys, E.M. Nanocomposites of gold nanoparticles and graphene oxide towards an stable label-free electrochemical immunosensor for detection of cardiac marker troponin-I. *Anal. Chim. Acta* **2016**, *909*, 1–8. [CrossRef] [PubMed]
49. Peng, D.; Liang, R.P.; Huang, H.; Qiu, J.D. Electrochemical immunosensor for carcinoembryonic antigen based on signal amplification strategy of graphene and Fe3O4/Au NPs. *J. Electroanal. Chem.* **2016**, *761*, 112–117. [CrossRef]
50. Malarkodi, C.; Rajeshkumar, S.; Vanaja, M.; Paulkumar, K.; Gnanajobitha, G.; Annadurai, G. Eco-friendly synthesis and characterization of gold nanoparticles using Klebsiella pneumoniae. *J. Nanostructure Chem.* **2013**, *3*, 1–7. [CrossRef]
51. Jarocka, U.; Sawicka, R.; Góra-Sochacka, A.; Sirko, A.; Dehaen, W.; Radecki, J.; Radecka, H. An electrochemical immunosensor based on a 4,4′-thiobisbenzenethiol self-assembled monolayer for the detection of hemagglutinin from avian influenza virus H5N1. *Sens. Actuators B Chem.* **2016**, *228*, 25–30. [CrossRef]
52. Jarocka, U.; Wasowicz, M.; Radecka, H.; Malinowski, T.; Michalczuk, L.; Radecki, J. Impedimetric immunosensor for detection of plum pox virus in plant extracts. *Electroanalysis* **2011**, *23*, 2197–2204. [CrossRef]
53. Wasowicz, M.; Viswanathan, S.; Dvornyk, A.; Grzelak, K.; Kłudkiewicz, B.; Radecka, H. Comparison of electrochemical immunosensors based on gold nano materials and immunoblot techniques for detection of histidine-tagged proteins in culture medium. *Biosens. Bioelectron.* **2008**, *24*, 284–389. [CrossRef]
54. Wasowicz, M.; Milner, M.; Radecka, D.; Grzelak, K.; Radecka, H. Immunosensor incorporating Anti-His (C-term) IgG F(ab′) fragments attached to gold nanorods for detection of His-tagged proteins in culture medium. *Sensors* **2010**, *10*, 5409–5424. [CrossRef] [PubMed]
55. Rubira, R.J.G.; Camacho, S.A.; Martin, C.S.; Mejía-Salazar, J.R.; Gómez, F.R.; da Silva, R.R.; de Oliveira Junior, O.N.; Alessio, P.; Constantino, C.J.L. Designing silver nanoparticles for detecting levodopa (3,4-dihydroxyphenylalanine, l-dopa) using surface-enhanced raman scattering (SERS). *Sensors* **2020**, *20*, 15. [CrossRef] [PubMed]
56. Bhalla, N.; Di Lorenzo, M.; Pula, G.; Estrela, P. Protein phosphorylation detection using dual-mode field-effect devices and nanoplasmonic sensors. *Sci. Rep.* **2015**, *5*, 1–8. [CrossRef]
57. Formisano, N.; Bhalla, N.; Wong, L.C.C.; Di Lorenzo, M.; Pula, G.; Estrela, P. Multimodal electrochemical and nanoplasmonic biosensors using ferrocene-crowned nanoparticles for kinase drug discovery applications. *Electrochem. Commun.* **2015**, *57*, 70–73. [CrossRef]
58. Li, J.; Wu, Z.; Wang, H.; Shen, G.; Yu, R. A reusable capacitive immunosensor with a novel immobilization procedure based on 1,6-hexanedithiol and nano-Au self-assembled layers. *Sens. Actuators B Chem.* **2005**, *110*, 327–334. [CrossRef]
59. Kausaite-Minkstimiene, A.; Ramanaviciene, A.; Kirlyte, J.; Ramanavicius, A. Comparative study of random and oriented antibody immobilization techniques on the binding capacity of immunosensor. *Anal. Chem.* **2010**, *82*, 6401–6408. [CrossRef] [PubMed]

60. Bonroy, K.; Frederix, F.; Reekmans, G.; Dewolf, E.; De Palma, R.; Borghs, G.; Declerck, P.; Goddeeris, B. Comparison of random and oriented immobilisation of antibody fragments on mixed self-assembled monolayers. *J. Immunol. Methods* **2006**, *312*, 167–181. [CrossRef] [PubMed]
61. Matula, R.A. Electrical resistivity of copper, gold, palladium, and silver. *J. Phys. Chem. Ref. Data* **1979**, *8*, 1147–1298. [CrossRef]
62. Ruiz, G.; Tripathi, K.; Okyem, S.; Driskell, J.D. PH Impacts the Orientation of Antibody Adsorbed onto Gold Nanoparticles. *Bioconjug. Chem.* **2019**, *30*, 1182–1191. [CrossRef] [PubMed]
63. Sharma, H.; Mutharasan, R. Half antibody fragments improve biosensor sensitivity without loss of selectivity. *Anal. Chem.* **2013**, *85*, 2472–2477. [CrossRef] [PubMed]
64. Brett, C. Electrochemical Impedance Spectroscopy for Characterization of Electrochemical Sensors and Biosensors. *ECS Trans.* **2019**, *13*, 67. [CrossRef]
65. Luo, Y.; Packard, R.; Abiri, P.; Tai, Y.C.; Hsiai, T.K. Flexible intravascular EIS sensors for detecting metabolically active plaque. *Interfacing Bioelectron. Biomed. Sens.* **2020**, 143–162. [CrossRef]
66. Pejcic, B.; De Marco, R. Impedance spectroscopy: Over 35 years of electrochemical sensor optimization. *Electrochim. Acta* **2006**, *51*, 6217–6229. [CrossRef]
67. Halliwell, J.; Savage, A.C.; Buckley, N.; Gwenin, C. Electrochemical impedance spectroscopy biosensor for detection of active botulinum neurotoxin. *Sens. Bio-Sensing Res.* **2014**, *2*, 12–15. [CrossRef]
68. Manickam, P.; Vashist, A.; Madhu, S.; Sadasivam, M.; Sakthivel, A.; Kaushik, A.; Nair, M. Gold nanocubes embedded biocompatible hybrid hydrogels for electrochemical detection of H2O2. *Bioelectrochemistry* **2020**, *131*, 107373. [CrossRef]
69. Ahangar, L.E.; Mehrgardi, M.A. Amplified detection of hepatitis B virus using an electrochemical DNA biosensor on a nanoporous gold platform. *Bioelectrochemistry* **2017**, *131*, 107373. [CrossRef]
70. Xuan, J.; Jia, X.D.; Jiang, L.P.; Abdel-Halim, E.S.; Zhu, J.J. Gold nanoparticle-assembled capsules and their application as hydrogen peroxide biosensor based on hemoglobin. *Bioelectrochemistry* **2012**, *84*, 32–37. [CrossRef] [PubMed]
71. Park, W.; Emoto, K.; Jin, Y.; Shimizu, A.; Tamma, V.A.; Zhang, W. Controlled self-assembly of gold nanoparticles mediated by novel organic molecular cages. *Opt. Mater. Express* **2013**, *3*, 205–215. [CrossRef]
72. Khlebtsov, B.N.; Khlebtsov, N.G. On the measurement of gold nanoparticle sizes by the dynamic light scattering method. *Colloid J.* **2011**, *73*, 118–127. [CrossRef]
73. Philip, D. Synthesis and spectroscopic characterization of gold nanoparticles. *Spectrochim. Acta Part A Mol. Biomol. Spectrosc.* **2008**, *71*, 80–85. [CrossRef]
74. Stroth, N. A surface plasmon resonance-based method for monitoring interactions between G protein-coupled receptors and interacting proteins. *J. Biol. Methods* **2016**, *3*, 155–181. [CrossRef]
75. Locatelli-Hoops, S.; Yeliseev, A.A.; Gawrisch, K.; Gorshkova, I. Surface plasmon resonance applied to G protein-coupled receptors. *Biomed. Spectrosc. Imaging* **2013**, *2*, 155–181. [CrossRef] [PubMed]
76. Bhardwaj, S.K.; Basu, T. Study on binding phenomenon of lipase enzyme with tributyrin on the surface of graphene oxide array using surface plasmon resonance. *Thin Solid Films* **2018**, *645*, 10–181. [CrossRef]
77. Zhao, H.; Gorshkova, I.I.; Fu, G.L.; Schuck, P. A comparison of binding surfaces for SPR biosensing using an antibody-antigen system and affinity distribution analysis. *Methods* **2013**, *59*, 328–335. [CrossRef] [PubMed]
78. Wang, X.; Lv, W.; Wu, J.; Li, H.; Li, F. In situ generated nanozyme-initiated cascade reaction for amplified surface plasmon resonance sensing. *Chem. Commun.* **2020**. [CrossRef]
79. Wang, X.; Hou, T.; Lin, H.; Lv, W.; Li, H.; Li, F. In situ template generation of silver nanoparticles as amplification tags for ultrasensitive surface plasmon resonance biosensing of microRNA. *Biosens. Bioelectron.* **2019**, *39*, 124–132. [CrossRef]
80. Li, H.; Chang, J.; Hou, T.; Li, F. HRP-Mimicking DNAzyme-Catalyzed in Situ Generation of Polyaniline to Assist Signal Amplification for Ultrasensitive Surface Plasmon Resonance Biosensing. *Anal. Chem.* **2017**, *89*, 673–680. [CrossRef] [PubMed]
81. Gu, C.; Gai, P.; Hou, T.; Li, H.; Xue, C.; Li, F. Enzymatic Fuel Cell-Based Self-Powered Homogeneous Immunosensing Platform via Target-Induced Glucose Release: An Appealing Alternative Strategy for Turn-On Melamine Assay. *ACS Appl. Mater. Interfaces* **2017**, *9*, 35721–35728. [CrossRef]
82. De Juan-Franco, E.; Caruz, A.; Pedrajas, J.R.; Lechuga, L.M. Site-directed antibody immobilization using a protein A-gold binding domain fusion protein for enhanced SPR immunosensing. *Analyst* **2013**, *138*, 2023–2031. [CrossRef] [PubMed]
83. Soh, N.; Tokuda, T.; Watanabe, T.; Mishima, K.; Imato, T.; Masadome, T.; Asano, Y.; Okutani, S.; Niwa, O.; Brown, S. A surface plasmon resonance immunosensor for detecting a dioxin precursor using a gold binding polypeptide. *Talanta* **2003**, *60*, 733–745. [CrossRef]
84. Li, G.; Li, X.; Yang, M.; Chen, M.M.; Chen, L.C.; Xiong, X.L. A gold nanoparticles enhanced surface plasmon resonance immunosensor for highly sensitive detection of Ischemia-modified albumin. *Sensors* **2013**, *13*, 12794–12803. [CrossRef] [PubMed]
85. Wu, S.; Liu, H.; Liang, X.M.; Wu, X.; Wang, B.; Zhang, Q. Highly sensitive nanomechanical immunosensor using half antibody fragments. *Anal. Chem.* **2014**, *86*, 4271–4277. [CrossRef] [PubMed]
86. Lin, D.; Tang, T.; Jed Harrison, D.; Lee, W.E.; Jemere, A.B. A regenerating ultrasensitive electrochemical impedance immunosensor for the detection of adenovirus. *Biosens. Bioelectron.* **2015**, *68*, 129–134. [CrossRef]
87. Swartz, M.E.; Krull, I.S. *Handbook of Analytical Validation*; CRC Press: Boca Raton, FL, USA, 2012; p. 384. [CrossRef]
88. Srivastava, A.K.; MacFarlane, G.; Srivastava, V.P.; Mohan, S.; Baylink, D.J. A new monoclonal antibody ELISA for detection and characterization of C-telopeptide fragments of type I collagen in urine. *Calcif. Tissue Int.* **2001**, *69*, 327–336. [CrossRef]

89. Sun, X.; Fan, J.; Ye, W.; Zhang, H.; Cong, Y.; Xiao, J. A highly specific graphene platform for sensing collagen triple helix. *J. Mater. Chem. B* **2016**, *4*, 1064–1069. [CrossRef] [PubMed]
90. Sankiewicz, A.; Lukaszewski, Z.; Trojanowska, K.; Gorodkiewicz, E. Determination of collagen type IV by Surface Plasmon Resonance Imaging using a specific biosensor. *Anal. Biochem.* **2016**, *515*, 40–46. [CrossRef]
91. Leeming, D.J.; He, Y.; Veidal, S.S.; Nguyen, Q.H.T.; Larsen, D.V.; Koizumi, M.; Segovia-Silvestre, T.; Zhang, C.; Zheng, Q.; Sun, S.; et al. A novel marker for assessment of liver matrix remodeling: An enzyme-linked immunosorbent assay (ELISA) detecting a MMP generated type I collagen neo-epitope (C1M). *Biomarkers* **2011**, *16*, 616–628. [CrossRef]
92. Nielsen, M.J.; Nedergaard, A.F.; Sun, S.; Veidal, S.S.; Larsen, L.; Zheng, Q.; Suetta, C.; Henriksen, K.; Christiansen, C.; Karsdal, M.A.; et al. The neo-epitope specific PRO-C3 ELISA measures true formation of type III collagen associated with liver and muscle parameters. *Am. J. Transl. Res.* **2013**, *5*, 303.
93. Hua, X.; Wang, Y.Y.; Jia, P.; Xiong, Q.; Hu, Y.; Chang, Y.; Lai, S.; Xu, Y.; Zhao, Z.; Song, J. Multi-level transcriptome sequencing identifies COL1A1 as a candidate marker in human heart failure progression. *BMC Med.* **2020**, *18*, 1–16. [CrossRef]
94. Rega, R.; Mugnano, M.; Oleandro, E.; Tkachenko, V.; del Giudice, D.; Bagnato, G.; Ferraro, P.; Grilli, S.; Gangemi, S. Detecting collagen molecules at picogram level through electric field-induced accumulation. *Sensors* **2020**, *18*, 3567. [CrossRef] [PubMed]
95. Chen, E.T.; Thornton, J.T.; Kissinger, P.T.; Duh, S.H. Discovering of collagen-1's role in producing superconducting current in nanobiomimetic superlattice structured organometallic devices at room temperature enabled direct quantitation of sub pg/mL collagen-1. *Inform. Electron. Microsyst. TechConnect Briefs.* **2018**, *1*, 43–46.
96. Lisdat, F.; Schäfer, D. The use of electrochemical impedance spectroscopy for biosensing. *Anal. Bioanal. Chem.* **2008**, *391*, 1555–1567. [CrossRef] [PubMed]
97. Pal, K.; Asthana, N.; Aljabali, A.A.; Bhardwaj, S.K.; Kralj, S.; Penkova, A.; Thomas, A.; Zaheer, T.S.N.; Souza, F.G. A critical review on multifunctional smart materials 'nanographene' emerging avenue: Nano-imaging and biosensor applications. *Crit. Rev. Solid State Mater. Sci.* **2021**, *122*, 1–18. [CrossRef]

biosensors

Article

Electrochemical Biosensor for Markers of Neurological Esterase Inhibition

Neda Rafat [1,2], Paul Satoh [1] and Robert Mark Worden [1,2,3,*]

[1] Department of Chemical Engineering and Materials Science, Michigan State University, 428 S. Shaw Lane, East Lansing, MI 48824, USA; rafatned@msu.edu (N.R.); satoh@msu.edu (P.S.)
[2] The Institute for Quantitative Health Science and Engineering, Michigan State University, 775 Woodlot Dr, East Lansing, MI 48824, USA
[3] Department of Biomedical Engineering, Michigan State University, 775 Woodlot Dr, East Lansing, MI 48824, USA
* Correspondence: worden@msu.edu; Tel.: +1-(517)-242-8117

Abstract: A novel, integrated experimental and modeling framework was applied to an inhibition-based bi-enzyme (IBE) electrochemical biosensor to detect acetylcholinesterase (AChE) inhibitors that may trigger neurological diseases. The biosensor was fabricated by co-immobilizing AChE and tyrosinase (Tyr) on the gold working electrode of a screen-printed electrode (SPE) array. The reaction chemistry included a redox-recycle amplification mechanism to improve the biosensor's current output and sensitivity. A mechanistic mathematical model of the biosensor was used to simulate key diffusion and reaction steps, including diffusion of AChE's reactant (phenylacetate) and inhibitor, the reaction kinetics of the two enzymes, and electrochemical reaction kinetics at the SPE's working electrode. The model was validated by showing that it could reproduce a steady-state biosensor current as a function of the inhibitor (PMSF) concentration and unsteady-state dynamics of the biosensor current following the addition of a reactant (phenylacetate) and inhibitor phenylmethyl-sulfonylfluoride). The model's utility for characterizing and optimizing biosensor performance was then demonstrated. It was used to calculate the sensitivity of the biosensor's current output and the redox-recycle amplification factor as a function of experimental variables. It was used to calculate dimensionless Damkohler numbers and current-control coefficients that indicated the degree to which individual diffusion and reaction steps limited the biosensor's output current. Finally, the model's utility in designing IBE biosensors and operating conditions that achieve specific performance criteria was discussed.

Keywords: amperometric biosensor; neural esterase; acetylcholinesterase; inhibition; organophosphate; design; optimization; mathematical model; flux control; dimensionless

Citation: Rafat, N.; Satoh, P.; Worden, R.M. Electrochemical Biosensor for Markers of Neurological Esterase Inhibition. *Biosensors* **2021**, *11*, 459. https://doi.org/10.3390/bios11110459

Received: 30 August 2021
Accepted: 8 November 2021
Published: 16 November 2021

Publisher's Note: MDPI stays neutral with regard to jurisdictional claims in published maps and institutional affiliations.

1. Introduction

Electrochemical biosensors are analytical devices that detect analytes by transforming a biochemical reaction into a quantitative, electrical signal. They integrate the specificity of biological recognition molecules (e.g., antibodies) with the advantages of electrochemical detection techniques [1,2]. Electrochemical biosensors benefit from several advantages, such as low cost, ease of use, portability, and simplicity of construction. These advantages make electrochemical biosensors great options for the development of analytical devices in different fields [3,4]. Some of the limitations for electrochemical biosensors are limited shelf life, narrow or limited temperature range for operation, and sometimes high sensitivity of detection results in false-positive results [5]. The electrochemical biosensors can be divided into four major categories based on the electrochemical technique that is used to measure the electrical signal produced by the biochemical mechanism: amperometric biosensors, potentiometric biosensors, conductometric biosensors, and impedimetric biosensors [6].

Amperometric biosensors detect chemicals at a constant electrochemical potential by measuring the oxidation or reduction current produced by electroactive products of a biochemical reaction [7]. Their low cost, high sensitivity, fast response time, simplicity of design, compactness, and potential for miniaturization make amperometric biosensors well suited for detecting a wide range of chemicals and biochemical agents, including disease markers [8,9].

Amperometric biosensors that measure analytes indirectly by their inhibition of target enzymes have been developed for environmental and healthcare applications [10]. Such inhibition-based biosensors can be very sensitive when the target enzyme is inhibited by a very low concentration of its inhibitor [11]. For that reason, significant research has been devoted to developing amperometric biosensors that measure markers of neurological disease processes that inhibit neural esterases, such as acetylcholinesterase (AChE) [12–17].

Some organophosphate compounds (OPs) are potent inhibitors of neural esterases and, for that reason, are used as pesticides and as chemical weapons [18]. The well-known neural esterase acetylcholinesterase (AChE) breaks down the neurotransmitter acetylcholine, which chemically relays an impulse across the synapse between two neurons [19]. The inhibition of AChE by OPs prevents acetylcholine hydrolysis, resulting in continuous nerve firing, which can cause severe, acute health issues, including death [20]. Each year, approximately 3 million people are poisoned by organophosphates, accounting for 300,000 deaths worldwide [21].

The gold standard analytical method for OPs is gas/liquid chromatography combined with mass spectroscopy [22]. This method is sensitive, specific, and reliable. However, it is not well suited for many on-site applications because it requires bulky, expensive equipment and involves complicated and time-consuming sample processing by trained technicians [22]. In contrast, inhibition-based amperometric biosensors offer the potential to measure OPs on-site rapidly, inexpensively, with minimal sample processing using a miniature electronic device similar to a personal blood-glucose meter [23].

When an enzyme is strongly inhibited by a specific substance, it may be possible to develop an inhibition-based enzyme biosensor that can specifically detect the presence of the inhibitor in a complex mixture that may include unknown chemicals or pollutants. However, for enzymes that are sensitive to multiple inhibitors, this approach cannot discern which inhibitor(s) is present in the mixture.

Although amperometric biosensors might not offer the same sensitivity and specificity of detection that gas/liquid chromatography-based techniques offer, the fact that they can be developed as portable diagnostic devices for quick and cost-effective initial analysis makes them valuable for initial screening and monitoring. Commercialized miniaturized potentiostats and screen-printed electrodes (SPEs) can be used to develop portable amperometric biosensor systems. SPEs include one or more printed working electrodes, a reference electrode, and a counter electrode printed on a solid substrate. The assay chemistry is performed on the working electrode, and the electrochemical assay is conducted by contacting the SPE with a sample solution. SPEs can replace bulky convention electrochemical cells with a miniaturized system that can be used for simple and quick electrochemical measurements. However, because SPEs are designed to minimize the required space and reagent volume, their measurements are often not as stable and accurate as those conducted in a conventional electrochemical cell.

Research to rationally design and optimize amperometric biosensors for detecting inhibitors of AChE or other neural esterases (e.g., butyrylesterase) has been hampered by the lack of a comprehensive mathematical model able to predict the rates of potentially rate-limiting mass-transfer and chemical reaction steps that produce the amperometric signal. Zhang et al. developed a theoretical model for immobilized-enzyme-inhibition biosensors under the assumption that the inhibition process is diffusion-limited [24]. Choi et al. developed a mathematical model for a fiber-optic biosensor to detect OPs. This model, which simulated both AChE inhibition kinetics and diffusion, was able to optimize the concentrations of AChE and its substrate [25].

We recently developed a novel, integrated experimental and modeling framework that includes a steady-state, mechanistic mathematical model that describes the rate of key mass-transfer and reaction steps and a novel dimensional-analysis approach to assess the degree to which individual mass-transfer and reaction steps limit the biosensor's amplitude and sensitivity [26]. We then demonstrated the framework's utility using a novel amperometric electrochemical immunosensor.

In this paper, we apply the framework to an inhibition-based bi-enzyme (IBE) amperometric biosensor assembled on a s SPE. The IBE interface contained a neural esterase (AChE) and an oxidase enzyme (tyrosinase) that generates a redox-reaction loop to amplify the biosensor's output [27–29]. We present a novel, unsteady-state model of the IBE biosensor that consists of unsteady-state mass balance equations describing the mass-transfer and reaction steps that govern the biosensor's signal. We use experimental results to validate the model and discuss the utility of dimensionless groups based on the model, including current-control coefficients, sensitivity coefficients, and Damkohler numbers, to rationally design and optimize IBE biosensors.

2. Materials and Methods

2.1. Materials

Sodium phosphate (monobasic and dibasic), AChE (C2888, from Electrophorus electricus), tyrosinase (T3824, from mushroom), bovine serum albumin (BSA), glutaric dialdehyde (50 wt.% solution in water), PMSF, and phenylacetate were obtained from Sigma Aldrich (St. Louis, MO, USA). Ultrapure water (18.2 MΩ) was produced by a Nanopure-UV four-stage purifier (Barnstead International, Dubuque, IA, USA); the purifier was equipped with a UV source and a final 0.2 μm filter. Ultrapure water was used to prepare all aqueous solutions. Screen-printed electrodes were obtained from Conductive Technologies Inc. (New York, NY, USA). and Metrohm DropSens (models DRP-250AT, Asturias, Spain).

2.2. Enzyme Electrode Preparation

SPEs were selected as the platform for conducting the experiments for two reasons. First, SPEs are small, inexpensive, and disposable, making them well-suited for POC applications. Second, SPEs are often used in the development of commercialized electrochemical biosensors. SPEs were cleaned by sonication in pure ethanol for 2 min followed by rinsing with ultrapure water. Different types of SPEs, including carbon (DPR-C110), low temperature cured gold (DRP-220BT), high temperature cured gold SPEs (DRP-250AT), and carbon nanotube-modified (DRP-10SWCNT), were tried for the fabrication of the biosensor. The immobilization technique used in this work was based on the crosslinking of two enzymes with glutaraldehyde and bovine serum albumin (BSA) [30]. This technique resulted in an efficient and rapid comobilization of two enzymes. Although this technique worked on all types of SPEs, DPR-250AT resulted in a better repeatability of data. To optimize the immobilization method, a variety of BSA concentrations, glutaraldehyde concentrations, and ratios of AChE to tyrosinase were studied.

To prepare the enzyme solution, 40 μL of 50 mM phosphate buffer pH 7, 20 μL of 20 mg/mL tyrosinase in phosphate buffer, 20 μL of 1 mg/mL AChE in phosphate buffer, 10 μL of 2.7 mg/mL BSA in phosphate buffer, and 10 μL of 4 wt.% glutaraldehyde in water were mixed together just before starting the preparation procedure. To obtain the optimized concentration of the two enzymes, BSA, and glutaraldehyde, 3 μL of enzyme solution (in the case of DropSens SPEs) or 1 μL of enzyme solution (in the case of CTI SPEs) were deposited on the working electrode, and the SPEs were left at 4 °C to dry overnight. The next day, the prepared bi-enzyme-modified SPEs were rinsed with ultrapure water and then stored in phosphate buffer at 4 °C.

2.3. PMSF Detection and Electrochemical Measurements

PMSF is used as a model AChE inhibitor because it is less toxic to humans than many OPs. Its reaction mechanism is similar to that of OPs, but its sulfonamide bond with serine's hydroxyl group in the AChE active site is more stable than a typical OP linkage.

To conduct the electrochemical measurements, the desired electrochemical potential was applied on the SPE's working electrode relative to the SPE's printed pseudo-Ag/AgCl reference electrode. The SPE's counter electrode served as the anode, so the biosensor's current would not flow through the reference electrode and change its potential. In experiments to detect AChE inhibition by PMSF, 30 μL of 50 mM phosphate buffer (pH 7) was added to the IBE SPE biosensors. A potential of −200 mV relative to an Ag/AgCl reference electrode was maintained on the working electrode using a potentiometer (CHI 660, C.H. Instruments, Austin, TX, USA). An aliquot of phenylacetate solution was added to initiate the IBE's amperometric signal. Then, after a stable electrochemical signal was obtained, a known amount of PMSF was added while continuously recording the electrochemical current as a function of time. The experiments were repeated in triplicate, and steady-state current values were reported as the mean ± standard deviation of three replicates.

2.4. Mechanistic Mathematical Model of the IBE Biosensor Interface

The biosensor's conceptual model (Figure 1) includes a working electrode onto which an enzyme-containing layer of thickness L is bound, a diffusion layer having thickness δ, and the bulk solution. AChE (E_1) hydrolyzes the reactant phenylacetate (S_1) to give phenol (S_2) (Figure 2), which is then oxidized twice by tyrosinase (E_2)–first to catechol (S_4) and then to o-quinone (S_3). The S_4 can then be reduced back to S_3 at the electrode, generating the biosensor's output current. This current is amplified by a redox-recycle loop in which each molecule of S_4 produced by the combined actions of E_1 and E_2 may be sequentially oxidized by E_2 and then reduced at the electrode many times, with additional current being produced in each cycle.

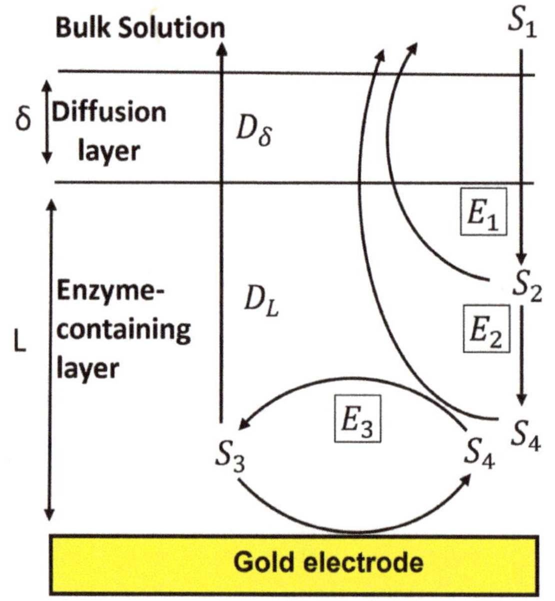

Figure 1. Schematic representation of reactions in the IBE biosensor interface. S_1, S_2, S_3, and S_4 denote phenylacetate, phenol, catechol, and o-quinone, respectively. E_1, E_2, and E_3 denote acetylcholinesterase, tyrosinase's phenolase activity, and tyrosinase's catecholase activity, respectively.

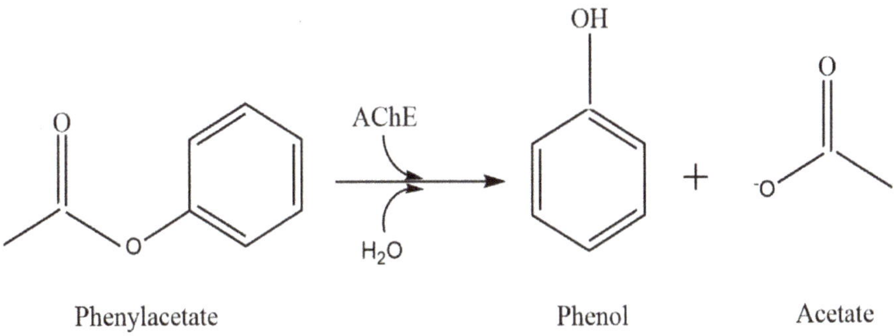

Figure 2. Hydrolysis of phenylacetate with AChE.

The concentration of PMSF (I, Figure 3) in a sample was determined from the drop in the biosensor's current following addition and exposure to PMSF.

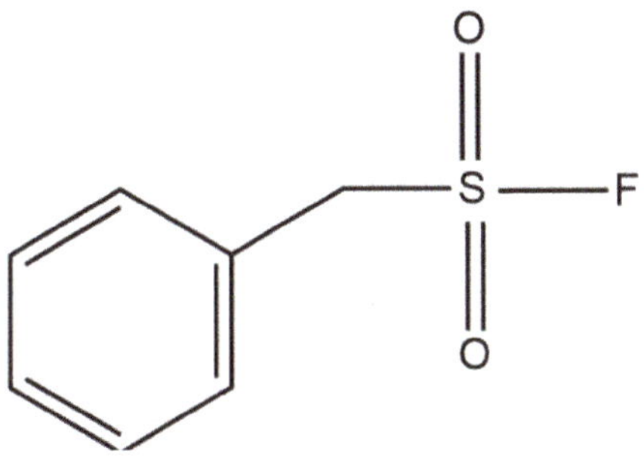

Figure 3. Molecular structure of PMSF.

The biosensor's mathematical model consists of a set of coupled, unsteady-state, differential mass-balance equations that take into account: (1) the rate of mass transfer of phenylacetate, phenol, catechol, O-quinone, and PMSF in the x-direction through the diffusion layer ($L < x < L + \delta$) and the enzyme-containing layer ($0 < x < L$); (2) the kinetics of the enzyme-catalyzed chemical reactions by AChE and tyrosinase within the enzyme-containing layer; and (3) the kinetics of electrochemical reduction of o-quinone at the gold electrode. The enzymes' concentrations are assumed to be uniform across the enzyme-containing layer [31,32]. The bulk solution is assumed to be well-mixed, with the concentrations of all chemical species remaining constant at their initial values [33]. The PMSF bulk concentration is assumed to be zero before the addition time ($t = T_0$).

2.4.1. AChE Inactivation and Enzyme Kinetics

PMSF inhibits AChE's reaction rate (E_1) by binding at AChE's active site [34]. The sulfonyl group of PMSF (Figure 3) mimics the carbonyl group of phenylacetate's transition state. As a result, the hydroxyl group of the serine residue in AChE's active site nucleophilically attacks the sulfonyl group, which can lead to irreversible, covalent sulfonylation of AChE [35]. In this model, we assumed that the rate of PMSF (I) consumption is equal to the rate of AChE inactivation.

The general scheme for inactivation of AChE with PMSF (I) in the presence of the substrate (S_1) is shown in Figure 4.

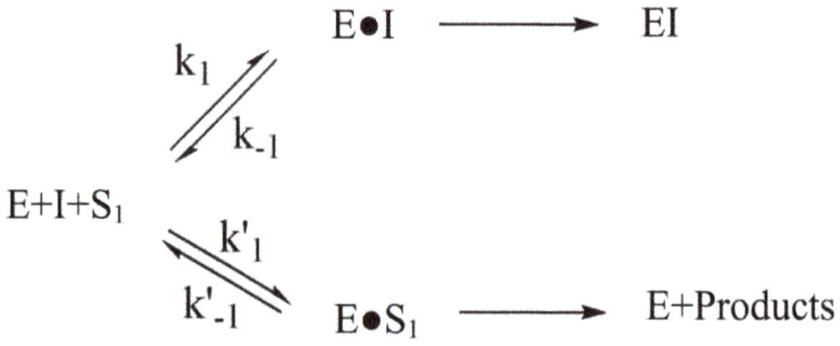

Figure 4. Inhibition mechanism of AChE (E) with PMSF (I) in the presence of substrate (S_1).

Studies have shown that AChE inhibition with PMSF follows pseudo-first-order kinetics [35] (Equation (1)):

$$\ln \frac{V'_{max,1}}{V_{max,1}} = -k't' \tag{1}$$

where $V_{max,1}$ and $V'_{max,1}$ are the maximum reaction rates for AChE in the absence of the inhibitor and when incubated with inhibitor for a time of t', respectively. k' is the pseudo-first-order rate constant for the inactivation of AChE by PMSF (Equation (2)):

$$k' = \frac{k_2[I]}{\frac{1}{(1-\gamma)}k_I + [I]} \tag{2}$$

The affinity of PMSF for AChE is given by the Michaelis–Menten type constant, k_I [35]:

$$k_I = \frac{k_{-1} + k_2}{k_{+1}} \tag{3}$$

where k_{+1} and k_{-1} are the forward and backward rate constants for the formation of the Michaelis–Menten type complex, and k_2 is the sulfonylation rate constant (Figure 4). The value of γ is given by Equation (4), where $K_{m,1}$ is the Michaelis–Menten constant for phenylacetate hydrolysis.

$$\gamma = \frac{[S_1]}{[S_1] + K_{m,1}} \tag{4}$$

PMSF competes with phenylacetate for the active site of AChE, thereby changing $K_{m,1}$ to an the apparent value $K'_{m,1}$ (Equation (5)) [25].

$$K'_{m,1} = K_{m,1}\left(1 + \frac{[I]}{k_I}\right) \tag{5}$$

Equations (6)–(8) describe the enzymatic kinetics of AChE in the presence of PMSF, where $k_{cat,1}$ is the turnover number of AChE for phenylacetate. By assuming that the rate of PMSF (I) consumption equals the rate of enzyme inactivation, Equation (9) was derived to describe the rate of PMSF (I) consumption.

$$v_1 = \frac{V'_{max,1}[S_1]}{K'_{m,1} + [S_1]} \tag{6}$$

$$V'_{max,1} = V_{max,1}e^{-k/t} \tag{7}$$

$$V_{max,1} = k_{cat,1}E_1 \tag{8}$$

$$\frac{dI}{dt} = -k'E_1e^{-k't} \tag{9}$$

2.4.2. Tyrosinase Enzyme Kinetics

Tyrosinase exhibits two enzymatic activities: monophenolase activity, which catalyzes the hydroxylation of phenol to produce o-diphenol (catechol) and catecholase activity, which catalyzes the oxidation of catechol to o-quinone. Figure 5 shows the scheme for the two-step oxidation of phenol with tyrosinase.

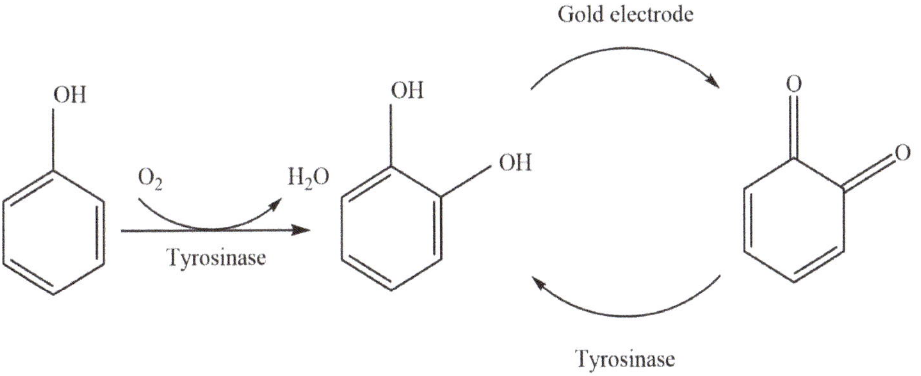

Figure 5. Scheme of phenol oxidation with tyrosinase to produce o-quinone.

Studies have shown that the hydroxylation step (monophenolase activity) is much slower than the oxidation step (catecholase activity), and therefore limits the o-quinone production rate [36]. Therefore, we assumed that the rate (v_2) of o-quinone (S_4) production from phenol (S_2) can be obtained from Equations (11)–(12), where E_2 corresponds to phenolase activity of tyrosinase. The rate (v_3) of conversion of catechol (S_3) to o-quinone (S_4) can be given by Equations (12) and (13), where E_3 denotes the catecholase activity of tyrosinase [29]

$$v_2 = \frac{V_{max,2}[S_2]}{K_{m,2} + [S_2]} \tag{10}$$

$$V_{max,2} = k_{cat,2}\, E_2 \tag{11}$$

$$v_3 = \frac{V_{max,3}[S_3]}{K_{m,3} + [S_3]} \tag{12}$$

$$V_{max,3} = k_{cat,3}\, E_3 \tag{13}$$

The molecules of o-quinone produced by tyrosinase are assumed to be reduced back to catechol at the working electrode at a rate described by the Butler–Volmer equation (Equation (14)):

$$J = nFD_L \left[\frac{\partial Q}{\partial x}\right]_{x=0} = nFK_0[Q]_{x=0}\, e^{\left(-\frac{\alpha nF(E-E_h)}{RT}\right)} - nFK_0[C]_{x=0}\, e^{\left(\frac{(1-\alpha)nF(E-E_h)}{RT}\right)} \tag{14}$$

where J is the electric current density, n is the number of electrons transferred (e.g., n = 2 for the electrochemical reduction of Q), α is the charge transfer coefficient (assumed to be 0.4), F is the Faraday constant (96,485 C mol^{-1}), K_0 is the apparent electron transfer rate constant for Q, R is the universal gas constant (8.314 J K^{-1} mol^{-1}), T is the absolute temperature (298 K), and E_h is the redox potential for electrochemical reduction of Q to C under the experimental conditions. An E_h value of 0.15 V was determined as the midpoint between the cathodic peak and anodic peak of cyclic voltammogram obtained under the same conditions.

2.4.3. Mass Balance Equations

The mass balance equations including diffusion and enzymatic reaction for S_1, S_2, S_3, S_4, and I across the enzyme-containing layer (0 < x < L) can be derived (Equations (15)–(19)).

$$\frac{\partial S_1}{\partial t} = D_L \frac{\partial^2 S_1}{\partial x^2} - \frac{V'_{max,1}[S_1]}{K'_{m,1} + [S_1]} \tag{15}$$

$$\frac{\partial S_2}{\partial t} = D_L \frac{\partial^2 S_2}{\partial x^2} - \frac{V_{max,2}E_2[S_2]}{K_{m,2} + [S_2]} + \frac{V'_{max}[S_1]}{K'_{m,1} + [S_1]} \tag{16}$$

$$\frac{\partial S_3}{\partial t} = D_L \frac{\partial^2 S_3}{\partial x^2} - \frac{V_{max,3}E_3[S_3]}{K_{m,3} + [S_3]} \tag{17}$$

$$\frac{\partial S_4}{\partial t} = D_L \frac{\partial^2 S_4}{\partial x^2} + \frac{V_{max,3}[S_3]}{K_{m,3} + [S_3]} \tag{18}$$

$$\frac{\partial I}{\partial t} = D_L \frac{\partial^2 I}{\partial x^2} + k'E_1 e^{-k't} \tag{19}$$

2.4.4. Boundary Conditions

Because Q reduction at the electrode generates C in equimolar amounts, the fluxes of Q and C at x = 0 were assumed to be equal in magnitude but opposite in sign (Equation (20)).

$$D_L[\frac{\partial S_4}{\partial x}]_{x=0} = -D_L[\frac{\partial S_3}{\partial x}]_{x=0} \tag{20}$$

At x = 0, S_1, S_2, S_3, and I are assumed not to be consumed or produced at the electrode (Equation (21)):

$$[\frac{\partial S_1}{\partial x}]_{x=0} = 0, [\frac{\partial S_2}{\partial x}]_{x=0} = 0, [\frac{\partial S_3}{\partial x}]_{x=0} = 0, [\frac{\partial I}{\partial x}]_{x=0} = 0 \tag{21}$$

Partitioning kinetics of all reactants were assumed to be rapid enough that the interfacial concentrations at the boundaries of the diffusion layer and enzyme-containing layer remained at equilibrium. Identical partition coefficients ($k_p = 1$) were assumed for all reactants (Equations (22)–(26)).

$$[S_1]_{L+} = k_p[S_1]_{L+} \tag{22}$$

$$[S_2]_{L+} = k_p[S_2]_{L+} \tag{23}$$

$$[S_3]_{L+} = k_p[S_3]_{L+} \tag{24}$$

$$[S_4]_{L+} = k_p[S_4]_{L+} \tag{25}$$

$$[I]_{L+} = k_p[S_4]_{L+} \tag{26}$$

The bulk solution (where x = ∞) contained S_1 at a concentration of $S_1(\infty)$ but negligible concentrations of S_2, S_3, and S_4 (Equations (27)–(31)).

$$[S_1]_{x=\infty} = C(\infty) \tag{27}$$

$$[S_2]_{x=\infty} = 0 \tag{28}$$

$$[S_3]_{x=\infty} = 0 \tag{29}$$

$$[S_4]_{x=\infty} = 0 \tag{30}$$

$$[I]_{x=\infty,\ t<T0} = 0,\ [I]_{x=\infty,\ T0<t} = I(\infty) \tag{31}$$

Because no reaction is assumed to occur in the diffusion layer, the flux of species entering this layer was assumed to equal that exiting it (Equations (32)–(36)).

$$D_L[\frac{\partial S_1}{\partial x}]_{x=L-} = \frac{D_\delta}{k_p\,\delta}\{k_p\,S_1(\infty) - [S_1]_{x=L-}\} \tag{32}$$

$$D_L[\frac{\partial S_2}{\partial x}]_{x=L-} = -\frac{D_\delta}{\delta}\{[S_2]_{x=L+} - 0\} = -\frac{D_\delta}{k_p\,\delta}[S_2]_{x=L-} \tag{33}$$

$$D_L[\frac{\partial S_3}{\partial x}]_{x=L-} = -\frac{D_\delta}{\delta}\{[S_3]_{x=L+} - 0\} = -\frac{D_\delta}{k_p\,\delta}[S_3]_{x=L-} \tag{34}$$

$$D_L[\frac{\partial S_4}{\partial x}]_{x=L-} = -\frac{D_\delta}{\delta}\{[S_4]_{x=L+} - 0\} = -\frac{D_\delta}{k_p\,\delta}[S_4]_{x=L-} \tag{35}$$

$$D_L[\frac{\partial I}{\partial x}]_{x=L-} = \frac{D_\delta}{k_p\,\delta}\{k_p\,I(\infty) - [I]_{x=L-}\} \tag{36}$$

2.4.5. Initial Conditions

Initial conditions of phenylacetate at injection time (t = 0) are given in Equation (37):

$$[S_i]_{\,i=2:4,0\leqslant x\leqslant L} = 0,\ [S_1]_{0\leqslant x<L} = 0, [S_1]_{x=L} = S_1(\infty) \tag{37}$$

The inhibitor concentration (I) was assumed to be zero before it was injected at (T_0) and was assumed to be constant throughout the enzyme-containing layer and solution afterward (Equation (38)):

$$[I]_{0<t<T_0,} = 0,\ [I]_{T_0<t} = I(\infty) \tag{38}$$

A splitting-finite-difference algorithm was programmed in MATLAB and used to solve the mass balance equations (Equations (15)–(19)) numerically using the parameters given in Table 1 and the boundary and initial conditions given in Equations (20)–(38).

Table 1. Parameters and variables used in the numerical simulation.

Parameter/Variable	Dimensional Parameter	Variation Range	Value Used to Fit Experimental Data
Time	t, s	0–300	–
Distance from electrode surface	x, cm	3.0×10^{-4}–3.0×10^{-2}	3.0×10^{-3}
Phenylacetate concentration	(S_1), mM	0–1.5	0.9
PMSF concentration	(I), mM	0–0.5	–
Acetylcholinesterase concentration	(E_1), μM	0–100	30
Tyrosinase Concentration (phenolase activity)	(E_2), mM	0–5	1.45
Tyrosinase Concentration (catecholase activity)	(E_3), mM	0–5	1.65
Michaelis–Menten constant of phenylacetate	$K_{m,1}$, μM	0–100	50.5
Michaelis–Menten constant of phenol	$K_{m,2}$, μM	0–10	0.25
Michaelis–Menten constant of catechol	$K_{m,3}$, μM	0–10	0.22
Acetylcholinesterase turnover number for phenylacetate	$k_{cat,1}$, s^{-1}	2.0×10^2–2.0×10^5	2.3×10^4
Tyrosinase turnover number for phenol	$k_{cat,2}$, s^{-1}	2.0–2.0×10^3	20
Tyrosinase turnover number for catechol	$k_{cat,3}$, s^{-1}	2.0–2.0×10^3	760
Dissociation constant of PMSF	k_I, mM	0.02–2.0	0.25

Table 1. *Cont.*

Parameter/Variable	Dimensional Parameter	Variation Range	Value Used to Fit Experimental Data
Reaction constant of deactivation of acetylcholinesterase with PMSF	k_2, s^{-1}	0.001–0.1	0.005
Enzyme-containing layer thickness	L, nm	10–100	25
Diffusion layer thickness	δ, μm	10–200	30
Diffusion coefficient in diffusion layer	D_δ, $cm^2\ s^{-1}$	1×10^{-6}–9×10^{-5}	2.2×10^{-5}
Diffusion coefficient in enzyme-containing layer	D_L, $cm^2\ s^{-1}$	1×10^{-8}–9×10^{-6}	2.28×10^{-8}
Standard redox electrochemical potential of O-quinone	E^0, V	0.15	0.15
Heterogeneous electron transfer rate constant	K_0, cm s^{-1}	1×10^{-7}–1×10^{-4}	1×10^{-5}

3. Results and Discussion

3.1. Biosensor's Response to PMSF

Figure 6 shows a typical amperometry experiment to detect PMSF. Phenylacetate was added at about 35 s, and PMSF was added at about 190 s. As soon as a buffer sample containing PMSF was added, the biosensor's current rapidly declined and then returned to a relatively stable value whose magnitude varied with the PMSF concentration in the sample. A first-order time constant for the IBE biosensors' response to PMSF (defined as 63% toward the relatively stable current value) was typically about 20 s.

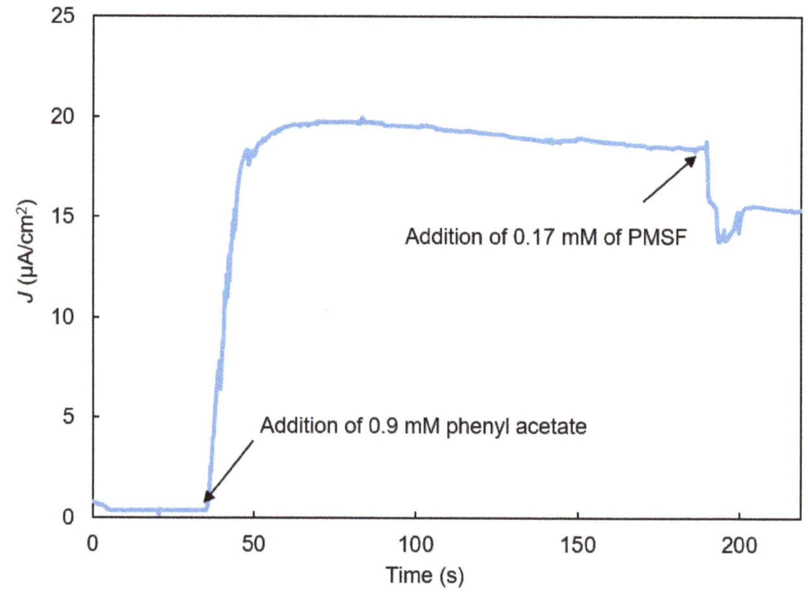

Figure 6. Current vs. time response of the bi-enzyme biosensor to the addition of phenylacetate (S_1) to obtain a final phenylacetate (S_1) concentration of 0.9 mM followed by the addition of inhibitor PMSF to obtain a final PMSF concentration of 0.17 mM.

Control experiments were conducted to characterize the IBE biosensor's response to blank samples with the addition of a bolus of the buffer without PMSF (Figure 7). As soon as a buffer sample without PMSF was added, the biosensor's signal rapidly declined and then returned to a relatively stable current very close to that before the blank sample was added.

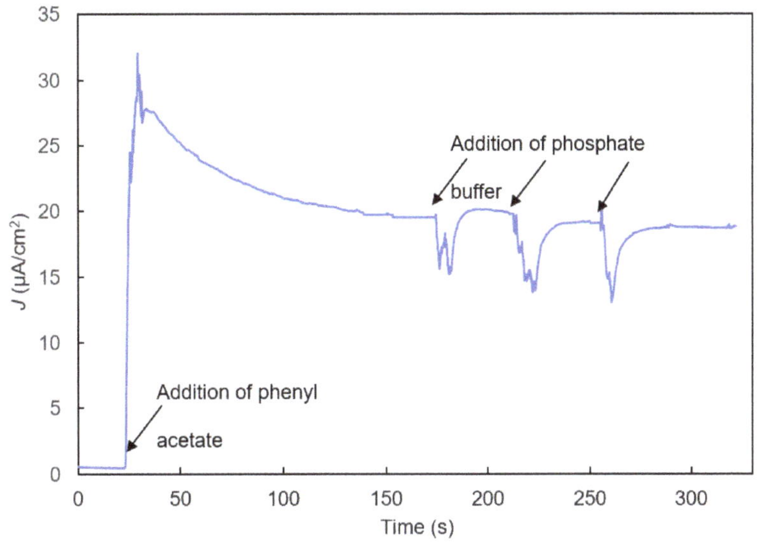

Figure 7. Control experiment to study the effect of phosphate buffer addition on the bi-enzyme biosensor's signal.

The PMSF-challenge experiments described above were repeated for samples containing a variety of PMSF concentrations. Figure 8 shows the current to which the signal returned after the initial decline as a function of the PMSF concentration in the sample. The calibration curve had a sensitivity (slope) of 18.4 µA cm^{-2} (mM PMSF)$^{-1}$ and an R^2 value for a linear fit of 0.995.

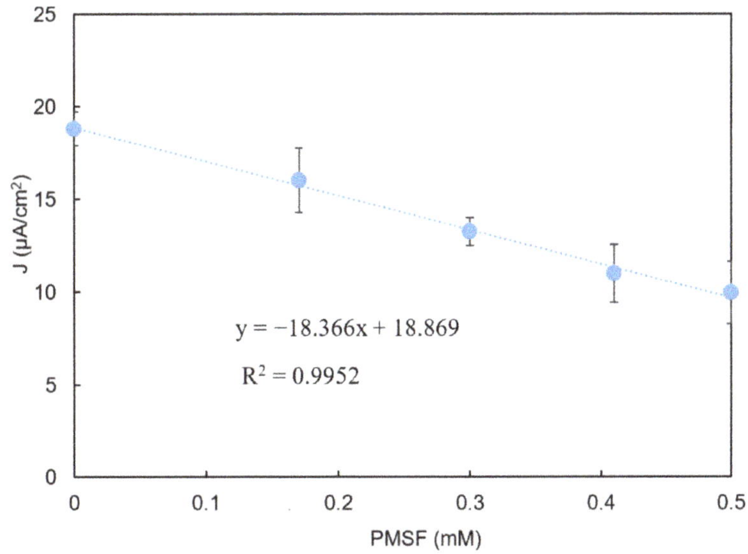

Figure 8. Current vs. PMSF concentration. Error bars indicate the mean ± standard deviation of three replicates. Phenylacetate: 0.9 mM. $y = -18.366x + 18.869$, $R^2 = 0.9952$.

3.2. Validation of the Mathematical Model and Simulation of the Biosensor's Response

The numerical model successfully simulated the biosensor's behavior shown in Figures 6–8. To explain the initial, rapid signal decline triggered by sample addition, we hypothesized that the increase in convective mass transfer while the sample was being pipetted into the solution on the SPE altered the pseudo-steady-state concentration gradients of the reacting chemical intermediates (S_2, S_3, and S_4) in the enzyme-containing layer. To simulate this effect in the model, we decreased the concentrations of these intermediates in the enzyme-containing layer by some fraction (e.g., 20%) at t = T_0 (Equations (39)–(41)):

$$[S_2]_{0<x<L,\ t=T_0^+} = 0.8\ [S_2]_{0<x<L,\ t=T_0^-} \quad (39)$$

$$[S_3]_{0<x<L,\ t=T_0^+} = 0.8\ [S_3]_{0<x<L,\ t=T_0^-} \quad (40)$$

$$[S_4]_{0<x<L,\ t=T_0^+} = 0.8\ [S_4]_{0<x<L,\ t=T_0^-} \quad (41)$$

This change enabled the model to predict the biosensors observed dynamics following sample addition, including the sudden drop in the biosensor's signal, followed by a return to a stable current (Figure 9A), providing support for the hypothesis.

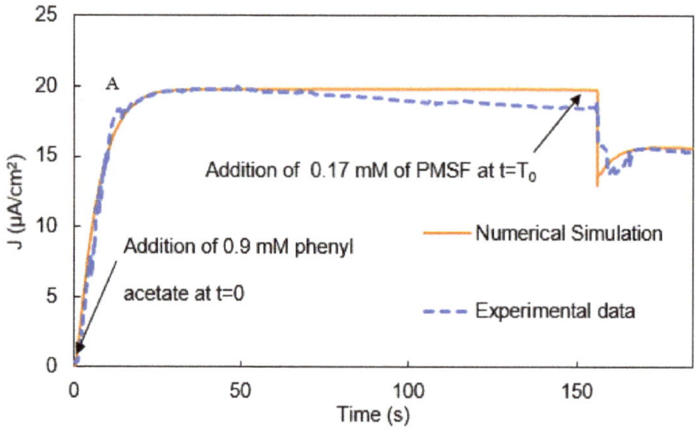

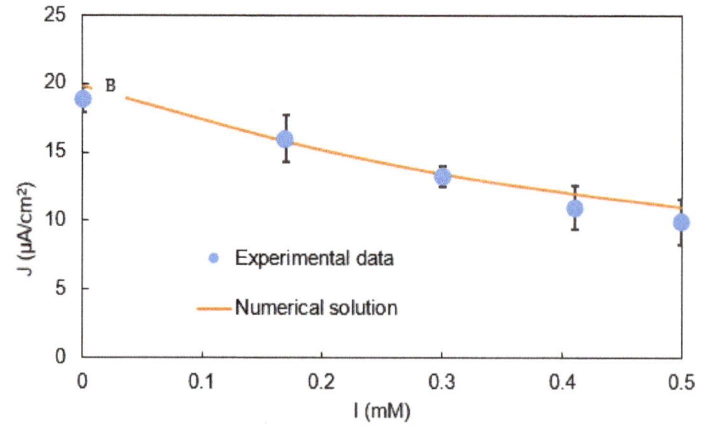

Figure 9. (**A**): Simulated the bi-enzyme biosensor's signal vs. time. (**B**): Simulated current density vs. PMSF concentration (I). Error bars indicate the mean ± standard deviation of three replicates.

The model was also able to accurately predict the relatively stable current that resulted after the initial biosensor-response dynamics as a function of the PMSF concentration in the sample (Figure 9B).

Figures 6, 7 and 9B show that after phenylacetate was added, the biosensor's current increased rapidly, went through a maximum, and then exhibited a gradual decay. The mechanism responsible for the decay is unknown, but it may result from the formation of byproducts of o-quinone reduction at the electrode that are not re-oxidized as rapidly by tyrosinase as catechol. The result of such a reaction would be a gradual increase in the byproduct concentration, and decrease in the catechol and o-quinone concentrations, and, consequently, a gradual decrease in the biosensor's current.

Signal Amplification by Redox-Recycle Loop

The degree of biosensor signal amplification due to the redox-recycle loop involving catechol and O-quinone (Figure 5) activity can be quantified using an amplification factor (AF), which is defined as the ratio of the biosensor's current density (J) in the presence of catecholase activity to that in the absence of the catecholase activity (Equation (42)) [29]:

$$AF = \frac{J|_{E_3 \neq 0}}{J|_{E_3 = 0}} \tag{42}$$

After validating the biosensor model (Figure 9A,B), we used it to explore the extent of signal amplification under a variety of operating conditions. Figure 10A shows the model-predicted output current both in the presence and absence of the amplification system. To predict the absence of amplification system zero, catecholase activity of tyrosinase was set to zero in the model. The predicted AF of about three across the range of [I] simulated indicates that redox amplification increases the biosensor's current roughly three-fold under the experimental conditions.

The effect of catecholase concentration (E3) on the predicted AF was also explored with the model (Figure 10B). This result shows an increasing tyrosinase concentration would increase the biosensor's output by increasing the redox amplification.

3.3. *Biosensor Sensitivity*

Biosensor sensitivity (S) with respect to PMSF concentration [I] is defined in Equation (43):

$$S = \frac{dJ}{d[I]} \tag{43}$$

To calculate S for a given set of experimental conditions, the incremental change in J (ΔJ) resulting from an incremental change in [I] ($\Delta[I]$) was calculated by the model. Then the asymptotic value of the ratio $\Delta J/\Delta[I]$ as $\Delta[I]$ approached zero was determined and used as the S value for those conditions. The resulting S values were plotted as function of a dimensionless phenylacetate concentration ($[S_1]/K_{m,1,app}$) for several [I] values (Figure 11A).

All the sensitivity curves exhibited a maximum value for the following reasons. At low $[S_1]/K_{m,1,app}$ values, the S_1 hydrolysis rate, and thus the J value, is so low that the maximum possible drop in J due to an increase on PMSF concentration is also small. At large $[S_1]/K_{m,1,app}$ values, almost all AChE active sites are occupied with S_1 values, and are unavailable to bind to PMSF molecules; thus the addition of PMSF has little effect on J.

For all $[S_1]/K_{m,1,app}$ values shown, sensitivity values increased as the PMSF concentration decreased. The lower the PMSF concentration, the higher the S_1 hydrolysis rate, the J value, and the maximum possible drop in J as the PMSF concentration is increased.

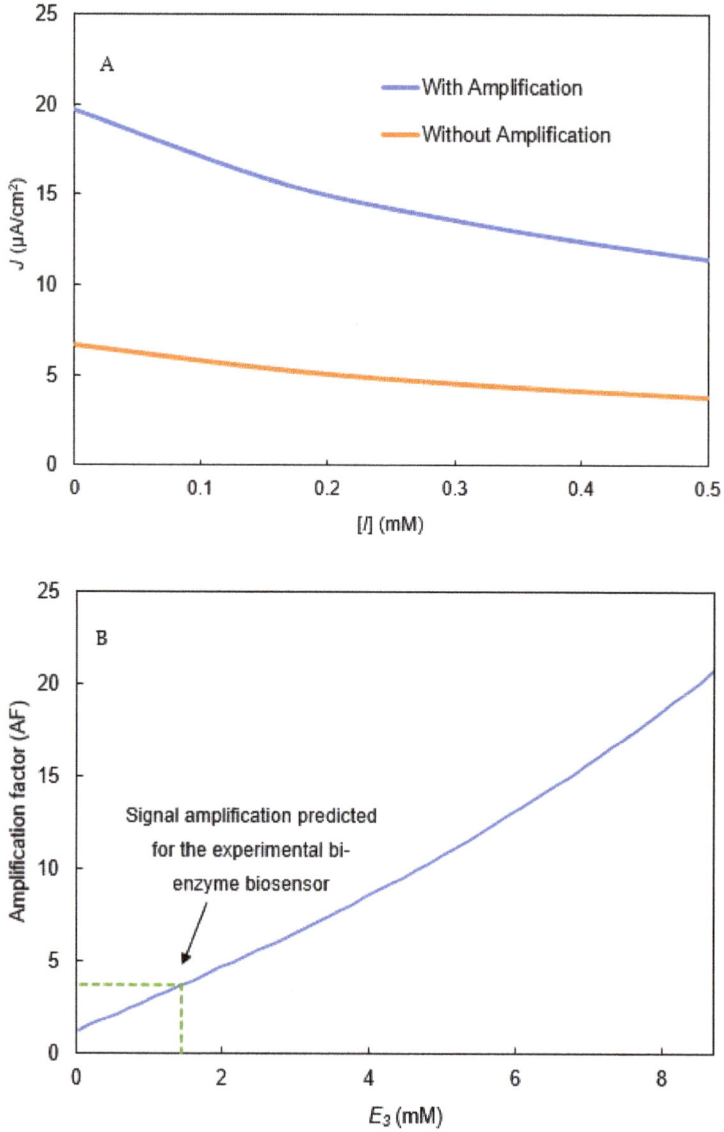

Figure 10. (**A**): Simulated current density with and without ($E_3 = 0$) the amplification system in the bi-enzyme biosensor. (**B**): Signal amplification in bi-enzyme biosensor due to S_3 recycling caused by catecholase activity (E_3).

The calculated S values were also plotted as a function of dimensionless AChE concentration for several dimensionless tyrosinase concentrations (Figure 11B).

For all tyrosinase concentrations, plots of sensitivity vs. (AChE)/(AChE*) exhibited a maximum. At low [AChE]/[AChE*] values, they are equal to the S_1 hydrolysis rate, and thus the J value is so low that the [AChE]/[AChE*] values are different from the S_1 hydrolysis limits, J; therefore, the inhibition of AChE by PMSF addition has little effect on J.

For all of the [AChE]/[AChE*] values shown, sensitivity values increased as the tyrosinase concentration increased. This effect is attributed to the catecholase activity, and thus greater amplification and J values that occur at higher tyrosinase concentrations (Figure 11B).

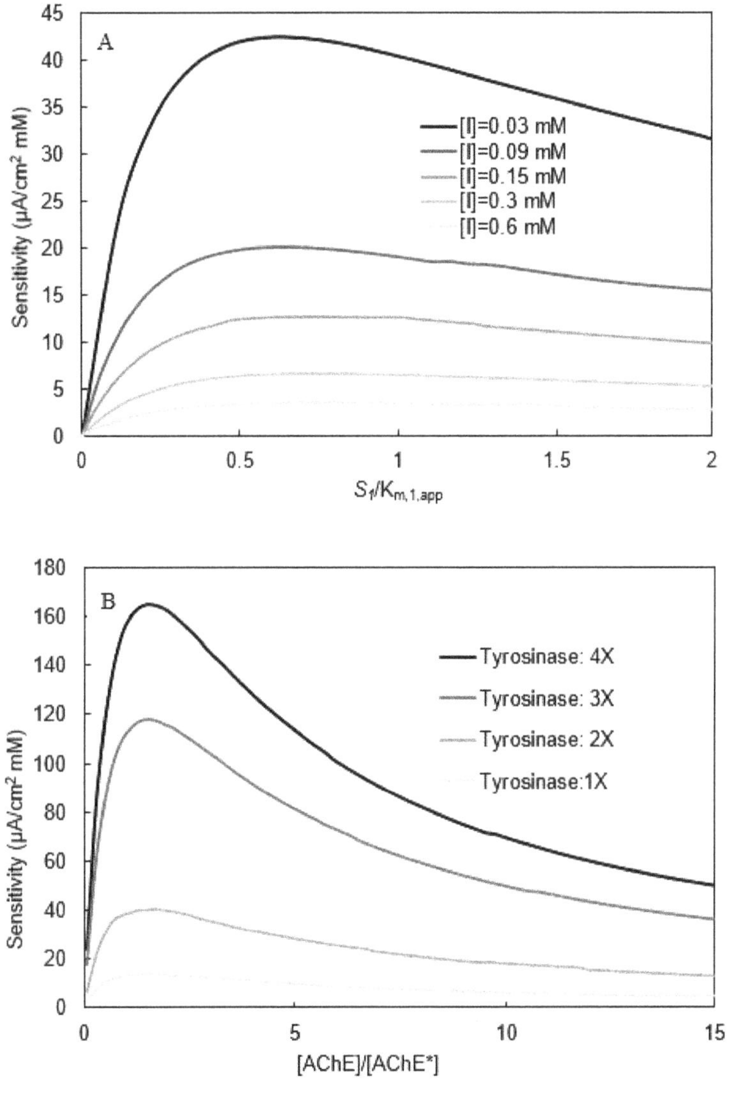

Figure 11. (**A**): Sensitivity vs. phenylacetate concentration (S_1). S_1 has been normalized with $K_{m,1,app}$. (**B**): Sensitivity vs. [AChE] at different tyrosinase concentrations. [AChE] has been normalized with [AChE*] = 3 μM. [I] = 0.3 mM.

3.4. Identification of Rate Limiting Step

In a recent publication, we described the use of dimensionless groups to assess the rate-limiting step(s) in amperometric biosensors. The biosensor's current results from the interplay of multiple mass transfer and reaction steps, each of which has the potential to be rate-limiting (i.e., control the biosensor current output) to some extent. Because the mechanistic model predicts the rate of each step, it enables the extent to which each step is rate-limiting to be calculated.

We used Equation (44) and parameter values from Table 1 to calculate the Damkohler number (σ), defined as the square root of the dimensionless ratio of the relative rates of enzymatic reaction ($\frac{V_{max}}{K_M}$) and diffusional mass transfer ($\frac{D_L}{L^2}$) within the enzyme-containing layer [37].

$$\sigma^2 = \frac{V_{max}L^2}{D_L K_M} \quad (44)$$

The σ values for AChE and tyrosinase were in the order of 10^{-5}, indicating that the diffusion steps are many orders of magnitude faster than the reaction steps [32,38].

Flux-control analysis has been used to determine the extent to which the rates of individual enzymatic reactions limit the overall mass flux through a metabolic pathway [39]. We extended this approach to assess to what extent both individual enzymatic reactions and electrochemical reactions limited current production by the biosensor. We defined a current-control coefficient (C^J_{Vi}) for a given reaction step (V_i) as the ratio of the percent change in the biosensor's output current (J) to the percent change in a given V_i while holding all other independent variables constant (Equation (45)). We used the validated model to calculate C^J_{Vi} values for each of the three reaction rates involved in generating that current: the AChE reaction rate (V_1), the tyrosinase reaction rate (V_2), or the electrochemical reaction rate (V_3). The mechanistic model allowed the enzymatic reaction rates (V_1 and V_2) to be varied by adjusting the assumed AChE and tyrosinase concentrations, respectively, and the electrochemical reaction rate (V_3) to be varied by adjusting the assumed working-electrode overpotential ($E\text{-}E_h$). Figure 12A–C show calculated C^J_{V1} values as a function of the AChE concentration, C^J_{V2} values as a function of the tyrosinase concentration, and C^J_{V3} values as a function of overpotential ($E–E_h$), respectively.

Figure 12A shows the effect of normalized AChE concentration C^J_{V1} values. The curve declines monotonically from a value of 1 as the AChE concentration increases. For the AChE concentration used in the validated biosensor mathematical model (3 µM), a current-control coefficient of 0.52 is predicted.

$$\frac{dJ}{J} \Big/ \frac{dV_i}{V_i} = C^J_{Vi} \quad (45)$$

Figure 12B shows the effect of tyrosinase concentration (normalized by a constant [AChE] value of 3 µM) on C^J_{V2} values. The curve exhibits a maximum at very low tyrosinase concentrations and then declines monotonically at the tyrosinase concentration increases. Similar curve shapes were predicted for three applied working-electrode overpotentials, with C^J_{Vi} values increasing as the overpotential increases in magnitude (i.e., the working electrode becomes more negative).

Figure 12C shows the effect of applied overpotential on C^J_{V3} values appear to decrease monotonically from a maximum value as overpotential values increase in magnitude (i.e., the working electrode becomes more negative). Similar curve shapes were predicted for the three tyrosinase concentrations studied, with C^J_{V3} values increasing as the tyrosinase concentration increases.

Once validated, the IBE model's predictive power has utility for guiding future biosensor design and optimization efforts. For example, Figure 8 indicates that the IBE biosensor has a sensitivity for detecting PMSF of 18.4 µA cm^{-2} (mM PMSF)$^{-1}$. To increase that sensitivity, researchers might consider whether it would be possible to increase the percent change in biosensor output per percent change in AChE activity due to PMSF inhibition (i.e., increase C^J_{V1}). Figure 12A predicts that the C^J_{V1} value under the experimental conditions was 0.52, and that the C^J_{V1} value could be increased by about a factor of two by decreasing the AChE concentration. The potential utility of other strategies to increase the sensitivity could be evaluated quickly and inexpensively in silico using the model. For example, the effects of changing the thickness of the enzyme-containing layer, the concentrations and ratios of the two enzymes, the working electrode's overpotential on the sensitivity could be rapidly assessed using the model.

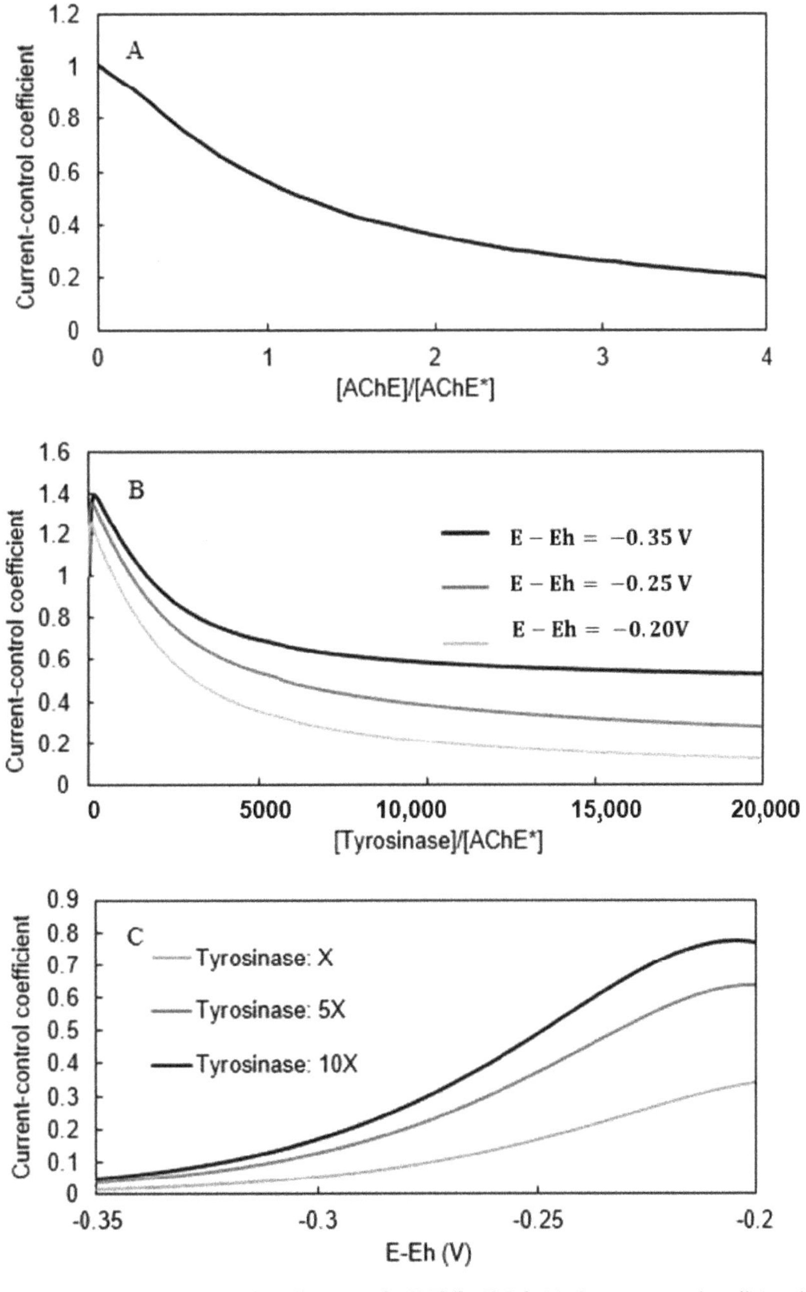

Figure 12. (**A**): Current-control coefficient vs. [AChE]/[AChE*]. (**B**): Current-control coefficient for tyrosinase. Tyrosinase concentration was normalized using [AChE*] = 3 μM. (**C**): Current-control coefficient based on the electrochemical reaction vs. working-electrode overpotential ($E–E_h$).

4. Conclusions

This study demonstrated the utility of a novel experimental and modeling framework to characterize and optimize IBE electrochemical biosensors to detect markers of neurological diseases (e.g., inhibitors of neural esterases). The experimental system was an amperometric biosensor with an oxidase (tyrosinase) and a neural esterase (AChE) co-immobilized on the working electrode of a commercially available SPE array to detect markers of neurological disease. The mechanistic model included a system of coupled, partial-differential, mass-balance equations that described the simultaneous reaction and diffusion of reactants and products between the bulk solution, the enzyme-containing layer, and the working electrode. These equations, together with their boundary and initial conditions, were solved numerically using a splitting-finite-difference algorithm. The model was able to reproduce several trends in the experimental results, including a steady-state biosensor current as a function of the inhibitor (PMSF) concentration, as well as unsteady-state dynamics of the biosensor current following the addition of a reactant (phenylacetate) and an ACE inhibitor (PMSF).

The successful application of our integrated experimental and modeling framework in this paper for IBE biosensors and in a previous paper for a novel amperometric electrochemical immunosensor [26] has demonstrated that the approach is generic and has wide utility for mechanistic modeling of the key mass-transfer and reaction steps that determine the biosensor's amplitude and sensitivity. Moreover, the novel dimensional-analysis approach (e.g., current-control coefficients, sensitivity coefficients, and Damkohler numbers) has been shown to be capable of determining the degree to which various steps limit the biosensor's signal magnitude and sensitivity to the target analyte. These capabilities enable the framework to be used for in silico design of biosensors having performance properties that are customized for the target application, whether that might be the maximum sensitivity at low analyte concentrations or a linear response over a very wide analyte range. The framework can also predict which independent variable(s) (e.g., the thickness of the enzyme-containing layer, the concentrations and ratios of the two enzymes, the working electrode's overpotential) would be most effective in obtaining the desired dependent performance variable(s) (e.g., signal magnitude, analyte sensitivity). Finally, this paper's extension of the modeling capability to predict unsteady-state IBE biosensor responses provides a novel capability to design biosensors having desired dynamic properties, thereby providing the capability for a new dimension of experimental characterization using electrochemical biosensors.

Author Contributions: Conceptualization, N.R., R.M.W., and P.S.; methodology, N.R., R.M.W., and P.S.; software, N.R.; validation, N.R., R.M.W., and P.S. formal analysis, N.R., R.M.W., and P.S.; investigation, N.R., R.M.W., and P.S.; resources, N.R., R.M.W., and P.S.; data curation, N.R.; writing—original draft preparation, N.R. and R.M.W.; writing—review and editing, N.R., R.M.W., and P.S.; supervision, R.M.W.; project administration, R.M.W.; funding acquisition, R.M.W. All authors have read and agreed to the published version of the manuscript.

Funding: This material is based on work supported by the National Science Foundation under Grant No. 1444991, a Michigan State University MTRAC for the Bio-Economy grant, and a grant from the USDA National Institute of Food and Agriculture (Hatch project 1018025).

Institutional Review Board Statement: Not applicable.

Informed Consent Statement: Not applicable.

Data Availability Statement: Not applicable.

Acknowledgments: We gratefully acknowledge Matthew Musho and Jeff Culver of Conductive Technologies Incorporated (CTI) for their helpful discussions and donation of CTI electrode arrays for research related to this project. We also gratefully acknowledge Mohsen Zayernouri in the MSU's Computational Mathematics, Science, and Engineering Department for his assistance in developing the splitting–finite-difference algorithm and Marissa Beatty, Kelly Potts, and Patrick Goughler for their participation in the research while they were undergraduate research assistants at MSU.

Conflicts of Interest: The authors declare no conflict of interest.

References

1. Zhang, S.; Wright, G.; Yang, Y. Materials and techniques for electrochemical biosensor design and construction. *Biosens. Bioelectron.* **2000**, *15*, 273–282. [CrossRef]
2. Uniyal, S.; Sharma, R.K. Technological advancement in electrochemical biosensor based detection of Organophosphate pesticide chlorpyrifos in the environment: A review of status and prospects. *Biosens. Bioelectron.* **2018**, *116*, 37–50. [CrossRef]
3. Kucherenko, I.; Soldatkin, O.; Dzyadevych, S.; Soldatkin, A. Electrochemical biosensors based on multienzyme systems: Main groups, advantages and limitations—A review. *Anal. Chim. Acta* **2020**, *1111*, 114–131. [CrossRef]
4. Ronkainen, N.J.; Halsall, H.B.; Heineman, W.R. Electrochemical biosensors. *Chem. Soc. Rev.* **2010**, *39*, 1747–1763. [CrossRef]
5. Menon, S.; Mathew, M.R.; Sam, S.; Keerthi, K.; Kumar, K.G. Recent advances and challenges in electrochemical biosensors for emerging and re-emerging infectious diseases. *J. Electroanal. Chem.* **2020**, *878*, 114596. [CrossRef]
6. Grieshaber, D.; MacKenzie, R.; Vörös, J.; Reimhult, E. Electrochemical biosensors—Sensor principles and architectures. *Sensors* **2008**, *8*, 1400–1458. [CrossRef]
7. Gerard, M.; Chaubey, A.; Malhotra, B. Application of conducting polymers to biosensors. *Biosens. Bioelectron.* **2002**, *17*, 345–359. [CrossRef]
8. Worsfold, P.; Townshend, A.; Poole, C.F.; Miró, M. *Encyclopedia of Analytical Science*; Elsevier: Amsterdam, The Netherlands, 2019.
9. Meena, A.; Rajendran, L. Mathematical modeling of amperometric and potentiometric biosensors and system of non-linear equations—Homotopy perturbation approach. *J. Electroanal. Chem.* **2010**, *644*, 50–59. [CrossRef]
10. Honeychurch, K.C.; Piano, M. Electrochemical (bio) sensors for environmental and food analyses. *Biosensors* **2018**, *8*, 57. [CrossRef]
11. Upadhyay, L.S.B.; Verma, N. Enzyme inhibition based biosensors: A review. *Anal. Lett.* **2013**, *46*, 225–241. [CrossRef]
12. Trojanowicz, M.; Hitchman, M.L. Determination of pesticides using electrochemical biosensors. *TrAC Trends Anal. Chem.* **1996**, *15*, 38–45. [CrossRef]
13. Barceló, D.; Hennion, M. Sampling of polar pesticides from water matrices. *Anal. Chim. Acta* **1997**, *338*, 3–18. [CrossRef]
14. Kumaran, S.; Morita, M. Application of a cholinesterase biosensor to screen for organophosphorus pesticides extracted from soil. *Talanta* **1995**, *42*, 649–655. [CrossRef]
15. Gahlaut, A. Electrochemical biosensors for determination of organophosphorus compounds. *Open J. Appl. Biosens.* **2012**, *1*, 1. [CrossRef]
16. Pundir, C.; Malik, A. Preety Bio-sensing of organophosphorus pesticides: A review. *Biosens. Bioelectron.* **2019**, *140*, 111348. [CrossRef]
17. Dhull, V.; Gahlaut, A.; Dilbaghi, N.; Hooda, V. Acetylcholinesterase biosensors for electrochemical detection of organophosphorus compounds: A review. *Biochem. Res. Int.* **2013**, *2013*, 731501. [CrossRef]
18. Yongliang, Z.; Lifang, L.; Yuanyuan, F.; Jianping, G.; Jianping, F.; Weibin, J.; Zheng, Y.; Long, L.; Fan, Y.; Gan, J.; et al. A review on the detoxification of organophosphorus compounds by microorganisms. *Afr. J. Microbiol. Res.* **2013**, *7*, 2127–2134. [CrossRef]
19. Pohanka, M. Acetylcholinesterase inhibitors: A patent review (2008–present). *Expert Opin. Ther. Patents* **2012**, *22*, 871–886. [CrossRef]
20. Pundir, C.S.; Chauhan, N. Acetylcholinesterase inhibition-based biosensors for pesticide determination: A review. *Anal. Biochem.* **2012**, *429*, 19–31. [CrossRef]
21. Robb, E.L.; Baker, M.B. Organophosphate toxicity. *Nurse Pract.* **2017**, *46*, 18–21. [CrossRef]
22. Xu, M.-L.; Gao, Y.; Han, X.X.; Zhao, B. Detection of pesticide residues in food using surface-enhanced Raman spectroscopy: A review. *J. Agric. Food Chem.* **2017**, *65*, 6719–6726. [CrossRef]
23. Palchetti, I.; Laschi, S.; Mascini, M. Electrochemical biosensor technology: Application to pesticide detection. In *Biosensors and Biodetection*; Springer: Berlin/Heidelberg, Germany, 2009; pp. 115–126.
24. Zhang, S.; Zhao, H.; John, R. A theoretical model for immobilized enzyme inhibition biosensors. *Electroanal. Int. J. Devoted Fundam. Pract. Asp. Electroanal.* **2001**, *13*, 1528–1534. [CrossRef]
25. Choi, J.-W.; Min, J.; Lee, W.-H. Signal analysis of fiber-optic biosensor for the detection of organophosphorus compounds in the contaminated water. *Korean J. Chem. Eng.* **1997**, *14*, 101–108. [CrossRef]
26. Rafat, N.; Satoh, P.; Barton, S.C.; Worden, R. Integrated Experimental and Theoretical Studies on an Electrochemical Immunosensor. *Biosensors* **2020**, *10*, 144. [CrossRef]
27. Kohli, N.; Srivastava, D.; Sun, J.; Richardson, R.J.; Lee, I.; Worden, R.M. Nanostructured Biosensor for measuring neuropathy target esterase activity. *Anal. Chem.* **2007**, *79*, 5196–5203. [CrossRef] [PubMed]
28. Richardson, R.J.; Fink, J.K.; Worden, R.M.; Wijeyesakere, S.J.; Makhaeva, G.F. Neuropathy target esterase as a biomarker and biosensor of delayed neuropathic agents. In *Handbook of Toxicology of Chemical Warfare Agents*; Elsevier: Amsterdam, The Netherlands, 2020; pp. 1005–1025.
29. Kohli, N.; Lee, I.; Richardson, R.J.; Worden, R.M. Theoretical and experimental study of bi-enzyme electrodes with substrate recycling. *J. Electroanal. Chem.* **2010**, *641*, 104–110. [CrossRef]
30. Ruan, C.; Li, Y. Detection of zeptomolar concentrations of alkaline phosphatase based on a tyrosinase and horse-radish peroxidase bienzyme biosensor. *Talanta* **2001**, *54*, 1095–1103. [CrossRef]

31. Kulys, J.; Baronas, R. Modelling of amperometric biosensors in the case of substrate inhibition. *Sensors* **2006**, *6*, 1513–1522. [CrossRef]
32. Baronas, R.; Kulys, J.; Lančinskas, A.; Žilinskas, A. Effect of diffusion limitations on multianalyte determination from biased biosensor response. *Sensors* **2014**, *14*, 4634–4656. [CrossRef]
33. Baronas, D.; Ivanauskas, F.; Baronas, R. Mechanisms controlling the sensitivity of amperometric biosensors in flow injection analysis systems. *J. Math. Chem.* **2011**, *49*, 1521–1534. [CrossRef]
34. Irie, T.; Fukushi, K.; Iyo, M. Evaluation of phenylmethanesulfonyl fluoride (PMSF) as a tracer candidate mapping acetylcholinesterase in vivo. *Nucl. Med. Biol.* **1993**, *20*, 991–992. [CrossRef]
35. Kraut, D.; Goff, H.; Pai, R.K.; Hosea, N.A.; Silman, I.; Sussman, J.; Taylor, P.; Voet, J.G. Inactivation studies of acetylcholinesterase with phenylmethylsulfonyl fluoride. *Mol. Pharmacol.* **2000**, *57*, 1243–1248.
36. Coche-Guerente, L.; Labbé, P.; Mengeaud, V. Amplification of Amperometric Biosensor Responses by Electrochemical Substrate Recycling. 3. Theoretical and Experimental Study of the Phenol−Polyphenol Oxidase System Immobilized in Laponite Hydrogels and Layer-by-Layer Self-Assembled Structures. *Anal. Chem.* **2001**, *73*, 3206–3218. [CrossRef] [PubMed]
37. Parthasarathy, P.; Vivekanandan, S. A numerical modelling of an amperometric-enzymatic based uric acid biosensor for GOUT arthritis diseases. *Inform. Med. Unlocked* **2019**, *16*, 100233. [CrossRef]
38. Ismail, I.; Oluleye, G.; Oluwafemi, I. Mathematical modelling of an enzyme-based biosensor. *Int. J. Biosens. Bioelectron.* **2017**, *3*, 265–268.
39. Kacser, H.; Burns, J.A.; Fell, D.A. *The Control of Flux*; Portland Press Limited: London, UK, 1995.

biosensors

MDPI

Review

Electrochemical Biosensors for Detection of MicroRNA as a Cancer Biomarker: Pros and Cons

Maliana El Aamri [1,†], Ghita Yammouri [1,†], Hasna Mohammadi [1], Aziz Amine [1,*] and Hafsa Korri-Youssoufi [2]

1 Laboratory of Process Engineering & Environment, Faculty of Sciences and Techniques, Hassan II, University of Casablanca, B.P.146, Mohammedia 28806, Morocco; maliana.elaamri@etu.fstm.ac.ma (M.E.A.); ghita.yammouri-etu@etu.univh2c.ma (G.Y.); hasna2001fr@yahoo.fr (H.M.)

2 Université Paris-Saclay, CNRS, Institut de Chimie Moléculaire et des Matériaux d'Orsay (ICMMO), Equipe de Chimie Biorganique et Bioinorganique (ECBB) , Bât 420, 2 Rue du Doyen Georges Poitou, 91400 Orsay, France; hafsa.korri-youssoufi@universite-paris-saclay.fr

* Correspondence: azizamine@yahoo.fr

† These authors contributed equally to this work.

Received: 26 October 2020; Accepted: 18 November 2020; Published: 20 November 2020

Abstract: Cancer is the second most fatal disease in the world and an early diagnosis is important for a successful treatment. Thus, it is necessary to develop fast, sensitive, simple, and inexpensive analytical tools for cancer biomarker detection. MicroRNA (miRNA) is an RNA cancer biomarker where the expression level in body fluid is strongly correlated to cancer. Various biosensors involving the detection of miRNA for cancer diagnosis were developed. The present review offers a comprehensive overview of the recent developments in electrochemical biosensor for miRNA cancer marker detection from 2015 to 2020. The review focuses on the approaches to direct miRNA detection based on the electrochemical signal. It includes a RedOx-labeled probe with different designs, RedOx DNA-intercalating agents, various kinds of RedOx catalysts used to produce a signal response, and finally a free RedOx indicator. Furthermore, the advantages and drawbacks of these approaches are highlighted.

Keywords: microRNA; electrochemical biosensor; catalysts; RedOx indicator; cancer biomarker

1. Introduction

Cancer has been the focus of intense scientific research in recent decades because it includes more than 14 million new cancer cases as well as 8.2 million deaths annually, which makes it one of the most fatal diseases in the world. It is a complex disease characterized by abnormally large cell proliferation, or malignant tumor, formed from the transformation by mutation or genetic instability of an initially normal cell [1]. Attacking some tumor cells that are the source of the disease requires early diagnosis to control and treat them.

The detection of cancer in the early stage of its evolution greatly increases the chances of the treatment success [2]. Indeed, it is based on screening, and on educating patients about early diagnosis. There are many methods of detecting cancer, but the challenge is whether these tests are used to help identify cancer and give an appropriate treatment at an early stage. Among these methods, the most effective ones include imaging exams [3,4] including, radiography, echography, computed tomography scan, magnetic resonance imaging, and positron emission tomography. However, biochemical methods based on the detection and quantification of biomarkers could give an early diagnosis. Biomarkers are defined as substances found naturally in the cells, tissues, or fluids of the human body and present in abnormal amounts in people with cancer or a precancerous condition [5]. Cancer biomarkers could be specific to a single type of cancer or associated with more than one type of cancer [6]. Various cancer biomarkers are known and some of the associated ones with cancer diagnosis are summarized in Table 1.

Table 1. Biomarkers associated with the diagnosis and prognosis of cancer.

Cancer	Biomarkers	Reference
Breast	BRCA1, BRCA2, MUC1, CEA, CA 15-3, CA 27, CA29, EGFR, EpCAM, HER2; miRNA-21, miRNA-373, miRNA-182, miRNA-1246 and miRNA-105	[7–10]
Prostate	PSA, Sarcosine; TEMPRSS2; miRNA-21, miRNA-141, miRNA-375	[11–13]
Brain	MDM2;	[14]
Pancreas	CA 19-9, PAM4; miRNA-21, miRNA-155, miRNA-196	[15,16]
Gastric/Stomach	CA72-4, CA19-9, CEA, IL-6; PVT1; miRNA-21, miRNA-331, miRNA-421	[17,18]
Liver	AFP, DCP, GP73; miRNA-21, miRNA-122, miRNA-16	[19]
Ovarian	CA 125 (MUC-16), CEA, Claudin-4;	[20,21]
Lung	ANXA2, CEA, Chromogranin A, CA 19-9, CYFRA 21-1 (CA-19 fragment), NSE, SCC, SAA1, HER1; P53, P16, Ras genes, Telomere length and telomere-related genes, EGFR gene (c-ErbB-1 and c-ErbB-2); miRNA-21 (in sputum)	[22–26]
Neck	MGMT gene	[27]

Abbreviations: BRCA1, breast cancer 1 gene; BRCA2, breast cancer 2 gene; MUC1, mucin1; CEA, carcinoembryonic antigen; CA, cancer antigen; EGFR, epidermal growth factor receptor; EpCAM, epithelial cell adhesion molecule; HER, human epidermal growth factor receptor; miR, micro-RNA; PSA, prostate-specific antigen; PAP, prostatic acidic phosphatase; MDM2, murine double minute 2; AFP, α-1-fetoprotein; DCP, des-γ-carboxyprothrombin; GP73, golgi protein 73; ANXA2, annexin A2; NSE, neuron-specific enolase; SCC, squamous cell carcinoma antigen; SAA1, serum amyloid A1; P53, protein suppressor gene; MGMT, o^6-methylguanine DNA methyltransferase.

In recent decades, researchers have focused on microRNA (miRNA) as a cancer biomarker. According to Scopus, and over the years, miRNAs have generated a high amount of interest in the cancer research area, as described in Scheme 1. The number of papers related to miRNA detection as a cancer biomarker was about 650 in 2019, showing the high interest in miRNA analysis.

The interest in targeting miRNAs as cancer biomarkers is related to their biochemical properties and their large amount in biological fluids; they allow easy detection avoiding sample treatment complications.

MiRNAs are small non-coding single-stranded sequences constituted of 18–25 nucleotides [28]. The expression level of the miRNAs is strongly correlated with the onset and development of diseases, including cancer, diabetes, and heart disease [29,30].

The conventional methods used for the quantification and identification of miRNAs are real-time quantitative polymerase chain reaction (RT-qPCR), DNA microarray, Northern blot techniques, and deep sequencing [31]. In general, they have good sensitivity and high specificity, but the methods are complex and need a high level of technology that requires costly equipment and materials, qualified personnel for the assay, and is time consuming [32].

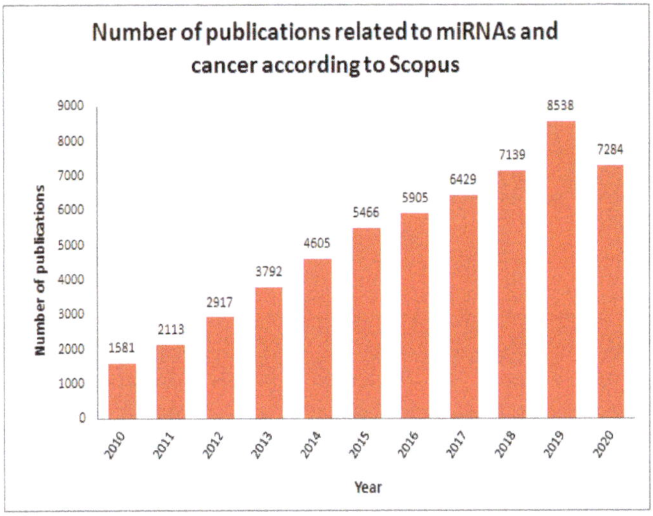

Scheme 1. Number of publications in the field of micro-RNAs and cancer in the period between 2010 and 2020 (www.scopus.com, analyzed by years) (consulted 25 October 2020) (Keywords: micro-RNAs, cancer).

For this reason, the development of other more efficient and less expensive emerging techniques is important and vital for cancer diagnosis and therapy. A variety of methods providing high sensitivity and specificity, and that are easy to handle have been recently developed based on various direct detection methods such as photoelectrochemical, localized surface plasmon resonance, and electrochemical biosensors [33].

Electrochemical biosensors present interest because they can be easily miniaturized, and allow mass-production at a low cost. They could be modified with various recognition elements and are greatly used as versatile devices for nucleic acids-based biosensors development (E-DNA). In addition, such biosensors have demonstrated convincing results with versatile approaches based on newly developed materials and nanomaterials, natural organic and bioorganic polymers, electroactive molecules, catalysts, and biocatalysis, etc. [34–36].

In recent years, reviews of electrochemical miRNA biosensors at various viewpoints have been published. Therefore, various strategies based on multi-functional nanomaterials in miRNA biosensors were reported [37,38]. For example, Chen et al. [31] discussed the use of nanomaterials and oligonucleotides as amplification strategies for miRNA detection. Besides, Michael et al. [39] focused more on electrochemical biosensors based on using various combinations of oligonucleotide strategies. Furthermore, Mohammadi et al. [40] reviewed the various amplification strategies based on nanomaterials, oligonucleotides, and enzymes for miRNA analysis and their different possible combinations.

In this review, we provide a compressive overview of various detection approaches of miRNA detection in the literature from 2015 to 2020 following their prevalence. The review focuses on direct miRNA electrochemical biosensing systems based on the RedOx marker. These approaches are based on the RNA biosensors with (i) an electroactive labeled DNA probe sequence, (ii) the use of a catalyst that generates RedOx specie, (iii) the system with DNA RedOx intercalating agent, (iv) the employment of free RedOx indicator and finally, other methods of detection free of the RedOx marker. Various detection approaches are discussed in terms of analytical performances, particularly sensitivity and limit of detection (LOD). We highlight the advantages and drawbacks of these detection approaches. The challenges and successes of these assays are discussed.

2. Electrochemical Biosensor Based on Electroactive Labeled Probe Sequence

Electroactive species-labeled DNA probe sequence strategies are widely used for miRNA detection. They provide direct RedOx current response related to the signal variation after the miRNA hybridization. These electroactive species can be inorganic molecules as well as organic ones. For example, metals such as gold nanoparticles [41], silver nanoparticles [42], cadmium [43], and plomb [44] were employed as an inorganic RedOx probe. Organic molecules including, thionine (Thi) [45], ferrocene (Fc) [46], and methylene blue (MB) [47] were mostly used. Indeed, the RedOx molecule could be labeled to the probe sequence directly or with the help of a linker. These methods of labeling will be detailed in this section.

2.1. Direct Labeling

Biosensors with direct current response readout are based on short strand DNA probes complementary to the target sequence (miRNA) labeled with molecules of RedOx activity. These labeled probes are firstly immobilized at the surface of the electrode through surface chemistry. The recognition of the miRNA target sequence generates a variation in signal response of the RedOx molecule, which is proportional to miRNA concentration. The literature data show that the labeled DNA probes could be presented with different types of architecture (Figure 1) providing a decrease (ON-OFF signal) or increase (OFF-ON signal) in current response after the hybridization step, starting with a basic design (Figure 1A) and progressing to other more advanced designs based on the elimination of the labeled probe sequence (Figure 1B), the use of a secondary probe labeled with RedOx molecule (Figure 1C) and finally, the use of a two-probe labeled sequence (Figure 1D).

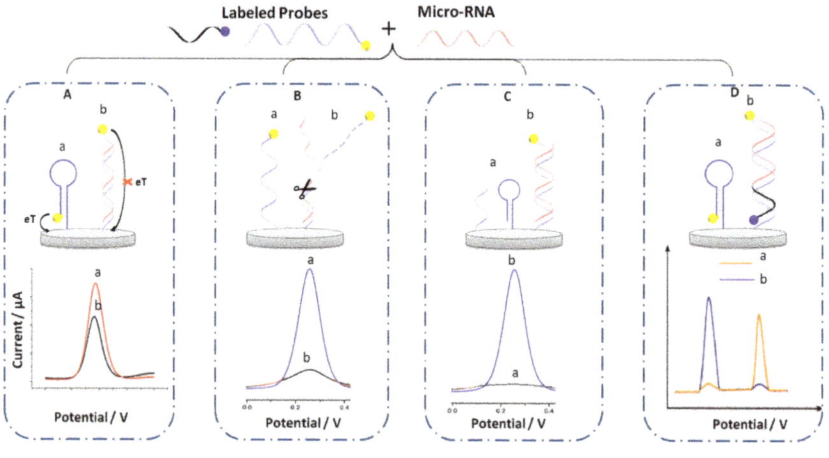

Figure 1. Different architecture of electrochemical biosensors based on labeled probe with RedOx molecules before and after hybridization. (**A**) Basic design; (**B**) elimination of labeled probe sequence; (**C**) the use of secondary probe labeled with RedOx molecule; (**D**) the use of two-probe labeled sequence, (**a**) before and (**b**) after hybridization.

2.1.1. Basic Design

This method is based on the use of a labeled capture DNA probe, which is immobilized at the electrode surface and labeled with a RedOx molecule at the other extremity. However, as shown in Figure 1A, the presence of target miRNA after a hybridization reaction leads to a variation of the distance from the RedOx molecule to the electrode surface, which hampers electron transfer and leads to a decrease in current response (ON-OFF systems). Following this approach, Jou et al. [48], immobilized hairpin DNA probes on a screen-printed carbon electrode (SPCE) modified with AuNPs. The hairpin was labeled at the 5′ end position with MB as a RedOx signal reporter. Before hybridization, the MB is near the electrode surface and thus the electron transfer between the MB and the electrode is possible, so the oxidation response of MB is very high. However, in the presence of the miRNA target, and after displacement amplification reaction and duplex-specific nuclease (DSN), the hairpin was opened indicating the presence of the target, which generates a distance between the RedOx molecule and the surface resulting in a decrease in MB oxidation signal. This method showed an LOD of 3.57 fM for miRNA-155 as a blood cancer biomarker. To improve the sensitivity of detection, Miao et al. [49] used a DNA hairpin immobilized directly on a gold surface electrode and marked with MB at the 5′ end. They introduced the tris (2-carboxyethyl) phosphine hydrochloride reducer (TCEP) providing an enhanced electrochemical signal of MB. The oxidation signal enhancement is based on the activation of MB by reducing its oxidized form in the presence of TCEP. This method allows an improvement of the LOD where 3.2 aM is demonstrated. Yammouri et al. [47] demonstrated a biosensor for miRNA cancer markers with LOD of 1 fM using a basic design where MB-labeled DNA probe sequences and well adapted surface chemistry based on pencil carbon were used. This allows a signal of readout after DNA hybridization without using TCEP as a mediator. The aforementioned methods based on ON-OFF systems lead to an increase in the error of the measurement at low miRNA concentrations. To overcome this problem, a specific architecture of DNA such as loop DNA or DNA stream could be used and the hybridization, in this case, brings the RedOx marker closer to the surface leading to an increase in current response (OFF-ON systems). Wang et al. [50] relied on the "OFF-ON" systems offering a femtomolar detection limit of miRNA-122. In this case, a triple-stem DNA-labeled MB was used. This structure locks MB away from the electrode, and thus blocks electron transfer pathways. Indeed, the signal is turned on only upon the recognition with the target miRNA, which leads to a significant signal response of MB after the hybridization reaction.

2.1.2. Response Based on the Elimination of the Labeled Probe

In this strategy, the labeled probes are released after their hybridization with miRNA targets as shown in Figure 1B. Various methods were employed to achieve this approach. The more popular method is the use of a cleaving agent such as endonucleases [51], duplex-specific nuclease [52], or calcium ions [53] to remove the hybridized duplexes and eliminate the labeled probe from the electrode surface.

The removal could also be obtained by desorption of dsDNA bearing the labeled probe after the hybridization reaction of miRNA due to lower affinity of dsDNA–RNA to the surface (Figure 2). In this case, biosensors based on carbon nanomaterials were demonstrated such as graphene oxide [42] or SWCNTs [46] where the adsorbed ssDNA probe has more affinity to the nanomaterial than dsDNA–RNA does.

Another method uses the competition of miRNA target with two DNA probes in which one is non-labeled and could be hybridized with an MB-labeled duplex reporter. When miRNA target is present, its hybridization reaction with a non-labeled attached probe takes place leading to the displacement of the labeled reporter from the surface [54].

A 2D DNA nanoprobe (DNP) and enzyme-free-target-recycling amplification method based on toehold-mediated strand displacement reactions (TSDRs) was also used to achieve the release of Fc-labeled DNA strands in the case of miRNA-21 detection. The method is based on the displacement of the Fc-labeled DNA strands from the glassy carbone electrode (GCE)/gold nanoparticles (AuNPs) surface after TSDRs, resulting in a decrease in the electrochemical signal. The proposed biosensor has an LOD of 0.31 fM and can be regenerated four times [55].

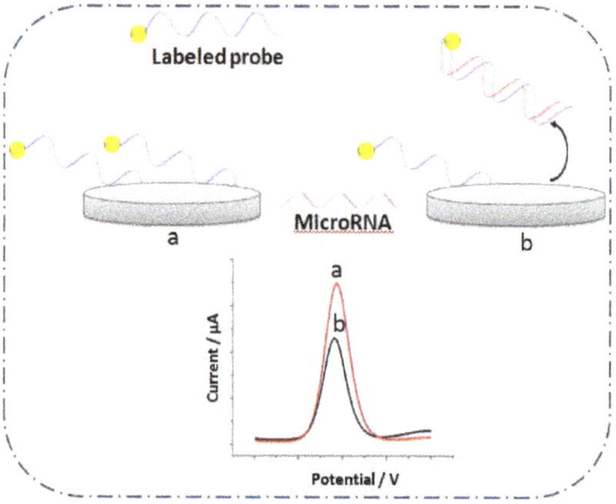

Figure 2. Architecture of electrochemical biosensor based on destroying the adsorption of the labeled probe after hybridization step on the electrode surface (**a**) before and (**b**) after hybridization.

The previous methods described are simple in the design of the biosensors but lead to a decrease in current signal upon miRNA hybridization with "On-OFF systems". The detection with increasing response signals based on "OFF-ON Signal" was also demonstrated in the case of the release of the labeled DNA probe. Thus, Fu et al. [56] developed a biosensor based on a homogenous system of detection without immobilization of the ssDNA probe, permitting the reduction in the preparation time of the biosensor. Indeed, the biosensor is based on the negatively charged probes marked with MB at the 3′ end and a negatively charged indium tinoxide (ITO) electrode surface where DNA cannot diffuse easily to the surface due to electrostatic repulsion and the low electrochemical signal of MB is detected. After hybridization, the duplex DNA probe-miRNA was cleaved by DSN hybridization and miRNA continue the second cycle of hybridization cleavage; in the end, this released many short fragments of MB-labeled oligonucleotides with less negative charges, which easily allowed the diffusion on the electrode surface, resulting in a high electrochemical signal.

2.1.3. The Use of Secondary Probe Labeled with RedOx Molecule

This strategy is based on the use of two DNA sequences, the first one is a DNA probe immobilized on the electrode surface, which is targeting a part of miRNA, and the second one is a DNA probe labeled with RedOx molecule targeting the other part of miRNA. After hybridization, the secondary probe labeled with the RedOx molecule leads to a positive signal readout. The principal of this strategy is presented in Figure 1C. This approach was demonstrated by Miao et al. [57] with a biosensor in which an miRNA opened a hairpin capture probe that was immobilized on a gold electrode, while a second probe labeled with silver nanoparticles (AgNPs) was hybridized with the capture probe. A Klenow fragment initiates polymerization of the labeled probe and leads to a release of miRNA. The obtained biosensor provides intense electrochemical signals reaching an LOD of 0.4 fM. Other groups used the same method and amplified the signal readout by the use of rolling circle amplification (RCA) and several probes labeled AgNPs. This leads to an increase in the number of AgNPs on the electrode surface reducing the LOD to 50 aM [58]. Otherwise, with the same principle of detection, other nanoparticles could be used such as CdTe quantum dots (CdTe QDs) instead of AgNPs. With CdTe, a biosensor of miRNA with a very low LOD of 33 aM was demonstrated [59].

An interesting approach was demonstrated for the simultaneous detection of miRNAs using the tetrahedron DNA (TDN) nanostructure (Figure 3A) [60]. This biosensor involved an advanced DNA structure such as TDN which is immobilized on the surface and hybridized with DNA circle as a capture probe presenting many target recognition domains. In the presence of two target miRNAs, and with the assistance of two DNA probes, the mimetic proximity ligation assay (mPLA) can be triggered. The last step is the capturing of two labeled DNA probes labeled with Fc and MB which generate two electrical signal responses. The LOD obtained is in an attomolar range for miRNA-21 and miRNA-155 of 18.9 aM and 39.6 aM, respectively.

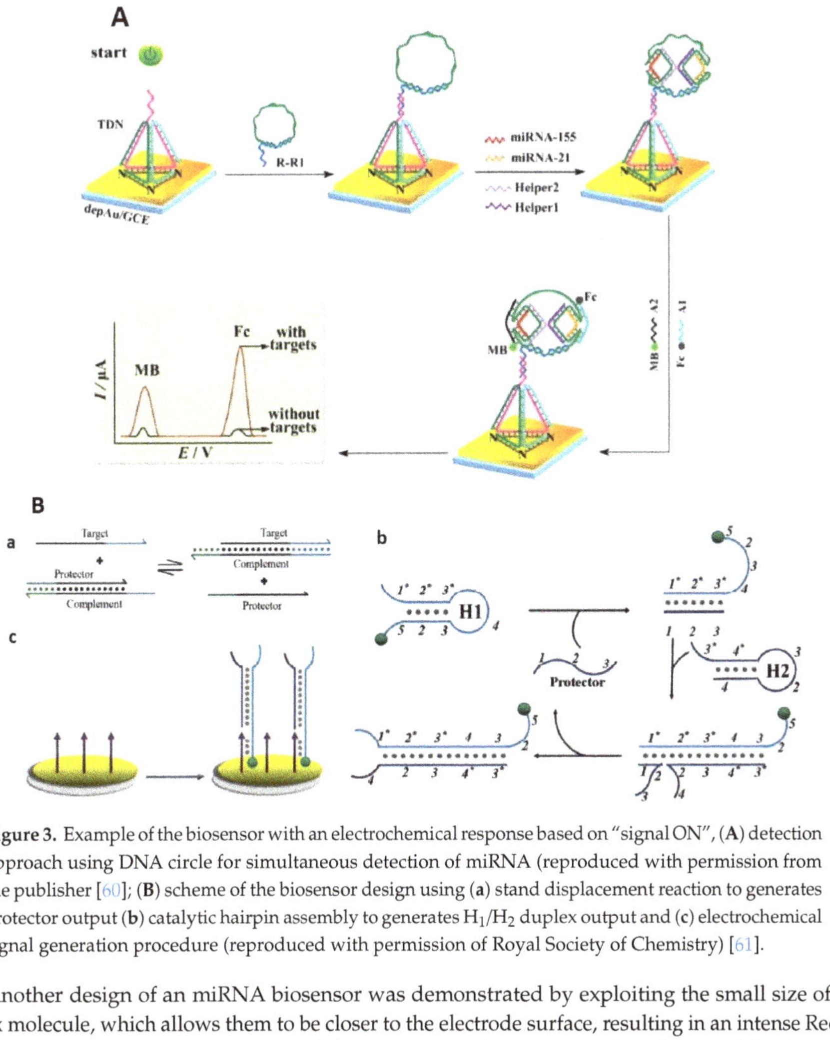

Figure 3. Example of the biosensor with an electrochemical response based on "signal ON", (**A**) detection approach using DNA circle for simultaneous detection of miRNA (reproduced with permission from the publisher [60]; (**B**) scheme of the biosensor design using (**a**) stand displacement reaction to generates protector output (**b**) catalytic hairpin assembly to generates H_1/H_2 duplex output and (**c**) electrochemical signal generation procedure (reproduced with permission of Royal Society of Chemistry) [61].

Another design of an miRNA biosensor was demonstrated by exploiting the small size of the RedOx molecule, which allows them to be closer to the electrode surface, resulting in an intense RedOx signal. This was obtained by sophisticated design strategies based on coupling the strand displacement reaction and catalytic hairpin assembly recycling (see Figure 3B) [61] or by using an isothermal target recycling amplification strategy [62].

2.1.4. Response Based on Two Labeled Probes

This strategy is based on two probes labeled with different RedOx molecules, in which one is placed near the surface electrode and the second is far from the surface. The signal obtained after RNA hybridization leads to a response where one of the RedOx molecules increases because it becomes closer to the surface and the second one decreases according to the concentration of the hybridized DNA. The final response is a ratio between the two responses (Figure 1D). Various biosensors for miRNA detection were developed following this method in addition to the amplification strategy [63] (see Figure 4A). Most of the developed biosensors used ratiometric electrochemical sensors to obtain a reliable experimental result, which is less sensitive to electrode surface conditions, the probe packing density, the environment, and artificial factors [64–67].

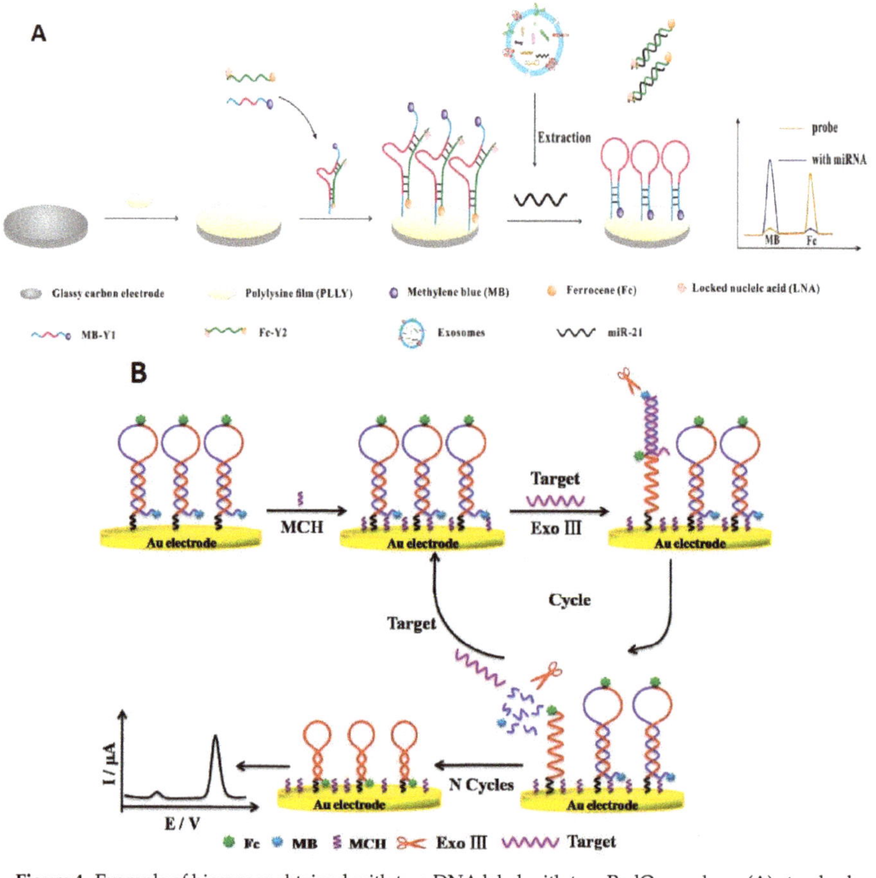

Figure 4. Example of biosensor obtained with two DNA label with two RedOx markers; (**A**) standard design reproduced from [68] with permission of publisher, (**B**) same approach using amplification strategy reproduced with permission of the publisher from [63].

Amplification strategy using exonuclease-assisted target recycling [63] (Figure 4B) or mismatched catalytic hairpin assembly (CHA) [65] can improve the signal-to-background ratio of the sensor. Using this type of ratiometric design, Zhang et al. [64] developed a more original biosensor based on bipedal DNA walkers for the detection of exosomal miRNA-21. Fc and MB RedOx probes produce a final ratiometric signal, allowing them to obtain an LOD up to 67 aM of miRNA-21. The biosensor developed was applied in a real sample and compared with other methods as RT-qPCR and was regenerated five times without signal decrease.

2.2. *RedOx Molecules Linker to Nanocarriers*

This strategy is based on the use of a RedOx molecule labeled to the probe through a linker such, nanomaterial, polymer, and streptavidin and leads to RedOx signal amplification leading to signal ON. This allows the immobilization of a large number of RedOx molecules after a hybridization reaction leading to the high sensitivity of the biosensor (Figure 5).

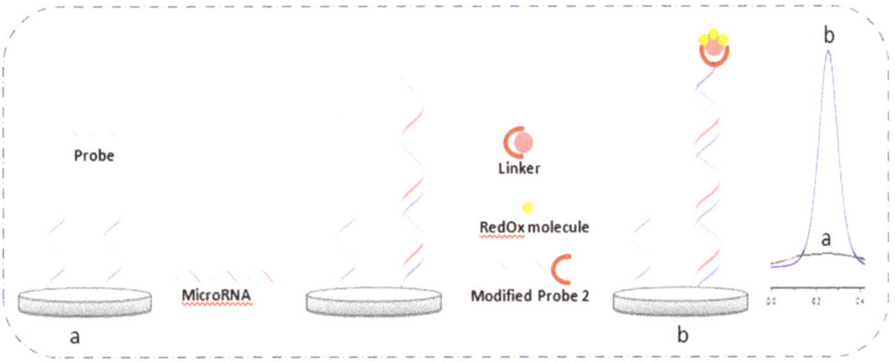

Figure 5. Architecture of electrochemical biosensor based on a RedOx molecule labeled probe via a linker molecule (**a**) before and (**b**) after hybridization.

Nanomaterials can be used as carriers of the RedOx molecule [44]. AuNPs are usually used in this case as they allow easy attachment through the thiol link. For example, AuNPs have demonstrated an amplification transducer signal conjugated to RedOx molecules such as doxorubicin [69] or cadmium sulfide nanoparticles [66], through sulfur interaction. Another example of a biosensor for miRNA-141 was demonstrated by Yuan et al. [70] where AuNPs were conjugated to Thi- and Fc-labeled hairpin capture probes immobilized on the electrode surface. In the presence of miRNA-141, an increase in the Thi signal is observed, causing a decrease in the Fc signal. The AuNPs-conjugated RedOx molecule could be linked to the capture probe sequence via streptavidin (SA). In this regard, Fc-AuNPs-SA can be used as a labeling nanocarrier for a sandwich biosensor structure. In this system, the capture DNA probes are immobilized on GCE modified with graphene oxide-AuNPs through thiol chemistry. After miRNA hybridization, a second biotinylated capture probe is hybridized. The probe bearing a nanohybrid was added for the quantization of hybridized miRNA-21. This biosensor gives a femtomolar LOD and presents good stability (63 days) [71].

Magnetic nanoparticles such as Fe_3O_4 were also employed as a reporter for RNA detection. As an example, a biosensor was developed with the objective of simultaneous detection of miRNA-141 and miRNA-21. In this case, two RedOx molecules, Thi and Fc are attached to the magnetic nanoparticle and the captured probe leading to a large number of RedOx molecules attached. In the presence of miRNAs, the hybridization chain reaction was performed, and then the DNA1/Fe_3O_4NPs/Thi and DNA2/Fe_3O_4NPs/Fc were captured by the formed dsDNA, which generate a large number of magnetic nanoprobes attached to the surface. A magnified response of currents is obtained with good stability for 4 weeks and was applied for the diagnosis of miRNA in human breast cancer cells [72].

Protein such as streptavidin could be also used as carriers of RedOx molecules. Indeed, AuNPs as RedOx molecules were conjugated to a probe sequence through streptavidin for miRNA-106a detection in the case of gastric cancer diagnosis, causing a lower LOD [41].

Most electrochemical biosensors based on electroactive species-labeled probe sequences for miRNA detection of cancer markers published from 2015 to 2020 are reviewed in Table 2 and their various analytical performances are highlighted.

Table 2. Current sensitive electrochemical biosensors using electroactive species-labeled probe sequence miRNA detection.

miRNA	labeled RedOx Molecule	Platform	Signal Amplification	Tech	Linear Range	LOD	Real-Samples Application	Ref
miRNA-141	MB	AuE	SDR	SWV	0.1fM–0.2 pM	23 aM	Human bladder cancer T24 cells	[53]
-	MB	GCE/PDDA/AuNPs	DSN	SWV	100 aM–1 nM	30 aM	human serum samples	[51]
miRNA-21	MB	GCE/CNNS/AuNPs	DSN	SWV	10 fM–1 nM	2.9 fM	Spiked human serum	[52]
MiRNA-21	MB	PtE/AuNFs	MB/barcode AuNPs	DPV	500 aM–50 pM	135 aM	spiked human serum	[73]
miRNA 21	Fc	AuE	SWCNTs	DPV	100 pM–3.5 fM	0.01 fM	Human serum	[46]
miRNA-155	Fc	GCE/Mo_2C/AuNPs	CHA	DPV	0.1 fM–1.0 nM	0.033 fM	Spiked human serum	[74]
miRNA-21	Fc	GCE/Mo_2C/NCS	SDR	Amperometric	1.0 fM–1.0 nM	0.34 fM	Spiked human serum	[75]
miRNA-21	AgNPs	GCE/GO	-	LSV	100 fM–1 nM	60 fM	serum samples from breast cancer patients	[42]
miRNA-155	AgNPs	AuE	SDR and nicking endonuclease	LSV	1 fM–1 pM	70 aM	HeLa cells, A549, human renal cubularepithelial	[76]
Hsa-miR-17-5p	AgNPs	AuE	AuNPs HCR	LSV	100 aM–0.1 nM	2 aM	HUVEC, HK-2, HeLa, MCF-7 cells	[77]
-	AgNCs	AuE	pDNA-AgDNCs@DNA/AgNCs	DPV	1 fM–1 nM	0.38 fM	spiked human serum	[78]
miRNA-21	AgNPs	AuE	SDR	SWV	200 pM–1 fM	0.4 fM	Blood sample	[79]
miRNA-155	PEIAgNPs	AuE	-	CV	200 zM–2 pM	20 zM	cancerous humann serum	[80]

Table 2. *Cont.*

miRNA	labeled RedOx Molecule	Platform	Signal Amplification	Tech	Linear Range	LOD	Real-Samples Application	Ref
miRNA-21	Thi	GCE/AuNPs	MWCNTs	DPV	0.1–12000 pM	0.032 pM	spiked human serum	[81]
miRNA-155	Thi	3D N-doped rGO/AuNPs	AuAgNR	DPV	10 pM–100 µM	1pM	Spiked serum samples	[45]
miRNA-21	TB	GCE/DpAu	-	SWV	1 fM–2 nM	0.3 fM	MCF-7, human breast cancer cell line	[82]
miRNA-21	Pd NPs	GCE/GO	Pd/NPs-DNALNR and CHA	DPV	1 fM–50 pM	63.1 aM	Spiked human serum	[83]
miRNA-21	Cd	GCE/Au-RGO	TPSs $Ru(NH_3)_6^{3+}$	SWV	1.0 aM–10.0 pM	0.76 aM	spiked human serum	[69]
miRNA	CdTe/QDs	AuE	CESA 3-QD@DNA NC	DPV	5 aM–5 fM	1.2 aM	Spiked human serum	[43]
miRNA-21	MB and Fc	AuE	-	SWV	5 fM–0.1 nM	1.1 fM	MCF-7 and HeLa	[65]
miRNA-16	MB and Fc	AuE	-	SWV	0.1 pM–100 nM	16 fM	MCF-7 cells	[84]
miRNA-21	MB and Fc	GCE/PLLy	LNA/structure"Y"shape	DPV	10–70 fM	2.3 fM	MCF-7 cells	[68]
let-7a	MB and Fc	NS-grafted ITO	-	DPV	80 aM–300 fM	25 aM	Spiked human serum	[85]
miRNA-21	MB and Fc	AuE	-	DPV	0.1–100.0 fM	67 aM	breast cancer cell line MCF-7	[64]
miRNA 21	Fc	AuE/AuNPs	-	DPV	100 pM to 1fM	0.36fM	serum	[86]
-	CdSNPs	GCE	AuNPS and DSN	ASV	1 f M–100 pM	0.48 fM	HeLa	[67]
miRNA-21 and miRNA-155	MB and Fc	SPCE	Fe_3O_4@Au@HHCR	SWV	5 fM–2 nM	1.5 fM 1.8 fM	Spiked human serum	[87]

Table 2. *Cont.*

miRNA	labeled RedOx Molecule	Platform	Signal Amplification	Tech	Linear Range	LOD	Real-Samples Application	Ref
miRNA-21 and miRNA-155	MB and Fc	AuE	-	SWV	10 fM–5 nM 50 fM–5 nM	2.49 fM 11.63 fM	HeLa, MCF-7 and MDA-MB-231 cells	[88]
miRNA-21 and miRNA-141	Au ion and Ag ion	GCE/Neutravidin	-	SSWV	0.5–1000 pM 50–1000 pM	0.3 pM 10 pM	Spiked Serum Sample	[89]
miRNA-21 and miRNA-141	MB and Fc	SPGE/MXene/AuNPs	-	DPV	500 aM–50 nM	204 aM 138 aM	human plasma cancer patients	[90]
miRNA-1246 and miRNA-4521	Pb (II) and Cd (II)	GCE/AuNPs	PbS@ZIF-8 CdS@ZIF-8	DPV	1 fM–1 mM	0.19 fM 0.28 fM	spiked human blood	[44]

Abbreviations: Au-disk microE, gold-disk microelectrode; MB, methylene blue; TCEP, tris(2-carboxyethyl) phosphine hydrochloride; SWV, square wave voltammetry; AuNPs, gold nanoparticles; DPV, differential pulse voltammetry; AuE, gold electrode; AgNPs, silver nanoparticles; LSV, linear sweep voltammetry; CdTe QDs, CdTe quantum dots; CESA, cyclic enzymatic signal amplification; 3-QD@DNA NC, triple-CdTe quantum dot-labeled DNA nanocomposites; GCE, glassy carbone electrode; HCR, hybridization chain reaction; Mo_2CNSs, molybdenum carbide nanosheets; Fc, ferrocene; Thio, thionine; CHA, catalytic hairpin assembly; GNF@Pt, gold nanoflower/platinum electrode; SDR, strand displacement reaction; DepAu; HeLa, human cervical cancer cell line; MCF-7, human breast adenocarcinoma cell line; SPCE, screen-printed carbone electrode; Strep, streptavidine; HUVEC, human umbilical vein endothelial cells; HK-2, human renal cubular epithelial cell; A549, human pulmonary carcinoma cell line; LNA, locked nucleic acid; NCS, N-carboxymethyl chitosan; PLLy, polylysine; NS, 1-naphthalenesulfonate; ZIF-8, Zeolitic imidazolate framework, Pb, Plomb sulfide, CdS, Cadmium sulfide; CdS NPs, cadmium sulfide nanoparticules; DSN, duplex-specific nuclease; ASV, anodic stripping voltammetry; AuAgNR, gold and silver nanorod; rGO, reduced graphene oxide; Pd NPs, palladium nanoparticules; SSWV, stripping square-wave voltammetry; SPGE, screen-printed gold electrode; PDDA, polydiallyldimethylammonium chloride; CNNS, carbon nitride nanosheet; SWCNTs, single-walled carbon nanotubes; MDA-MB-231: human breast cancer cells; MWCNTs, multi-walled carbon nanotubes; AgNCs, silver nanoclosters; RGO, polyethylenimine-grafted graphene; $Ru(NH_3)_6{}^{3+}$, hexaamine ruthenium(III); PtE, platinum electrode; TB, toluidine blue; AuNFs, gold nanoflowers; TPSs, titanium phosphate spheres; PEIAgNPs, polyethyleneimine-silver nanoparticles, HHCR, hyperbranched hybridization chain reaction.

Direct probe labeling is an approach in which the capture probe is ready to use, therefore it facilitates biosensor's construction and reduces the required time. The linker molecule labeled probe approach permitts amplification of the signal, but needs an additional step, resulting in an increase in the time and the cost of analysis.

In general, the electrochemical biosensor based on an electroactive species-labeled probe sequence is a commonly used method by researchers, due to the high stability and sensitivity. Indeed, these biosensors enable an LOD in femtomolar to attomolar range and are able to detect miRNA in a complex sample. However, most of the work on biosensors support include an additional amplification procedure or use a sophisticated electrode interface to reach high sensitivity. Additionally, this method is considered as a versatile one, permitting the development of various kinds of biosensor design with new properties. For example, it allows ratiometric dual-current signal responses that provide self-calibration. Consequently, this method can reduce the experimentally and environmental dependent factors/interferences and is effective for miRNA detection in a complex matrix. Moreover, the small size of some RedOx molecules and rational design allow them to be near the electrode surface, which could amplify the signal and detect a small amount of the biomarker. The simultaneous detection was also demonstrated with a simple approach where various biomarkers could be detected at the same time. The direct oxidation/reduction of these molecules without the need of adding other reagents or specific temperature conditions allows them to act as a point of care test. Despite, the above-mentioned advantages, there are a risk of contamination with these molecules and the use of toxic molecules such as cadmium as labeling probe sequence should be avoided for environmental pollution. Concerning the stability of the biosensor with such a design, few works describe these aspects and the stability time is demonstrated between 7 and 30 days depending on the design. Thus, more studies should be highlighted to demonstrate the long-term stability and conditions of storing to allow their actual application.

3. Electrochemical Biosensor Based on Catalysts

The catalysts including, enzymes, chemical catalysts, and DNAzyme have been used for miRNA detection (Figure 6). Enzymes are biomacromolecules with highly selective catalytic activities. More than 5000 biological processes have been established to be catalyzed by enzymes. Additionally, they can accelerate chemical reactions with tremendously high efficiency and selectivity, typically with 10^{10}–10^{15}-fold rate enhancements over uncatalyzed chemical reactions.

Nanomaterials as chemical catalysts can also mimic enzyme catalysis by their ability to act in catalytic processes and are potentially viable alternatives for enzymes. Thus, they attract a great deal of interest and have been actively researched over decades. Indeed, nanomaterials have unique physico-chemical properties, including a size comparable with natural enzymes, a high surface/volume ratio, a large number of catalytically active sites on their surface, as well as the availability of multifunctional reactive groups for subsequent modification and functionalization. The high surface/volume ratio and a large number of active sites should result in a high catalytic efficiency [91].

DNAzymes are ssDNA molecules that also exhibit a catalytic activity and are exploited in biology, medicine, and material sciences. Development in this field is related to the many advantages of DNAzymes over conventional protein enzymes, like simpler preparation and thermal stability [92]. In this section, electrochemical biosensors for miRNA detection based on the enzymes, chemical catalysts, and DNAzyme will be discussed.

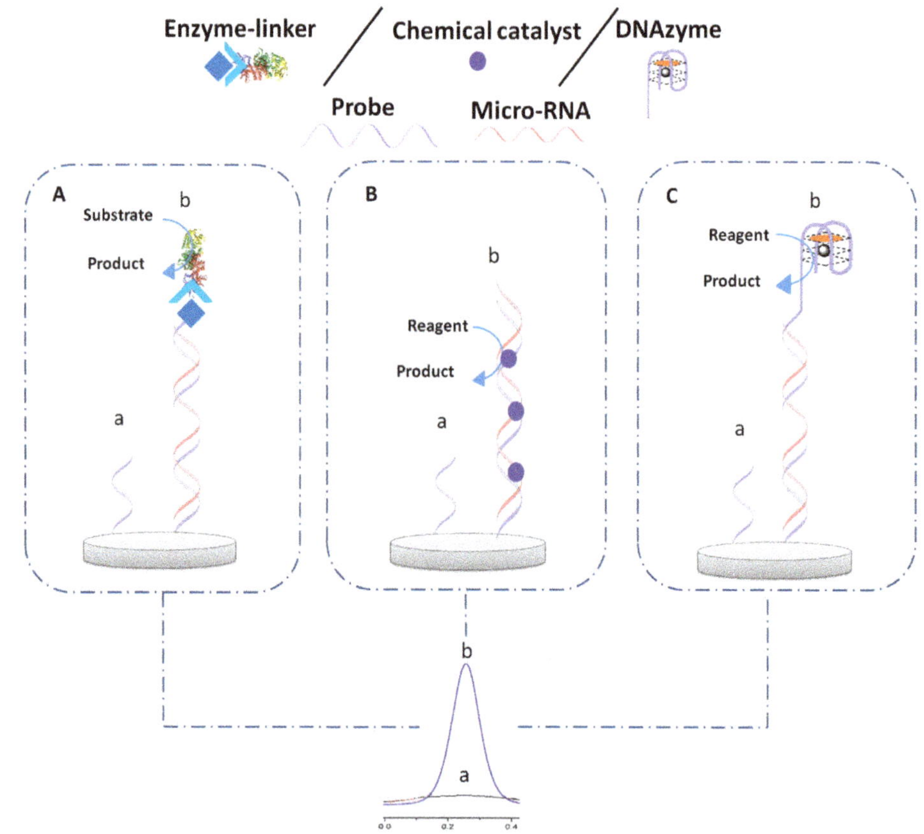

Figure 6. Principle of electrochemical biosensor based on different types of catalysts before (**a**) and after hybridization (**b**) with micro-RNA, (**A**) enzyme, (**B**) chemical catalyst, (**C**) DNAzyme.

3.1. *Enzyme*

The use of an enzyme in amplification strategies is widely used for miRNA detection. It includes various enzymes that lead to obtaining electroactive species which could be electrochemically detected. The most employed enzymes are alkaline phosphatase (ALP) and horseradish peroxidase (HRP). The binding strategy of the enzymes to the biosensors is the key to biosensors' success because it could affect the accessibility of the active site or lead to denaturation. In this regard, different works have been reported based on the different types of binding approach on the biosensor that will be discussed in this part. Some examples of enzyme binding approaches are presented in Figure 6A.

3.1.1. Enzyme–Steptavidin Binding

The binding of an enzyme on the biosensor via the interaction between biotin-modified probe sequence and streptavidin-modified enzyme is a habitually used method in the literature of enzyme binding employed for miRNA detection [93–96]. Using this type of interaction between a biotinylated capture probe and streptavidin-conjugated alkaline phosphatase (SA-ALP), Xia et al. [97] described an electrochemical–chemical–chemical (ECC) RedOx cycling system for miRNAs detection with Fc methanol, which acts as the RedOx mediator using TCEP as a reducing agent and L-ascorbic acid 2-phosphate as a subtract of ALP enzyme. With this system, one ALP enzyme captured by one target miRNA molecule favored the production of thousands of ascorbic acid (AA) enzymatic products, which allowed a sensitive detection with an LOD of 40 fM. This biosensor could be generated 10 times, which permits an increase in the sample throughput and reduces the sample analysis time. In another work based also on the ECC system, a sandwich biosensor was employed using a biotinylated DNA-linked GO-AuNPs hybrid as a signal probe, which was interacted with SA-ALP. A capture probe was immobilized on GCE/AuNPs/Magnesium oxide (MgO) for more sensitive miRNA detection of 50 aM [98]. Mandli et al. [99] developed an electrochemical miRNA biosensor based also on a sandwich system with the use of AuNPs as a biosensor platform that incorporates SA-ALP enzyme linked to a biotin-modified signaling probe, catalyzing α-naphthyl phosphate as a substrate to produce electroactive α-naphthol. The differential pulse voltammetry (DPV) technique was used for the measurement of α-naphthol oxidation.

A competitive RNA/RNA hybridization assay-based biosensor was developed by incorporation of SA-HRP linked to biotinylated capture probes for amperometric detection of miRNA using H_2O_2 as enzyme-substrate and hydroquinone (HQ) as RedOx mediator. Indeed, different platforms—one based on the screen-printed electrode (SPE)/AuNPS [100] and the other one based on GCE/tungsten diselenide/AuNPs [101]—were employed. A lower LOD of 0.06 fM was obtained using tungsten diselenide/AuNPs because tungsten diselenide displayed a large effective surface area. This allowed increased loading of AuNPs on its surface to act as an excellent sensing substrate, which therefore can immobilize more capture probe DNA to the electrode and in turn leads to a low LOD.

Using a new way for probe capture immobilization, Torrente-Rodríguez et al. [102] employed magnetic-beads (MBs) modified with a special DNA–RNA antibody as capture probe bioreceptor. The antibody recognized the hybridized microRNA and biotinylated capture probe linked to SA-HRP. Indeed, amperometric detection implying the H_2O_2/HQ system at disposable SPCE was performed. This methodology has been evaluated for the quantification of miRNA-205 and miRNA-21 in total RNA obtained from human breast tissues.

In another work, simultaneous detection of four miRNAs using DNA tetrahedral nanostructure-based sandwich-type assay and Poly-HRP40 was performed in a serum sample of pancreatic cancer patients. A biotinylated capture signaling probe linked to HRP-SA was hybridized with the immobilized DNA tetrahedral on the gold electrode surface. Indeed, the HRP enzyme catalyzed the reduction in H_2O_2 in the presence of microRNAs, with TMB employed as an electron mediator, and thus generated a quantitative amperometric signal in the presence of TMB substrate [103]. Despite, the advantages of simultaneous detection with the presented method, it is still unable to give a specific LOD of each analyzed miRNA because of the interaction of the enzyme with all of the biotinylated signal probe complementary sequences of each miRNA.

Enzyme reaction-based electrochemical biosensor-integrated hybridization chain reaction (HCR) amplification was used to enhance the sensitivity of detection. Using this method, a large amount of streptavidine enzyme binds to biotin labeled on the long-range HCR product, which could remarkably amplify electrochemical signals. Different electrochemical biosensor based HCR techniques and the interaction between biotin-modified probe sequence and streptavidin-modified enzyme were developed [104,105]. Indeed, Zhai et al. [104] developed an electrochemical biosensor based on HCR and ALP by measuring the oxidation of α-naphthol as the enzymatic product, which is proportional to the miRNA concentration, an LOD of 0.56 fM was obtained. This biosensor has a good stability of 2 weeks.

Otherwise, in other work, DSN was employed; indeed, biotinylated ssDNA capture probes were immobilized on gold electrodes allowing SA-ALP to be attached to the capture probe, facilitating the production of an electrochemically active p-aminophenol (p-AP) from p-aminophenyl phosphate (p-APP) substrate. The resulting p-AP was cycled by TCEP after its electro-oxidization, enabling an increase in the anodic current of p-AP, which is proportional to miRNA concentration. Due to the cleavage of the double-strand DNA (dsDNA) by DSN, a decrease in p-AP response was observed after hybridization indicating the presence of miRNA [106]. More sensitive biosensors were developed also using DSN and the introduction of nanomaterials as a biosensor platform. However, the detection of miRNA was performed by the evaluation of AA using ALP and ECC RedOx cycling, using different platforms such as GCE/molybdenum disulfide (MoS_2)/AuNPs and GCE/MWCNTs@graphene oxide nanoribbons (GONRs)/AuNPs [107,108].

Other works for miRNA detection based on enzymatic reaction reported the use of CHA, which is initiated by the presence of target miRNA [109–112]. CHA allows the infinite recycling of miRNA to create a mass of streptavidin-enzyme modified signal probes, leading to an enhancement of electrochemical response. Additionally, to further enhance the sensitivity for miRNA detection, nanomaterials linked to enzymes were used. In this regard, Chen et al. [109] proposed a sandwich system integrating CHA and carbon sphere-MoS_2 (CS-MoS_2)/AuNPs for the immobilization of capture DNA (see Figure 7). AuNP-modified biotinylated signaling probes were employed as carriers of Avidin-HRP, which catalyze the H_2O_2 + HQ system to produce a strong electrochemical response, used for sensitive miRNA detection, to achieve a lower LOD of 0.16 fM.

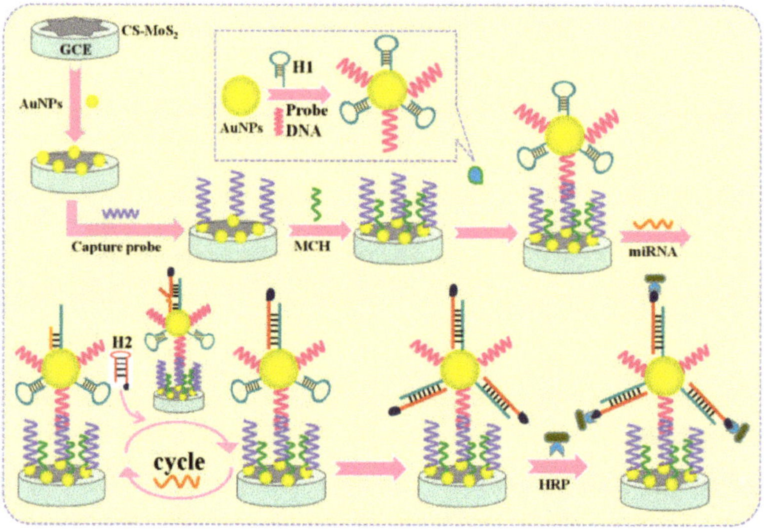

Figure 7. A sandwich-type electrochemical biosensing platform for microRNA-21 detection using carbon sphere-MoS2 and catalyzed hairpin assembly for signal amplification (reproduced with permission from the publisher) [109].

Zhang et al. [113] used DSN for miRNA-21 detection coupled with a capture probe labeled with biotin and SA-coated AuNPs, which were immobilized on the electrode surface due to the SA/biotin interaction. The numerous SA-coated AuNPs can subsequently immobilize a large number of biotin-labeled HRP molecules. Indeed, AuNPs were used as nanocarriers for HRP, helping to maintain their enzymatic activity. HRP was used to catalyze the reduction in H_2O_2 and in the presence of TMB, electrochemical current signals can be generated, which considerably enhances the electrochemical signal for miRNA-21 detection. The proposed biosensor permits an LOD of miRNA-21 down to 43.3 aM. The proposed biosensor allows an analysis of miRNA-21 in the human lung cancer cell line (A549 cells).

3.1.2. Enzyme–Protein Binding

The immobilization of enzymes is also possible by a protein. In this regard, Fang et al. [114] reported an electrochemical biosensor based on the immobilization of enzyme HRPs through zinc finger protein, which binds preferably to the DNA−RNA hybrid formed between an ssDNA capture probe and a target miRNA-21. For sensitive detection, ECC was used as an amplifier system based on the induction of a series of oxide-reduction reactions in the presence of HRP including $Ru(NH_3)_6^{3+}/Ru(NH_3)_6^{2+}$, BQ/HQ, and TCEP. The LOD for miRNA-21 in the buffer and diluted human serum were 2 and 30 fM, respectively.

Enzyme-conjugated protein was also employed for labeling an antibody that specifically recognizes DNA–RNA duplex [115]. In this view, Vargas et al. [116] involved the use of direct hybridization of miRNA-21 with a specific biotinylated DNA probe immobilized on streptavidin-modified MBs. A specific antibody labeled with a bacterial protein A conjugated with Poly-HRP40 recognized the capture probe/miRNA-21 duplex. Amperometric detection of miRNA-21 was performed upon the magnetic capture of the modified MBs onto the SPCEs using the H_2O_2/HQ system.

Zouari et al. [117] developed an electrochemical AuNP-based biosensor platform that was used for miRNA detection. Indeed, RNA/miRNA homoduplexes were recognized with the viral protein p19, labeled with a HRP-conjugated anti-maltose binding protein monoclonal antibody (see Figure 8). The bioplatforms present at least 2 months of storage stability. Additionally, the analysis of miRNA in total RNA extracted from healthy and cancerous breast cells was performed using the proposed biosensor.

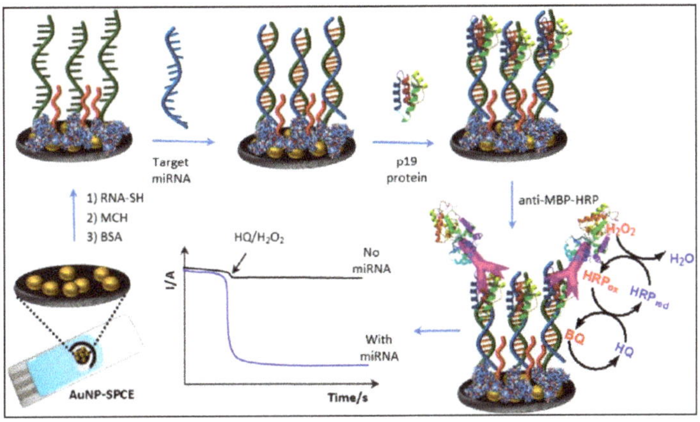

Figure 8. Schematic display of the amperometric integrated sensor developed for miRNA determination using a specific thiolated RNA probe, a direct RNA/miRNA hybridization assay and p19 viral protein as detector bioreceptor further labeled with anti-MBP-HRP (reproduced with permission from the publisher) [117].

3.1.3. Other Types of Enzyme Binding

There is another way for enzyme immobilization at the electrode surface for miRNA detection. Indeed, graphene quantum dots (GQDs) have a large surface-to-volume ratio, excellent compatibility of GQDs were used as a new platform for a large amount of HRP immobilization through the non-covalent assembly (see Figure 9). In this work, a sandwich system was employed for miRNA-155 detection integrating capture probe and signaling probe modified with NH_2 conjugated with QDs-HRP. The proposed biosensor is permitted to reach an LOD of 0.14 fM in a linear range from 1 fM to 100 pM [118]. Otherwise, an electrochemical biosensor for miRNA-221 detection using CHA and also a sandwich system based on the use of HRP directly labeled to signal probe was reported. HRP was used to catalyze the reaction of TMB/H_2O_2 for amperometric detection of miRNA-221 [119].

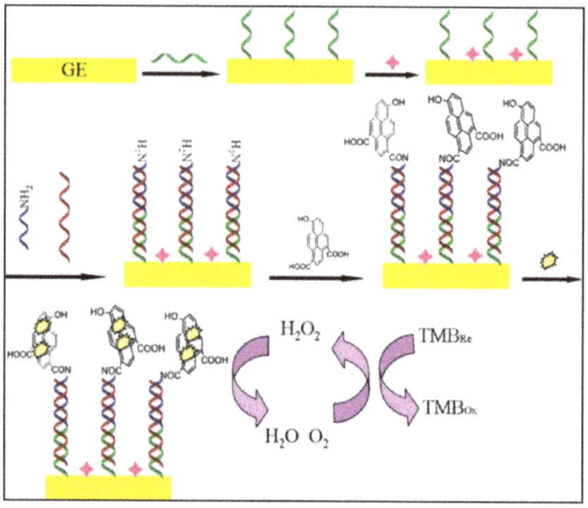

Figure 9. Principle of the enzyme catalytic amplification of miRNA-155 detection with graphene quantum dot-based electrochemical biosensor (reproduced with permission from the publisher) [118].

3.2. Chemical Catalysts

Different kinds of nanomaterials as chemical catalysts, including copper-based metal–organic framework (Cu-MOF), copper nanoclusters (CuNCs), Fe_3O_4NPs, platinum/tunable tin-doped indium oxide nanoparticles (Pt/Sn-In_2O_3) were utilized for miRNA detection and will be discussed in this part. An example of an electrochemical biosensor for miRNA detection based on the chemical catalyst is presented in Figure 6B.

Wang et al. [120] proposed a paper modified AuNP as a biosensor platform for miRNA-155 detection using a capture probe-AuNPs@Cu-MOF (see Figure 10). In the presence of glucose, Cu-MOFs and AuNPs as chemical catalysts cooperatively catalyzed the glucose oxidation, resulting in the wide linear detection range from 1.0 fM to 10 nM and the LOD of 0.35 fM for miRNA-155. The present biosensor showed stability of 30 days.

In other work, CuNCs as catalyst-based biosensor were employed for miRNA detection. CuNCs were synthesized at the electrode surface by taking DNA–RNA heteroduplexes as templates with the help of AA and Cu^{2+}. Besides, the formed CuNCs possessed the capability of catalyzing H_2O_2 reduction, resulting in steady and amplified electrochemical signals, which were used in miRNA analysis, reaching an LOD of 8.2 fM [121]. As other types of nanomaterial as a chemical catalyst, SA/Pt/Sn-In_2O_3 hybrids were employed for miRNA-21 biosensor development. Indeed, a SA/Pt/Sn-In_2O_3 was attached to a biotinylated hairpin capture probe by the presence of miRNA-21, producing an electrochemical signal of oxygen reduction for detection in O_2-saturated solution. SA/Pt/Sn-In_2O_3 as the amplifier led to an LOD of 1.92 fM [122].

Otherwise, a mixing of enzyme and nanomaterial as enzyme–nanomaterials composite was reported to enhance the sensitivity for miRNA detection [123–126]. This is obtained by the synergetic effect of the catalyst and nanomaterials that improve the electrochemical response. However, the LOD of miRNAs obtained with this composite could be also obtained using just one type of catalyst; consequently, the use of enzyme and nanomaterials as catalysts together increases the cost and the time of biosensor construction without significant signal amplification.

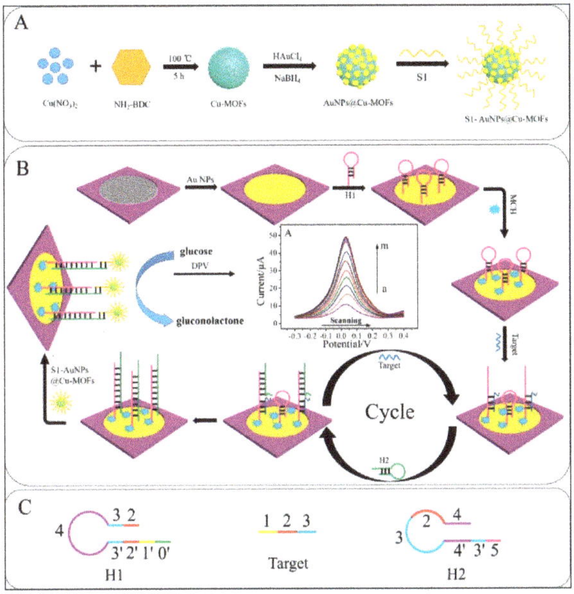

Figure 10. Schematic illustration of the fabrication of the biosensor: (**A**) preparation procedure of S1-AuNPs@Cu-MOFs; (**B**) the detection principle for glucose and the strategy of signal amplification; (**C**) structure of H1, target, and H2 (reproduced with permission from the publisher) [120].

3.3. *DNAzyme*

Recently, DNAzymes with peroxidase-like activity has aroused a high interest. To achieve such catalytic activity, the DNA probe requires a G-quadruplex structure, which is able to bind to hemin molecules. Such a system promotes a RedOx reaction between the target molecule and hydrogen peroxide, leading to the formation of an oxidized product. Indeed, hemin-G-quadruplex was employed for miRNA detection [127,128]. The principle of an electrochemical biosensor based on hemin-G-quadruplex as a DNAzyme is presented in Figure 6C. In this context, hemin-G-quadruplex was employed to catalyze H_2O_2 reduction, with coupling with HCR to fabricate long hemin-G-quadruplex DNAzyme nanowires (see Figure 11) [129]. In other work, hemin-G-quadruplex was also used for miRNA analysis by catalyzing the oxidation of TMB in the presence of H_2O_2 [130].

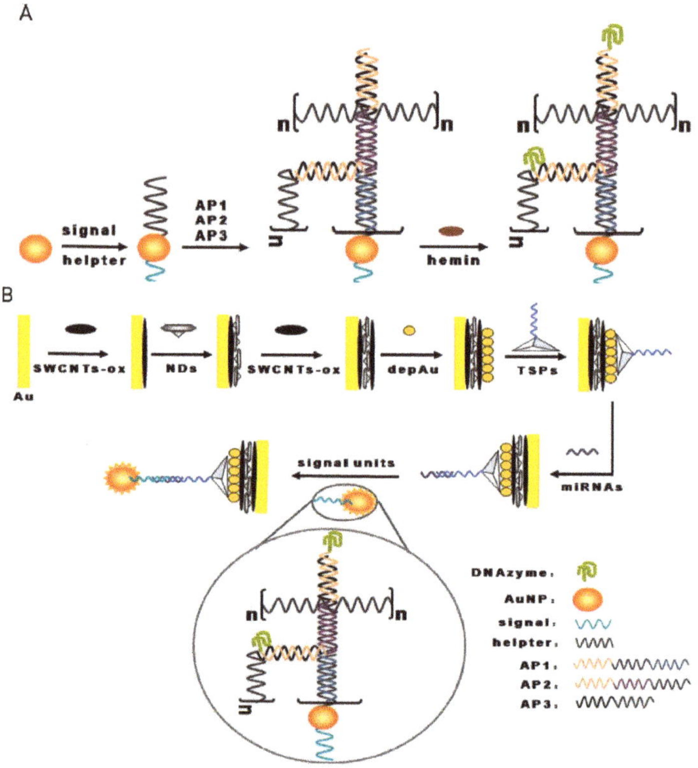

Figure 11. (**A**) DNA-functionalized AuNP based hybridization chain reaction, (**B**) Schematic illustration of miRNA biosensor using layered nanostructure of oxidized single-walled carbon nanotubes and nanodiamonds by hybridization chain reaction (reproduced with permission from the publisher) [129].

Electrochemical biosensors based on catalysts with the focus on their various analytical performances are summarized in Table 3.

Compared to DNAzyme and nanomaterials, enzymes generally display superior performance in terms of catalytic efficiency and specificity, as well as excellent activity in aqueous media under ambient conditions, thanks to their high turnover and high selectivity. On the other hand, the enzyme is influenced by the external environment, requires a specific reaction condition, the reaction time dependent on enzyme activity and finally we always need an additional molecule (substrate) for the detection of the enzymatic product. Otherwise, nanomaterials and DNAzyme present desired advantages including their high stability, a tunable structure, catalytic efficiencies, purely synthetic routes to their preparation, lower cost, and excellent tolerance to experimental conditions. Despite the above-mentioned advantages, there is a risk of contamination with these molecules.

Table 3. Current sensitive electrochemical biosensors using catalysts.

MicroRNA	Catalysts/Amplification Agents	Platform	Substrat or Reagent	Technique	Linear Range	LOD	Real-Samples Application	References
miRNA-21	ALP/DNA-linked GO–AuNPs	GCE/MgO/AuNPs	AAP	DPV	0.1–100 fM	50 aM	Spiked human serum	[98]
miRNA -21	ALP/HCR	AuE	α-NP	SWV	1 fM–100 pM	0.56 fM	Spiked HEK293T cells	[104]
miRNA-21	ALP/CHA-WO_3-Gr	GCE/WO_3-Gr/AuNPs	Ascorbic acid 2-phosphate	DPV	0.1 fM–100 pM	0.05 fM	Serum samples from breast cancer patients	[111]
miRNA -21	HRP/AuNPs	AuE	H_2O_2	Amperometry	0.1 fM–100 pM	43.3 aM	A549 tumor cells	[113]
miRNA-155	ALP/CHA	GCE/MWCNTs PtNPs	Phosphate ion Molybdophosphate anion	DPV	10 fM–1 nM	1.64 fM	Cervical cancer cells and human breast cancer cell lines	[131]
miRNA-155	ALP/-	SCPE/Fe_3O_4	AAP	DPV	0.6–9 ng/mL	29 pM	Spiked human serum	[132]
miRNA-21	HRP/-	SCPE/Fe_3O_4	H_2O_2	Amperometry	1.0–100 pM	10 aM	MCF-7 cells	[116]
miRNA -155	HRP/GQDs	AuE	TMB	Amperometry	1 fM–00 pM	0.14 fM	Spiked human serum	[118]
miRNA-21, let-7a & miRNA-31	HRP/HCR	SPCE/Fe_3O_4	H_2O_2	Amperometry	1.2–100 pM	0.66 pM	MCF-7 cells	[133]
miRNA-21	HRP/-	SPCE/Fe_3O_4	H_2O_2	Amperometry	3.0 to 100 nM	0.91 nM	MCF-7 cells	[134]
miRNA-21	Copper (II) complex/HCR	GCME/Fe3O4	TMB	DPV	100 aM–100 nM	33 aM	human serum samples from breast cancer	[135]
miRNA-155	Cu-MOFs/AuNPs	Au-PWE	Glucose	DPV	1 fM–10 nM	0.35 fM	Spiked human serum	[120]

Table 3. *Cont.*

MicroRNA	Catalysts/Amplification Agents	Platform	Substrat or Reagent	Technique	Linear Range	LOD	Real-Samples Application	References
miRNA-21	Sn-In_2O_3/-	AuE	O_2	DPV	5 pM–0.5 fM	1.92 fM	A549 and HeLa cell lines	[122]
miRNA-21	G-quadruplex−hemin/-	AuE	H_2O_2	DPV	0.1 fM–0.1 pM	0.04 fM	Human serum samples from breast cancer	[128]
miRNA-21	G-quadruplex−hemin /HCR	AuE/SWCNT-ox/NDs/SWCNTs-ox/AuNPs	H_2O_2	DPV	10 fM–1.0 nM	1.95 fM	Spiked human serum	[129]

Abbreviations: GCE, glassy carbone electrode; NDs, nanodiamonds; MB, magnetic beads; SWCNTs, single-walled carbon nanotubes; α-NP, α-naphtyl phosphate; AAP, ascorbic acid 2-phosphate; WO3-Gr, tungsten oxide-graphene composites; AA, ascorbic acid; ALP, alkaline phosphatase; CHA, catalytic hairpin assembly; DPV, differential pulse voltammetry; MgO, magnesium oxide; GO, graphene oxide, AuNPs, gold nanoparticles; AuE, gold electrode; HCR, hybridization chain reaction; SWV, square wave voltammetry; HEK293T cells, from human embryonic kidney 293T cells; SPCE, screen-printed carbon electrodes; H_2O_2, hydrogen peroxide; HRP, horseradish peroxidase; MCF-7 cells, human breast adenocarcinoma cell line; TMB, 3,3′,5,5′-tetramethylbenzidine; GQDs, graphene quantum dots; A549, human lung carcinoma cells; HeLa cells, human cervical cancer cells; Au-PWE, gold-paper working electrode; Cu-MOFs, copper-based metal–organic frameworks; G-quadruplex−hemin, Guanine-quadruplex−hemin; MDA-MB-231, human breast cancer cell lines, Sn-In2O3, tin-doped indium oxide particles. MWCNTs, multi-walled carbon nanotube, platinum nanoparticles, PtNPs; magnetic nanoparticles, Fe_3O_4.

4. Electrochemical Biosensor Based on RedOx Intercalating Agent

In chemistry, intercalation is the insertion of a molecule (or a group of molecules) between two other molecules (or groups). In the present approach, a RedOx molecule or a complex of RedOx molecules are employed for DNA strand binding via intercalation. The binding to ssDNA and dsDNA is obtained with different affinity regarding the nature of the intercalator. Different types of molecules were used as RedOx intercalating agents for miRNA analysis. This includes organic molecules such as the commonly used MB [136] as well as oracet blue (OB) [137] and toluidine blue [138]. Various other molecules and macromolecules could also be intercalated as an organometallic complex including $Ru(NH_3)_6^{3+}$ [139], cobalt phenanthroline, or metal intercalating agents such as palladium nanoparticles [140] and biomolecules as hemin [141]. The principle of the approaches is presented in Figure 12. The interlacing process on the biosensor could be direct to the target DNA strands (Figure 12A) [138] or indirect by the design of specific sites in the DNA probe called a template [142] (Figure 12B).

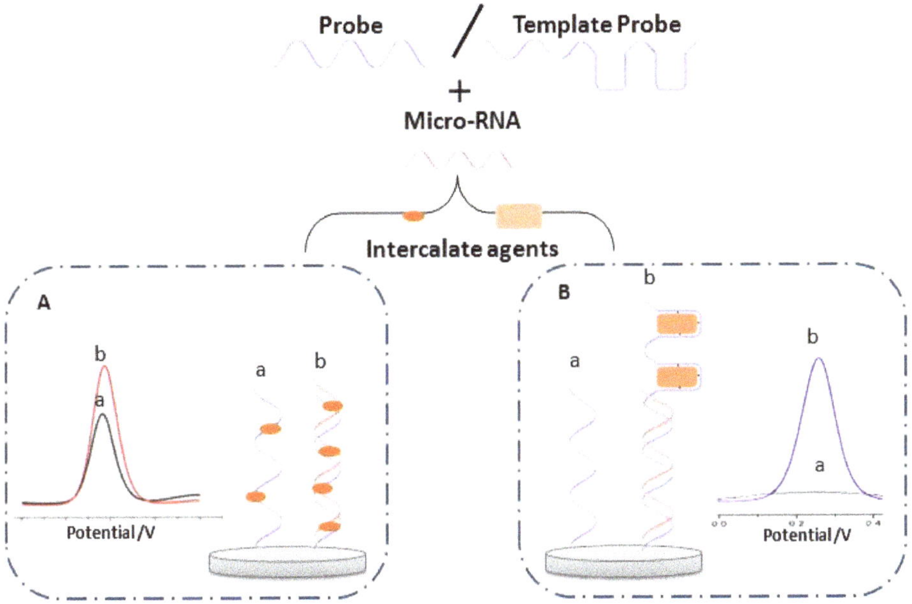

Figure 12. Principal of electrochemical biosensor based on RedOx intercalating agent before (**a**) and after hybridization (**b**) with micro-RNA, (**A**) direct intercalation, and (**B**) intercalation via the template.

4.1. Direct Intercalation

The direct intercalating of RedOx molecules between the DNA strands is based on an interaction of electroactive species on the formed double-strand DNA–DNA or DNA–RNA upon hybridization reaction (Figure 12A). Indeed, various kinds of RedOx molecules could be used in the case of electrochemical biosensors for miRNA that will be discussed in this part and they are divided into three kinds, electroactive molecules, and electroactive complex.

4.1.1. Electroactive Molecule

The MB is the popular electroactive indicator used as an intercalating DNA agent since MB interacts both with ss and ds DNA where the binding mode differs from each macromolecule. Thus MB and dsDNA interact by three binding modes: (i) intercalation between successive base pairs with the face-to-face binding of the bases and MB; (ii) insertion into the minor groove; and (iii) insertion into the major groove of the double helix. The interaction ssDNA with MB is obtained by face-to-face binding of the bases and MB. Thus, the affinity of MB regarding ssDNA and dsDNA is largely discussed. Regarding the literature, depending on the biosensors design, MB shows a higher affinity for ssDNA or dsDNA. In the case of miRNA detection, most biosensors published show less affinity of MB to DNA–RNA complex. Thus, it has been reported by Li et al. [143] that MB reacts easily with guanine present in ssDNA with high affinity due to the good accessibility of MB to the guanine of ssDNA. In this work, a transducer formed with GCE/MWCNTs/PAMAM modified with a DNA probe was used as a biosensors platform for miRNA-24 detection. The detection was followed through measuring the electroactivity of MB before and after hybridization. A decrease in the signal response is observed after the hybridization of miRNA-24 where LOD reached 0.5 fM. Furthermore, this biosensor was stable for 7 days and could be regenerated four times.

Nevertheless, a more complex biosensor design was performed using RedOx intercalator and amplification strategy in order to enhance the sensitivity of the detection. For example, a biosensor was developed for miRNA-155 detection, where HCR was used to amplify the number of intercalated MB molecules on the DNA strands, by creating a longer dsDNA and using a GCE modified with polypyrrole/reduced graphene oxide/AuNPs (Ppy/rGO/AuNPs) [144]. The amplification of MB response can also be performed by using a 3D DNA nanonet structure which is hybridized with the immobilized capture probe on a gold electrode by a sandwich system. In this case, a femtomolar detection of miRNA-21, was obtained [145]. Both presented biosensors were stable for 2 weeks and the analysis of miRNA was performed in spiked human serum.

Another approach involving nanomaterials as nanocatalysts which assisted the signal amplification strategy has been used to enhance the RedOx signal of MB intercalator. For example, the association of various kinds of nanomaterials as a catalyst was developed to improve the MB response. Thus, the synergetic effect of Fe_3O_4 and cerium dioxide (CeO_2) decorated with gold nanoparticles (Fe_3O_4/CeO_2@AuNPs) was demonstrated to improve the RedOx response of MB intercalator (Figure 13A). A labeled probe decorated with the nanocatalysts was employed in a sandwich system for the amplification of intercalated MB response by a direct catalyzation of MB reduction leading to LOD of 0.33fM [146]. Other nanomaterials such as carboxylate-reduced graphene oxide (COOH-rGO) have been reported as an amplification strategy. The nanomaterial can intercalate on the ssDNA, leading to an accumulation of electroactive MB (Figure 13B). In the presence of miRNA, a DSN cleave captures probe/miRNA duplex is obtained resulting in a decrease in MB response. A lower LOD of 0.01 fM was obtained [147].

Other approaches involving various innovative amplification strategies have also been published. For example, Guo et al. [148] reported an attomolar biosensor for the detection of miRNA-196a. The mechanism consists of after hybridization of miRNA and formation of a terminal deoxynucleotidyl, transferase will trigger a DNA extension reaction producing long ssDNA rich in guanine, in which MB is attached. The biosensor presents a very low sensitivity compared to other ones, used with other strategies due to obtained long ssDNA which can specifically adsorb positively charged MB via guanine bases, resulting in the attachment of a large amount of MB. However, this biosensor needs many steps after miRNA hybridization which can limit their application.

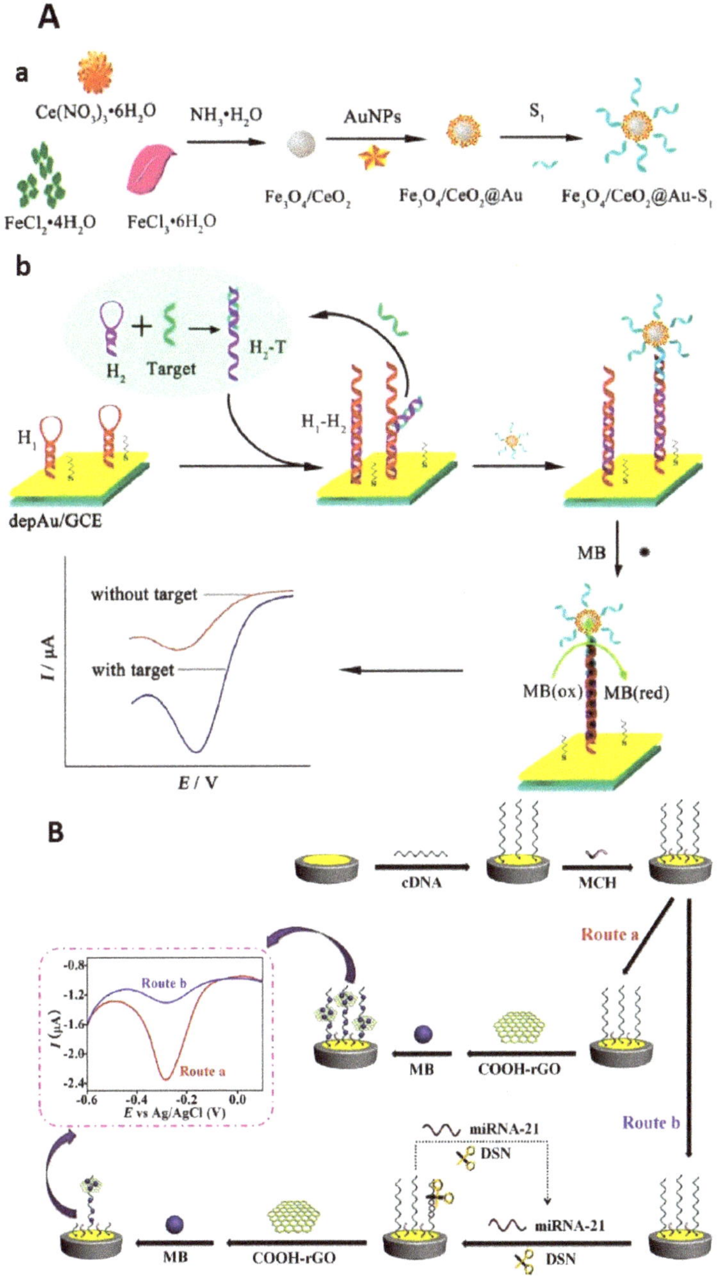

Figure 13. Example of biosensors using amplification strategy with nanomaterials as a non-nanocatalyst; (**A**) the nanomaterials are formed with Fe_3O_4 and cerium dioxide (CeO_2) decorated with gold nanoparticles (Fe_3O_4/CeO_2@AuNPs) reproduced from. (**a**) Preparation procedure of Fe_3O_4/CeO_2 @Au-S_1, (**b**) signal amplification strategy and the detection principle for microRNA [146] with permission of the publisher; (**B**) biosensors using graphene oxide and DSN as amplification method from [147] reproduced with permission of the publisher.

4.1.2. Electroactive Metals Complex

In the case of electroactive metal complex intercalator, hexaammineruthenium III chloride (RuHex) is used frequently as electroactive complex employed for miRNA detection. The RuHex is positively charged and could intercalate with DNA strand via the binding with the anionic phosphate of DNA through electrostatic interaction. Few studies have been published with this complex and the associated amplification strategies. For example, hierarchical flower-like gold nanostructures (HFGN) were developed as a biosensor platform and used for selective detection of miRNA-21 in the buffer and real sample; RuHex was employed as RedOx intercalator [149]. In other works and to increase the amount of intercalated RuHex, Yu et al. [150] and Chen et al. [151] used DNA nanostructures as probes immobilized on the gold electrode surface for enhancing the binding ability of RuHex. Thus, in the presence of miRNAs targets, these nanostructures provided an enhancement of RuHex intercalants. The analysis of miRNA in total RNA-extracted cancerous breast cells was performed using the proposed biosensors.

4.2. Intercalation via Template

The intercalation via template consists of the use of other molecules, which need to create recognition sites in DNA strands for their intercalation. The principal of this type of intercalation is presented in Figure 12B. Generally, the nanostructure of DNA is necessary to perform this method.

Starting with hemin that needs abundant guanines to form hemin/G-quadruplexes [152], an electrochemical biosensor was described by Wang et al. [153] for the quantification of miRNA-21 at fM level. The catching of hemin was enhanced by the integration of a sandwich system in which a signal probe is labeled with N-doped graphene/Au nanoparticles (NG-AuNPs) and works as a support for several strands of guanine-rich DNA.

Otherwise, Zhang et al. [140] described a label-free and attomolar electrochemical miRNA-21 biosensor based on a template for palladium nanoparticles witch lead to integration with the nitrogen of guanine. RCA amplification was used to produce a massive G-rich long ssDNA resulting in an enhanced electrochemical signal.

4.3. Other Type of Intercalation

Some other RedOx molecules able to intercalate poorly or that do not intercalate at all with the DNA strands have also been studied. However, their intercalation could be realized via a linker. In this regard, Asadzadeh et al. [154] used AgNPs as a RedOx molecule, which was intercalated to the ssDNA via single-walled carbon nanotube (SWCNT). The binding of the AgNPs/SWCNT nanohybrid to ssDNA was performed via interactions π–π between the nanohybrid and the nitrogenous bases of ssDNA. The proposed method was used for miRNA-25 detection as a lung cancer biomarker.

Wang et al. [155] used GO as support of Prussian blue (PB), which is the RedOx intercalant agent. The GO was adsorbed on the 3′ end of capture probe though π–π interaction. Then, the PB was attached to GO. In the presence of miRNA-122, the GO with the assembled PB was separated from the electrode surface due to the low affinity of the GO with the DNA/RNA hybrid, resulting in a decrease in electrochemical response of PB.

MiRNAs are characterized by cis-diol at the 3′-terminal, this propriety is employed by Liu et al. [156] for an attomolar detection of miRNA-21 using AgNP as a RedOx intercalate agent. Indeed, with the presence of miRNA-21, a 4-mercaptophenylboronic acid (MPBA) was attached in the 3′-terminal of miRNAs through the boronate ester bond formation and then captured AgNP via the Ag–Thiol interaction. Meanwhile, free MPBA molecules in solution induced the in situ assemblies of AgNPs on the electrode surface via the covalent interactions between α-hydroxycarboxylate of citrate and boronate of MPBA and the formation of Ag–Thiol bonds.

Electrochemical biosensors based on RedOx intercalating agents highlighting their various analytical performances are presented in Table 4.

Table 4. Current sensitive electrochemical biosensors using the RedOx intercalating agent.

MicroRNA	Intercalent Agent	Platform	Amplification of Signal Elements	Tech	Linear Range	LOD	Real-Samples Application	Ref
miRNA-155	OB	GCE/GO/GNR	-	DPV	2.0 fM–8.0 pM	0.6 fM	Spiked human plasma	[157]
miRNA-21	TB	GCE/AuNPs-Ppy	-	DPV	100 aM–1 nM	78 aM	Spiked human serum.	[138]
miRNA-196a	MB	AuE	DNA extension reaction	DPV	0.05 fM–50 pM	15 aM	Spiked plasma	[148]
miRNA-486-5p	Thinonine	GCE/FeCN/AuNPs	FeCN	DPV	1 fM–1000 pM	8.53 fM	Human lung A549 cells	[158]
miRNA-141	RuHex	AuE	HP-AuNPs	DPV	0–10 nM	25.1 aM	Human breast cancer cells MDA-MB-231	[150]
miRNA-21	RuHex	AuE	AuNPs enrichment by bridge DNA,	Chronocoulometry	0.1 fM–0.1 nM	68 aM	Serum samples from lung cancer patients	[159]
miRNA-21	RuHex	GCE/AuNPs@MoS_2	AuNPs@MoS_2	DPV	10 fM–1 nM	0.78 fM	Spiked human serum	[160]
miRNA-21	Molybdophosphate	AuE	HCR	SWV	1 fM–1 nM	0.78 fM	Spiked human serum	[161]
miRNA-21	CuNCs	AuE	HCR	DPSV	10 pM–0.1 fM	10 aM	Spiked blood sample	[162]
miRNA-21	Hemin	AuE	HCR	DPV	15 fM–250 pM	13.5 fM	Spiked human serum	[152]
miRNA-199 a	AgNPs	AuE	C-rich loop DNA templates	DPV	1.0 fM–0.1 nM	0.64 fM	Spiked human serum	[142]

Abbreviations: GCE, glassy carbon electrode; MB, methylene blue; DPV, differential pulse voltammetry; AuE, gold electrode; FeCN, iron-embedded nitrogen-rich carbon nanotubes; AuNPs, gold nanoparticles; A549 cells, adenocarcinoma cells; GO, graphene oxide; GNR, gold nanorods; Ppy, polypyrrole; RuHex, hexaammineruthenium III chloride; HP-AuNPs, hairpin-modified gold nanoparticles; MDA-MB-231: human breast cancer cells; HCR, hybridization chain reaction; SWV, square wave voltammetry; CuNCs, copper nanoclosters; DPSV, differential pulse stripping voltammetry; AgNPs, silver nanoparticles; C-rich loop DNA templates, cytosine-rich loop DNA templates; TB, toluidine blue; OB, oracet blue.

A comparison between different methods of intercalation used for miRNA detection shows that intercalation via a template presents some advantages such as good biocompatibility, good electrochemical properties facilitating a very low LOD of miRNA detection. Nevertheless, it still presents some limitations related to the complicated process of fabrication, which is considered time-consuming; and also, the need for an additional amplification step to obtain high sensitivity which is required for miRNA detection. Otherwise, direct intercalation of the RedOx molecules method is considered as an easy and fast method of intercalation since the used RedOx molecules could bind directly and specifically to DNA without the need of complicated preparation. Indeed, the LOD obtained using this method is slightly higher than the ones obtained with intercalation via the template method.

Overall, the intercalation strategy is easy to use on-site, but it does not allow simultaneous detection, because the interaction of the RedOx molecule is not specific and can intercalate on all DNA strands present at the surface of the electrode. Furthermore, the use of intercalation based on electrostatic interaction leads to a non-specific interaction and high background noise, especially using real samples.

5. Electrochemical Label-Free Biosensing

Label-free biosensor include the use of ferri–ferrocyanide complex or hexaammineruthenium (II)/(III) as RedOx-free indicators. The response is based on electrostatic repulsion or interaction depending on the marker. The ferri–ferrocyanide complex is negatively charged, thus after the hybridization of miRNA target, a repulsion effect is produced by the negatively charged phosphate leading to the variation of response. In the case of hexaammineruthenium (II)/(III) complex, it is positively charged and could undergo interaction with hybridized DNA. Another factor that could lead to the variation of the RedOx marker is its accessibility to the surface after DNA–RNA complex formation of a duplex preventing electron transfer to the surface. Various electrochemical methods could be used to follow such responses including electrochemical impedance spectroscopy (EIS), cyclic voltammetry (CV), DPV, and square wave voltammetry (SWV). The principle of electrochemical biosensors based on the free RedOx indicator is presented in Figure 14. In this section, electrochemical biosensors for miRNA detection based on the free RedOx indicator will be discussed.

5.1. Ferri/Ferrocyanide as Free RedOx Indicator

Ferri–ferrocyanide as a free RedOx indicator was widely employed for miRNA detection. The detection is based on the electrostatic repellence of two negatively charged DNA and $Fe(CN)_6^{3-/4-}$ molecules leading to the decrease in electrochemical reaction on the surface upon hybridization and decrease in current response or increase in impedance (Figure 14). In this regard, EIS as the detection method has been used extensively for miRNA monitoring in combination with various materials and nanomaterials as transducers [163–166]. In most research, the nature of materials attached to the surface plays an important role in the electrochemical response. In this respect, Yammouri et al. [167] used this approach in the association of transducer formed with a pencil graphite electrode (PGE) modified with a carbon black-bearing DNA probe. The miRNA-125a detection was monitored by EIS in the presence of this RedOx marker. The synergetic effect of negatively charged carbon black combined with the high surface ratio of PGE allows the detection with lower LOD and good determination in serum samples. In another work, the polythiophene film-modified screen-printed gold electrode was employed as a biosensor platform for miRNA-221detection from total RNA extracted from human lung and breast cancer cell lines. The proposed biosensor demonstrated the benefic effect of the conductive surface [168]. Mandli et al. [169] employed PGE modified with Ppy for microRNA-34a detection by EIS. Indeed, the immobilization of the probe was performed during Ppy electropolymerization on PGE and the hybridization was performed by the specific recognition sequence of miRNA-34a. This biosensor was functional for the analysis of miRNA-34a in human breast cancer cells samples.

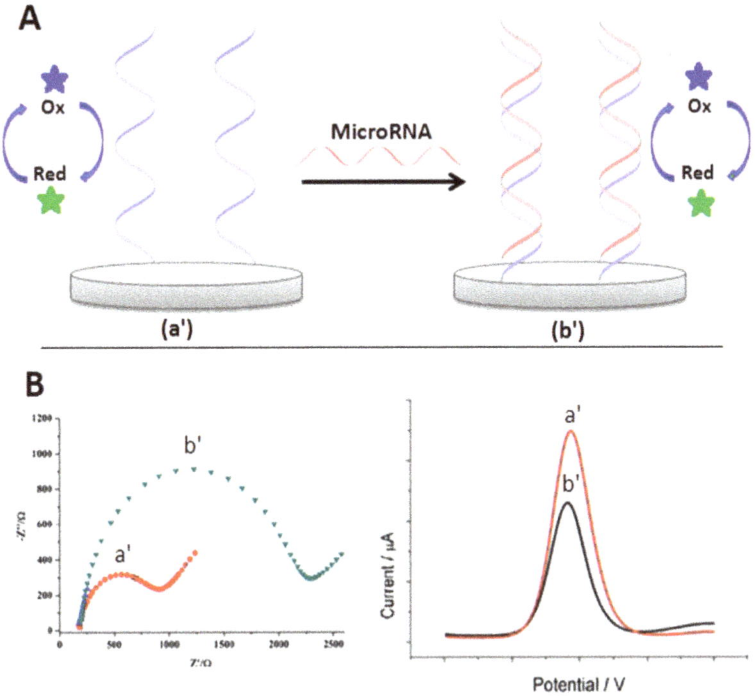

Figure 14. (**A**) Pricipale of electrochemical biosensors based on free RedOx indicator (**a′**) before and (**b′**) after hybridizition. (**B**) EIS and DPV response of the electrochemical biosensor based on free RedOx indicator (**a′**) before and (**b′**) after hybridization.

Association of this method with system amplification such as HCR was also performed. Indeed, Meng et al. [170] developed an electrochemical biosensor combining efficient HCR for signal amplification of oligonucleotides with negatively charged repelling $[Fe(CN)_6]^{3-/4-}$ ions inducing a spatial blockage to the electron transfer. In this biosensor, many linear DNA concatamers lead to a great increase in interfacial charge-transfer resistance (R_{ct}), which is positively correlated with miRNA-21 concentrations with an LOD of 4.63 fM with the stability of the biosensor lasting for 21 days. This strategy allowed the analysis of miRNA-21 in different cancer cells including breast, cervical, and non-small cell lung cancers.

Zhang et al. [171] employed a magnetic bead-modified glassy carbon electrode combined with a DSN amplification strategy for impedimetric miRNA-21 detection (see Figure 15). Due to the cleavage of the capture probe–miRNA-21 heteroduplex, after the hybridization steps the negatively charged layer could not be formed, resulting in a small R_{ct} in the presence of ferriferrocyanide, which was used for miRNA-21 detection, permitting an LOD of 60 aM.

Otherwise, DPV based on ferriferrocyanide was also employed for miRNA detection [172–174]. In this case, advanced surface modification was performed to obtain an efficient electron transfer. Indeed, a biosensor formed with fluorine-doped tin oxide electrode modified with nanomaterials composed with nitrogen-doped functionalized graphene associated with (AgNPs and polyaniline (PANI) nanocomposite modified, was developed for miRNA detection. The employed nanocomposite allowed more biomolecules to be immobilized at the surface of the electrode, which shortened the distance for electron transfer and ion diffusion paths from the capture probe to the nanomaterials. The nano-biosensor showed a wide dynamic detection range of 10 fM–10 μM and a low LOD of 0.2 fM [175].

Ferriferrocyanide as a free RedOx indicator was used for other strategies of detection based on the direct adsorption of miRNAs on the electrode surface. This strategy needs a preliminary step of target isolation mostly with capture probe-modified magnetic beads, then, a denaturation of the DNA–RNA hybrid is achieved by heating at 95 °C. Thereafter, researchers try different ways for adsorbing isolated miRNAs. For instance, a picomolar biosensor was reported by Boriachek's group based on gold electrode–miRNA affinity interaction [176]. Wan's group used a screen-printed graphene electrode, for miRNAs detection isolated and directly adsorbed on the surface of the graphene electrode via graphene–miRNA affinity interaction. This method showed an LOD of 10 fM [177]. According to the present two works, we can conclude that graphene–miRNA affinity is higher than the gold–miRNA affinity. Koo et al. [178] magnified the adsorption of miRNAs using a polyadenine extension, which has a high affinity with the gold surface. However, the miRNA was subjected to poly (A) extension on 3′ ends using poly(A) polymerase enzyme.

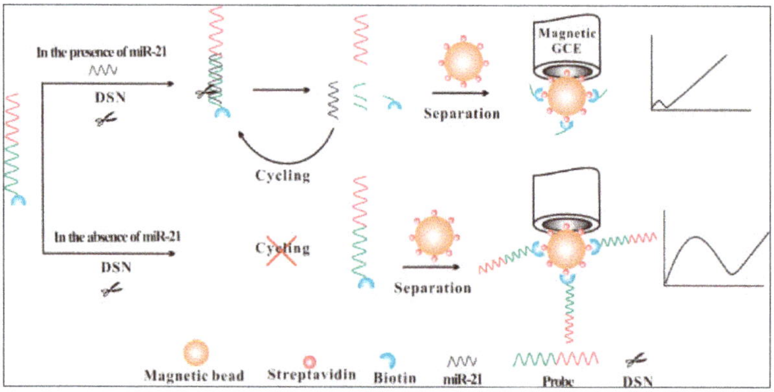

Figure 15. Experimental principle of the biosensor (reproduced with permission from the publisher) [171].

5.2. Hexaammineruthenium (II)/(III) Chloride as Free RedOx Indicator

Hexaammineruthenium (II)/(III) was also employed for miRNA detection. In this regard, nickel phosphate nanostructures (NiPNs) were used as a biosensor platform for the immobilization of the capture probe by coordination bonding between Ni and probe DNA especially phosphate groups. The constructed NiPNs-p-DNA surface acted as the amplified platform enabling efficient access to many target miRNA-21 sequences. The probe-DNA immobilization and the miRNA hybridization steps were supervised by EIS measurements in $[Ru(NH_3)_6]^{3+/2+}$. The proposed biosensor allowed reaching an LOD of 0.034 pM, and the analysis of miRNA-21 levels in human lung cancer cells [179].

Association of the two RedOx indicators ferricyanide and hexaammineruthenium (II)/(III) for miRNA detection was also explored. In this view, a ratiometric electrochemical miRNA biosensing platform based on the target-triggered ruthenium release and RedOx recycling was reported (see Figure 16). In this research, $[Ru(NH_3)_6]^{3+}$ was entrapped into the pores of mesoporous silica nanoparticles modified by an indium tin oxide electrode and was subsequently capped by a capture probe. Once the target miRNA was captured and hybridized into dsDNA/RNA, $[Ru(NH_3)_6]^{3+}$ was released and electroreduced into $[Ru(NH_3)_6]^{2+}$, which was then chemically oxidized back to $[Ru(NH_3)_6]^{2+}$ by $[Fe(CN)_6]^{3-}$. The consumed $[Fe(CN)_6]^{3-}$ and liberated $[Ru(NH_3)_6]^{3+}$ produced a significant ratiometric signal. Using this innovative approach, an LOD that decreased down to 33 aM was obtained. Additionally, the developed biosensor showed good stability over 20 days and permitted the analysis of miRNA-21 in different cancer cells including breast, cervical, and non-small cell lung cancers [180].

Electrochemical biosensors based on free RedOx indicator with the focus on their various analytical performances are exposed in Table 5.

The discussed methods in this section present some advantages including, higher sensitivity, easier signal quantification, direct conversion of the biological event into an electrical signal, and finally requiring fewer steps of fabrication since there is no need to use RedOx markers that interact with DNA strands. On the other hand, the inconvenience is that these methods suffer from some drawbacks such as the potential of non-specific adsorption of other biomolecules on the electrode surface, which may cause false-positive interference. Additionally, the results of this method were always easily disturbed by surface contamination and adsorption.

Table 5. Current sensitive electrochemical biosensors using free RedOx indicator.

MicroRNA	Free RedOx Indicator	Platform	Amplification Agent	Technique	Linear Range/LOD	LOD	Real-Samples Application	References
miRNA-21	$Fe(CN)_6^{3-/4-}$	AuE	biotin-FNPs	EIS	0.1–250 fM	0.1 fM	-	[181]
miRNA-21	$Fe(CN)_6^{3-/4-}$	GCE	AuNPs	EIS	1–1000 pM	0.3 pM	Spiked serum sample	[182]
miRNA-21	$Fe(CN)_6^{3-/4-}$	Magnetic GCE	DSN	EIS	-	60 aM	Human serum from breast cancer patients	[171]
miRNA-199a-5p	$Fe(CN)_6^{3-/4-}$	GCE/GO/GNR	GO and GNR	EIS	148 pM–15 fM	4.5 fM	Spiked human blood serum	[164]
miRNA-155	$Fe(CN)_6^{3-/4-}$	Pt wire/Ti_3C_2Tx@FePcQDs	Ti_3C_2Tx@FePcQDs	EIS	0.01 fM–10 pM	4.3 aM	Spiked human serum samples	[165]
miRNA-21	$Fe(CN)_6^{3-/4-}$	AuE	HCR	EIS	10 fM–50 pM	4.63 fM	A549, HeLa, MCF-7, RAW 264.7, and HUVEC cancer cells	[170]
miRNA-21	Fe(CN)63−/4-	SPE/rGO-Au	-	DPV	1 µM–1 pM	1 pM	Spiked artificial saliva	[183]
miRNA-319a	Fe(CN)63−/4-	GCE/AuNPs	nuclease S1	DPV	1000–5 pM	1.8 pM	-	[184]
miRNA-21	$Fe(CN)_6^{3-/4-}$	FTO/NFG/AgNPs/PANI	-	DPV	10 fM–10 µM	0.2 fM	Spiked blood samples	[175]
miRNA-21	$Fe(CN)_6^{3-/4-}$	FTO/CGO/Au-PtBNPs/SA	-	DPV	1 fM–1 µM	1 fM	spiked human serum	[174]
miRNA-21	$Fe(CN)_6^{3-/4-}$	GCE/MWCNTs	TRNEAS	DPV	0.1 fM–5 pM	56.7 aM	MDA-MB-231, MCF-7, HeLa, and L02 cell	[173]
hsa-miR-486-5p	$Fe(CN)_6^{3-/4-}$	Laser induced graphene	-	DPV		10 fM	-	[177]
miRNA-375	$Fe(CN)_6^{3-/4-}$	AuE	-	SWV	10–30 fM	11.7 aM	CaP cells (PC-3, DU145, and LNCaP)	[185]
miRNA	$[Ru(NH_3)_6]^{3+/2+}$	GCE/Ni PFNs	-	EIS	0.1–2500 pM	0.034 pM	A549 cancer cells	[179]
let-7a	$[Ru(NH_3)^6]^{3+/2+}$	GCE/CNTs	CNT based solid-phase RCA	DPV		1.2 fM	HeLa cells	[186]
miRNA-21	$Fe(CN)_6^{3-/4-}$/$[Ru(NH_3)_6]^{3+/2+}$	ITO	-	DPV	0.1–1500 fM	33 aM	HeLa, A549, MCF-7 cancer cells	[180]

Abbreviations: HCR, hybridization chain reaction; FTO, fluorine-doped tin oxide; NFG, nitrogen-doped functionalized graphene; AgNPs, silver nanoparticles; PANI, polyaniline; CGO, carboxylated graphene oxide; Au-PtBNPs, gold platinum bimetallic nanoparticles; SA, streptavidine; GCE, glassy carbon electrode; MWCNTs, multi-walled-carbone nanotube; AuE, gold electrode; MGCE, magnetic glassy carbon electrode; GO, graphene oxide; Fe(CN)63−/4, ferri/ferrocyanide; DPV, differential pulse voltammetry; MDA-MB-231, human breast cancer cell lines; MCF-7, human breast adenocarcinoma cell line; HeLa, human cervical cancer cell line; and L02 cell; SWV, square wave voltammetry; DSN, duplex-specific nuclease; EIS, electrochemical impedance spectroscopy; GNR, gold nanoroad; Pt wire/Ti3C2Tx@FePcQDs, platinium wire/iron phthalocyanine quantum dots; HUVEC, human umbilical vein endothelial; A549, non-small cell lung; RAW 264.7, mouse leukemia cells of monocyte-macrophage; biotin-FNPs, biotine-phenylalanine nanoparticles; Ni PFNs, nickel phosphate nanostructures; [Ru(NH3)6]3+/2+, hexaammineruthenium(III) chloride; TRNEAS, target-recycled non-enzymatic amplification strategy; ITO, indium tinoxide; PNT, peptide nanotube nanocomposite; biotin-FNPs, biotinylated phenylalanine nanoparticles; Au, gold; rGO, reduced graphene oxide; RCA, rolling-circle amplification.

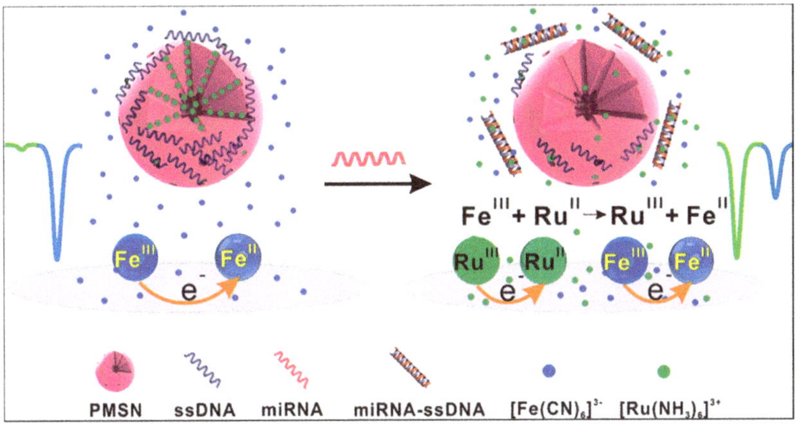

Figure 16. Scheme presenting the use of two free RedOx indicators reprinted from [180] with permission from (*Anal. Chem.***2017**, *89*, 12293–11298). Copyright (2017) American Chemical Society.

6. Other Methods of MicroRNA Electrochemical Detection

Other methods were employed in the electrochemical biosensor area for the detection of miRNAs as biomarkers of cancer, including the guanine oxidation method, RedOx current of the electrode surface, and labeled miRNA.

6.1. Oxidation of Guanine

The guanine is a purine nucleobase present in miRNAs strands, which have RedOx active groups employed in the construction of the electrochemical biosensors. The approach of following the oxidation of guanine presents the first approach used in the case of a DNA biosensor and could be used also for miRNA detection. Akbarnia et al. [187] proposed enzymatic digestion biosensors for femtomolar detection of miRNA-541as lung cancer biomarkers. Indeed, the probe is immobilized on the pencil graphite electrode modified graphene quantum dots (GQDs/PGE). Meanwhile, in the presence of miRNA-541, Hinf1 as a restriction enzyme cleaved the formed capture probe–miRNA-541 duplex. The oxidation of guanine was measured in the presence and absence of miRNA-541. After hybridization, a decrease in guanine's electrochemical signal was observed, because the DNA strands containing guanine were removed by the enzyme. In another use of the guanine oxidation method, Azab et al. [188] described a very sensitive biosensor at a zeptomolar level for miRNA let7-a detection using complementary sequence capture probe free-guanine bases. The capture probe was immobilized on the carbon paste electrode/carbon nanotubes/chrysine/gold nanoparticles (CPE/CNT/C/AuNPs) platform. The CNT/C film increases the surface area of the biosensor platform, increasing the conductivity, and thus is responsible for signal amplification.

The current method is very simple but has some limitations, especially considering that the oxidation of guanine bases as a free molecule is easier than in DNA strands and so could generate an unreliable result. As a matter of fact, the integration of a probe sequence without guanine, and its replacement with inosine that does not have the same potential for oxidation of guanine, is necessary in order to obtain only guanine oxidation response after the hybridization step (OFF-ON signal). Therefore, because the binding between cytosine and guanine is stronger than the binding of guanine with inosine, the use of such sequence does not provide a higher level of binding between the probe and miRNA compared to the sequence of the guanine-continuing DNA probe. Moreover, this method does not allow the regeneration of the biosensor because the oxidation of guanine is irreversible.

6.2. RedOx Current from Electrode Surface

Electrochemical biosensors designed for the detection of miRNAs based on RedOx current from the electrode surface were dismantled as a detection method. This method consists of modifying the electrode surface with an electroactive molecule before immobilizing the capture. The detection of miRNAs is done by electrochemical monitoring of the response of the redox molecule deposited on the electrode surface before and after the hybridization probe [189–191]. For this purpose, a simple model has recently been described by Zouari et al. [192] for the quantification of miRNA-21 at fM level, using screen-printed carbon electrode/pyrene carboxylic acid/rGO/AuNPs as biosensor platform. A 6-ferrocenylhexanethiol (Fc-SH) as a RedOx molecule was immobilized on the electrode surface.

6.3. Labeled MicroRNA

This method needs a labeled miRNA, which provides a hard step for the biosensor application in real samples. A labeled miRNA biosensor was recently described by Sabahi et al. [193] for the quantification of miRNA-21 at fM level. This was obtained by the use of cadmium ions (Cd^{2+}) which is linked to a phosphate group of miRNA via an electrostatic reaction. Then, the labeled miRNA hybridize with a capture probe immobilized on a fluorine-doped tin oxide electrode/SWCNTs/dendritic gold nanostructures through to Au–thiol interaction.

7. Conclusions and Future Perspectives

This work reviewed the progress in the development of electrochemical miRNAs biosensors using different approaches based on an electroactive species-labeled probe sequence, catalyst, RedOx intercalating agent, RedOx system, among others. In view of the various published papers, all miRNA strategies of detection based on electrochemical biosensors discussed in this review are presented according to their percentage of use (Figure 17). This distribution indicated clearly that the RedOx indicator as labeled, intercalant, or free RedOx indicator is widely used for miRNA detection with a percentage of 69% compared to catalytic detection, which presents 26%. In general, all approaches discussed in this review have almost equal use for miRNA detection, except the categories of other methods, which are still not developed yet compared to their employment in DNA biosensors. This is due probably to the lack of the association of these methods with the amplification approach generally used in the case of miRNA detection.

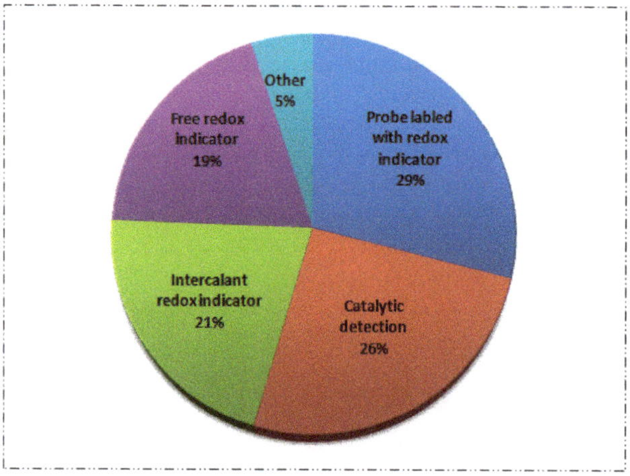

Figure 17. Distribution percentage of different microRNA strategies detection based on electrochemical biosensors.

The synthesis study clearly showed that electrochemical biosensors are efficient and practical approaches towards the analysis of miRNAs in the clinical field with high sensitivity. Nevertheless, the problem of miRNA analysis in the real sample cannot be neglected regarding the intercalating agent RedOx and the free RedOx indicator. These approaches have certain limitations, including the likely occurrence in the real sample of interferences, which could affect the results obtained. Otherwise, approaches based on electroactive species labeled with a probe sequence and a catalyst enable an accurate and precise analysis of miRNAs in a real sample. In addition, simultaneously detecting two miRNAs is more favorable with the RedOx-labeled probe sequence strategy, compared to the other strategies discussed. Although the LODs of the discussed biosensors are very low, most of the biosensors have not been tested and validated with a large number of samples from cancer patients and control groups. On the other hand, given the fact that, in general, known miRNAs are not specific to a single pathology, particular attention must also be paid to the development of electrochemical biosensors dedicated to the simultaneous quantification of a group of miRNAs to facilitate cancer diagnosis with improved reliability.

Although electrochemistry stands out due to its inherent miniaturization, mass production, and low cost, there are still significant challenges to meet before portable, robust, user-friendly point-of-care biosensors for cancer diagnosis through the detection of circulating miRNA expression profiles become a reality. Furthermore, because of these challenges, to date, to the best of our knowledge, no commercial electrochemical biosensor for circulating miRNA analysis is available; consequently, further effort should be devoted to validation, clinical assays, and the commercialization in the near future.

Author Contributions: The manuscript was written through contributions of all authors. All authors have read and agreed to the published version of the manuscript.

Funding: This research received no external funding.

Conflicts of Interest: The authors declare no conflict of interest.

References

1. Roointan, A.; Mir, T.A.; Wani, S.I.; Rehman, M.; Hussain, K.K.; Ahmed, B.; Abrahim, S.; Savardashtaki, A.; Gandomani, G.; Gandomani, M.; et al. Early detection of lung cancer biomarkers through biosensor technology: A review. *J. Pharm. Biomed. Anal.* **2019**, *164*, 93–103. [CrossRef] [PubMed]
2. Schootman, M.; Fuortes, L.; Aft, R. Prognosis of metachronous contralateral breast cancer according to stage at diagnosis: The importance of early detection. *Breast Cancer Res. Treat.* **2006**, *99*, 91–95. [CrossRef] [PubMed]
3. Lytras, D.; Connor, S.; Bosonnet, L.; Jayan, R.; Evans, J.; Hughes, M.; Garvey, C.; Ghaneh, P.; Sutton, R.; Vinjamuri, S.; et al. Positron Emission Tomography Does Not Add to Computed Tomography for the Diagnosis and Staging of Pancreatic Cancer. *Dig. Surg.* **2005**, *22*, 55–62. [CrossRef] [PubMed]
4. Portalez, D.; Mozer, P.; Cornud, F.; Renard-Penna, R.; Misrai, V.; Thoulouzan, M.; Malavaud, B. Validation of the European Society of Urogenital Radiology Scoring System for Prostate Cancer Diagnosis on Multiparametric Magnetic Resonance Imaging in a Cohort of Repeat Biopsy Patients. *Eur. Urol.* **2012**, *62*, 986–996. [CrossRef] [PubMed]
5. Wagner, P.D.; Verma, M.; Srivastava, S. Challenges for Biomarkers in Cancer Detection. *Ann. N. Y. Acad. Sci.* **2004**, *1022*, 9–16. [CrossRef] [PubMed]
6. Islam, N.; Masud, M.K.; Haque, H.; Hossain, S.A.; Yamauchi, Y.; Nguyen, N.-T.; Shiddiky, M.J. RNA Biomarkers: Diagnostic and Prognostic Potentials and Recent Developments of Electrochemical Biosensors. *Small Methods* **2017**, *1*, 1700131. [CrossRef]
7. Mittal, S.; Kaur, H.; Gautam, N.; Mantha, A.K. Biosensors for breast cancer diagnosis: A review of bioreceptors, biotransducers and signal amplification strategies. *Biosens. Bioelectron.* **2017**, *88*, 217–231. [CrossRef]
8. Mousa, S.A. Biosensors: The new wave in cancer diagnosis. *Nanotechnol. Sci. Appl.* **2010**, *4*, 1–10. [CrossRef]

9. Hasanzadeh, M.; Shadjou, N.; De La Guardia, M. Early stage screening of breast cancer using electrochemical biomarker detection. *TrAC Trends Anal. Chem.* **2017**, *91*, 67–76. [CrossRef]
10. Diaconu, I.; Cristea, C.; Harceaga, V.; Marrazza, G.; Berindan-Neagoe, I.; Săndulescu, R. Electrochemical immunosensors in breast and ovarian cancer. *Clin. Chim. Acta* **2013**, *425*, 128–138. [CrossRef]
11. Yang, H.; Wang, J.; Yang, C.; Zhao, X.; Xie, S.; Ge, Z. Nano Pt@ZIF8 Modified Electrode and Its Application to Detect Sarcosine. *J. Electrochem. Soc.* **2018**, *165*, H247–H250. [CrossRef]
12. Filella, X.; Fernández-Galán, E.; Bonifacio, R.F.; Foj, L. Emerging biomarkers in the diagnosis of prostate cancer. *Pharm. Pers. Med.* **2018**, *11*, 83–94. [CrossRef] [PubMed]
13. Vaarala, M.H.; Porvari, K.; Lukkarinen, O.; Vihko, P. TheTMPRSS2 gene encoding transmembrane serine protease is overexpressed in a majority of prostate cancer patients: Detection of mutatedTMPRSS2 form in a case of aggressive disease. *Int. J. Cancer* **2001**, *94*, 705–710. [CrossRef]
14. Elshafey, R.; Tlili, C.; Abulrob, A.; Tavares, A.C.; Zourob, M. Label-free impedimetric immunosensor for ultrasensitive detection of cancer marker Murine double minute 2 in brain tissue. *Biosens. Bioelectron.* **2013**, *39*, 220–225. [CrossRef] [PubMed]
15. Laocharoensuk, R. Development of Electrochemical Immunosensors towards Point-of-care Cancer Diagnostics: Clinically Relevant Studies. *Electroanalysis* **2016**, *28*, 1716–1729. [CrossRef]
16. Hasan, S.; Jacob, R.; Manne, U.; Paluri, R. Advances in pancreatic cancer biomarkers. *Oncol. Rev.* **2019**, *13*, 410. [CrossRef]
17. Matsuoka, T.; Yashiro, M. Biomarkers of gastric cancer: Current topics and future perspective. *World J. Gastroenterol.* **2018**, *24*, 2818–2832. [CrossRef]
18. Ashizawa, T.; Okada, R.; Suzuki, Y.; Takagi, M.; Yamazaki, T.; Sumi, T.; Aoki, T.; Ohnuma, S.; Aoki, T. Clinical significance of interleukin-6 (IL-6) in the spread of gastric cancer: Role of IL-6 as a prognostic factor. *Gastric Cancer* **2005**, *8*, 124–131. [CrossRef]
19. Lou, J.; Zhang, L.; Lv, S.; Zhang, C.; Jiang, S. Biomarkers for Hepatocellular Carcinoma. *Biomark. Cancer* **2017**, *9*, 1–9. [CrossRef]
20. Farzin, L.; Shamsipur, M. Recent advances in design of electrochemical affinity biosensors for low level detection of cancer protein biomarkers using nanomaterial-assisted signal enhancement strategies. *J. Pharm. Biomed. Anal.* **2018**, *147*, 185–210. [CrossRef]
21. Li, J.; Sherman-Baust, A.C.; Tsai-Turton, M.; Bristow, R.E.; Roden, R.B.S.; Morin, P.J. Claudin-containing exosomes in the peripheral circulation of women with ovarian cancer. *BMC Cancer* **2009**, *9*, 244. [CrossRef] [PubMed]
22. Altintas, Z.; Tothill, I. Biomarkers and biosensors for the early diagnosis of lung cancer. *Sens. Actuators B Chem.* **2013**, *188*, 988–998. [CrossRef]
23. Arya, S.K.; Bhansali, S. Lung Cancer and Its Early Detection Using Biomarker-Based Biosensors. *Chem. Rev.* **2011**, *111*, 6783–6809. [CrossRef] [PubMed]
24. Xie, Y.; Todd, N.W.; Liu, Z.; Zhan, M.; Fang, H.; Peng, H.; Alattar, M.; Deepak, J.; Stass, S.A.; Jiang, F. Altered miRNA expression in sputum for diagnosis of non-small cell lung cancer. *Lung Cancer* **2010**, *67*, 170–176. [CrossRef] [PubMed]
25. Lim, E.H.; Zhang, S.-L.; Li, J.-L.; Yap, W.-S.; Howe, T.-C.; Tan, B.-P.; Lee, Y.-S.; Wong, D.; Khoo, K.-L.; Seto, K.-Y.; et al. Using whole genome amplification (WGA) of low-volume biopsies to assess the prognostic role of EGFR, KRAS, p53, and CMET mutations in advanced-stage non-small cell lung cancer (NSCLC). *J. Thorac. Oncol.* **2009**, *4*, 12–21. [CrossRef] [PubMed]
26. Staden, R.-I.S.-V.; Comnea-Stancu, I.R.; Surdu-Bob, C.C. Molecular Screening of Blood Samples for the Simultaneous Detection of CEA, HER-1, NSE, CYFRA 21-1 Using Stochastic Sensors. *J. Electrochem. Soc.* **2017**, *164*, B267–B273. [CrossRef]
27. Carr, O.; Raymundo-Pereira, P.A.; Shimizu, F.M.; Sorroche, B.P.; Melendez, M.E.; Pedro, R.D.O.; Miranda, P.B.; Carvalho, A.L.; Reis, R.M.; Arantes, L.M.; et al. Genosensor made with a self-assembled monolayer matrix to detect MGMT gene methylation in head and neck cancer cell lines. *Talanta* **2020**, *210*, 120609. [CrossRef]
28. Lee, R.C.; Feinbaum, R.L.; Ambros, V. The C. elegans heterochronic gene lin-4 encodes small RNAs with antisense complementarity to lin-14. *Cell* **1993**, *75*, 843–854. [CrossRef]

29. Negrini, M.; Ferracin, M.; Sabbioni, S.; Croce, C.M. MicroRNAs in human cancer: From research to therapy. *J. Cell Sci.* **2007**, *120*, 1833–1840. [CrossRef]
30. Tang, X.; Tang, G.; Özcan, S. Role of microRNAs in diabetes. *Biochim. Biophys. Acta BBA Bioenergy* **2008**, *1779*, 697–701. [CrossRef]
31. Chen, Y.-X.; Huang, K.-J.; Niu, K.-X. Recent advances in signal amplification strategy based on oligonucleotide and nanomaterials for microRNA detection—A review. *Biosens. Bioelectron.* **2018**, *99*, 612–624. [CrossRef] [PubMed]
32. Keshavarz, M.; Behpour, M.; Rafiee-Pour, H.-A. Recent trends in electrochemical microRNA biosensors for early detection of cancer. *RSC Adv.* **2015**, *5*, 35651–35660. [CrossRef]
33. Aziz, N.B.; Mahmudunnabi, R.G.; Umer, M.; Sharma, S.; Rashid, A.; Alhamhoom, Y.; Shim, Y.-B.; Salomon, C.; Shiddiky, M.J. MicroRNAs in ovarian cancer and recent advances in the development of microRNA-based biosensors. *Analyst* **2020**, *145*, 2038–2057. [CrossRef] [PubMed]
34. Miodek, A.; Mejri-Omrani, N.; Khoder, R.; Korri-Youssoufi, H.; Mejri, N. Electrochemical functionalization of polypyrrole through amine oxidation of poly(amidoamine) dendrimers: Application to DNA biosensor. *Talanta* **2016**, *154*, 446–454. [CrossRef] [PubMed]
35. Wang, Y.; Hsine, Z.; Sauriat-Dorizon, H.; Mlika, R.; Korri-Youssoufi, H. Structural and electrochemical studies of functionalization of reduced graphene oxide with alkoxyphenylporphyrin mono- and tetra- carboxylic acid: Application to DNA sensors. *Electrochim. Acta* **2020**, *357*, 136852. [CrossRef]
36. Yazdanparast, S.; Benvidi, A.; Azimzadeh, M.; Tezerjani, M.D.; Ghaani, M.R. Experimental and theoretical study for miR-155 detection through resveratrol interaction with nucleic acids using magnetic core-shell nanoparticles. *Microchim. Acta* **2020**, *187*, 1–10. [CrossRef]
37. Masud, M.K.; Umer, M.; Hossain, S.A.; Yamauchi, Y.; Nguyen, N.-T.; Shiddiky, M.J. Nanoarchitecture Frameworks for Electrochemical miRNA Detection. *Trends Biochem. Sci.* **2019**, *44*, 433–452. [CrossRef]
38. Chen, C. Recent Advances in Nanomaterials-Based Electrochemical Biosensors for MicroRNAs Detection. *Int. J. Electrochem. Sci.* **2019**, *14*, 5174–5187. [CrossRef]
39. Mujica, M.L.; Gallay, P.A.; Perrachione, F.; Montemerlo, A.E.; Tamborelli, L.A.; Vaschetti, V.M.; Reartes, D.F.; Bollo, S.; Rodríguez, M.C.; Dalmasso, P.R.; et al. New trends in the development of electrochemical biosensors for the quantification of microRNAs. *J. Pharm. Biomed. Anal.* **2020**, *189*, 113478. [CrossRef]
40. Mohammadi, H.; Yammouri, G.; Amine, A. Current advances in electrochemical genosensors for detecting microRNA cancer markers. *Curr. Opin. Electrochem.* **2019**, *16*, 96–105. [CrossRef]
41. Daneshpour, M.; Omidfar, K.; Ghanbarian, H. A novel electrochemical nanobiosensor for the ultrasensitive and specific detection of femtomolar-level gastric cancer biomarker miRNA-106a. *Beilstein J. Nanotechnol.* **2016**, *7*, 2023–2036. [CrossRef]
42. Sun, E.; Wang, L.; Zhou, X.; Ma, C.; Sun, Y.; Lei, M.; Lu, B.; Han, R. Retracted Article: Graphene oxide/DNA-decorated electrode for the fabrication of microRNA biosensor. *RSC Adv.* **2015**, *5*, 69334–69338. [CrossRef]
43. Yang, B.; Zhang, S.; Fang, X.; Kong, J. Double signal amplification strategy for ultrasensitive electrochemical biosensor based on nuclease and quantum dot-DNA nanocomposites in the detection of breast cancer 1 gene mutation. *Biosens. Bioelectron.* **2019**, *142*, 111544. [CrossRef] [PubMed]
44. Rezaei, H.; Motovali-Bashi, M.; Radfar, S. An enzyme-free electrochemical biosensor for simultaneous detection of two hemophilia A biomarkers: Combining target recycling with quantum dots-encapsulated metal-organic frameworks for signal amplification. *Anal. Chim. Acta* **2019**, *1092*, 66–74. [CrossRef] [PubMed]
45. Tian, R.; Ning, W.; Chen, M.; Zhang, C.; Li, Q.; Bai, J. High performance electrochemical biosensor based on 3D nitrogen-doped reduced graphene oxide electrode and tetrahedral DNA nanostructure. *Talanta* **2019**, *194*, 273–281. [CrossRef]
46. Chen, Z.; Xie, Y.; Huang, W.; Qin, C.; Yu, A.; Lai, G. Exonuclease-assisted target recycling for ultrasensitive electrochemical detection of microRNA at vertically aligned carbon nanotubes. *Nanoscale* **2019**, *11*, 11262–11269. [CrossRef]
47. Yammouri, G.; Mohammadi, H.; Amine, A. A Highly Sensitive Electrochemical Biosensor Based on Carbon Black and Gold Nanoparticles Modified Pencil Graphite Electrode for microRNA-21 Detection. *Chem. Afr.* **2019**, *2*, 291–300. [CrossRef]

48. Jou, A.F.-J.; Chen, Y.-J.; Li, Y.; Chang, Y.-F.; Lee, J.-J.; Liao, A.T.; Ho, J.-A.A. Target-Triggered, Dual Amplification Strategy for Sensitive Electrochemical Detection of a Lymphoma-associated MicroRNA. *Electrochim. Acta* **2017**, *236*, 190–197. [CrossRef]
49. Miao, P.; Jiang, Y.; Zhang, T.; Huang, Y.; Tang, Y. Electrochemical sensing of attomolar miRNA combining cascade strand displacement polymerization and reductant-mediated amplification. *Chem. Commun.* **2018**, *54*, 7366–7369. [CrossRef]
50. Wang, T.; Viennois, E.; Merlin, D.; Wang, G. Microelectrode miRNA Sensors Enabled by Enzymeless Electrochemical Signal Amplification. *Anal. Chem.* **2015**, *87*, 8173–8180. [CrossRef]
51. Miao, P.; Wang, B.; Yu, Z.; Zhao, J.; Tang, Y. Ultrasensitive electrochemical detection of microRNA with star trigon structure and endonuclease mediated signal amplification. *Biosens. Bioelectron.* **2015**, *63*, 365–370. [CrossRef] [PubMed]
52. Ma, X.; Xu, H.; Qian, K.; Kandawa-Schulz, M.; Miao, W.; Wang, Y. Electrochemical detection of microRNAs based on AuNPs/CNNS nanocomposite with Duplex-specific nuclease assisted target recycling to improve the sensitivity. *Talanta* **2020**, *208*, 120441. [CrossRef] [PubMed]
53. Yang, D.; Cheng, W.; Chen, X.; Tang, Y.; Miao, P. Ultrasensitive electrochemical detection of miRNA based on DNA strand displacement polymerization and Ca^{2+}-dependent DNAzyme cleavage. *Analyst* **2018**, *143*, 5352–5357. [CrossRef] [PubMed]
54. Wang, W.; Jayachandran, S.; Li, M.; Xu, S.; Luo, X. Hyaluronic acid functionalized nanostructured sensing interface for voltammetric determination of microRNA in biological media with ultra-high sensitivity and ultra-low fouling. *Microchim. Acta* **2018**, *185*, 156. [CrossRef] [PubMed]
55. Zhang, X.; Yang, Z.; Chang, Y.; Qing, M.; Yuan, R.; Chai, Y. Novel 2D-DNA-Nanoprobe-Mediated Enzyme-Free-Target-Recycling Amplification for the Ultrasensitive Electrochemical Detection of MicroRNA. *Anal. Chem.* **2018**, *90*, 9538–9544. [CrossRef]
56. Fu, C.; Liu, C.; Wang, S.; Luo, F.; Lin, Z.; Chen, G. A signal-on homogeneous electrochemical biosensor for sequence-specific microRNA based on duplex-specific nuclease-assisted target recycling amplification. *Anal. Methods* **2016**, *8*, 7034–7039. [CrossRef]
57. Miao, P.; Wang, B.; Chen, X.; Li, X.; Tang, Y. Tetrahedral DNA Nanostructure-Based MicroRNA Biosensor Coupled with Catalytic Recycling of the Analyte. *ACS Appl. Mater. Interfaces* **2015**, *7*, 6238–6243. [CrossRef]
58. Miao, P.; Wang, B.; Meng, F.; Yin, J.; Tang, Y. Ultrasensitive Detection of MicroRNA through Rolling Circle Amplification on a DNA Tetrahedron Decorated Electrode. *Bioconjugate Chem.* **2015**, *26*, 602–607. [CrossRef]
59. Liu, H.; Bei, X.; Xia, Q.; Fu, Y.; Zhang, S.; Liu, M.; Fan, K.; Zhang, M.; Yang, Y. Enzyme-free electrochemical detection of microRNA-21 using immobilized hairpin probes and a target-triggered hybridization chain reaction amplification strategy. *Microchim. Acta* **2015**, *183*, 297–304. [CrossRef]
60. Xu, S.; Chang, Y.; Wu, Z.; Li, Y.; Yuan, R.; Chai, Y.-Q. One DNA circle capture probe with multiple target recognition domains for simultaneous electrochemical detection of miRNA-21 and miRNA-155. *Biosens. Bioelectron.* **2020**, *149*, 111848. [CrossRef]
61. Yao, J.; Zhang, Z.; Deng, Z.; Wang, Y.; Guo, Y. An enzyme free electrochemical biosensor for sensitive detection of miRNA with a high discrimination factor by coupling the strand displacement reaction and catalytic hairpin assembly recycling. *Analyst* **2017**, *142*, 4116–4123. [CrossRef] [PubMed]
62. Zhou, L.; Wang, J.; Chen, Z.; Li, J.; Wang, T.; Zhang, Z.; Xie, G. A universal electrochemical biosensor for the highly sensitive determination of microRNAs based on isothermal target recycling amplification and a DNA signal transducer triggered reaction. *Microchim. Acta* **2017**, *184*, 1305–1313. [CrossRef]
63. Xiong, E.; Zhang, X.; Liu, Y.; Zhou, J.; Yu, P.; Li, X.; Chen, J. Ultrasensitive Electrochemical Detection of Nucleic Acids Based on the Dual-Signaling Electrochemical Ratiometric Method and Exonuclease III-Assisted Target Recycling Amplification Strategy. *Anal. Chem.* **2015**, *87*, 7291–7296. [CrossRef] [PubMed]
64. Zhang, J.; Wang, L.-L.; Hou, M.-F.; Xia, Y.-K.; He, W.-H.; Yan, A.; Weng, Y.-P.; Zeng, L.-P.; Chen, J. A ratiometric electrochemical biosensor for the exosomal microRNAs detection based on bipedal DNA walkers propelled by locked nucleic acid modified toehold mediate strand displacement reaction. *Biosens. Bioelectron.* **2018**, *102*, 33–40. [CrossRef]
65. Li, X.; Dou, B.; Yuan, R.; Xiang, Y. Mismatched catalytic hairpin assembly and ratiometric strategy for highly sensitive electrochemical detection of microRNA from tumor cells. *Sens. Actuators B Chem.* **2019**, *286*, 191–197. [CrossRef]

66. Cheng, F.-F.; He, T.-T.; Miao, H.-T.; Shi, J.-J.; Jiang, L.-P.; Zhu, J. Electron Transfer Mediated Electrochemical Biosensor for MicroRNAs Detection Based on Metal Ion Functionalized Titanium Phosphate Nanospheres at Attomole Level. *ACS Appl. Mater. Interfaces* **2015**, *7*, 2979–2985. [CrossRef]
67. Li, X.-M.; Wang, L.-L.; Luo, J.; Wei, Q.-L. A dual-amplified electrochemical detection of mRNA based on duplex-specific nuclease and bio-bar-code conjugates. *Biosens. Bioelectron.* **2015**, *65*, 245–250. [CrossRef]
68. Luo, L.; Wang, L.; Zeng, L.; Wang, Y.; Weng, Y.; Liao, Y.; Chen, T.; Xia, Y.; Zhang, J.; Chen, J. A ratiometric electrochemical DNA biosensor for detection of exosomal MicroRNA. *Talanta* **2020**, *207*, 120298. [CrossRef]
69. Tao, Y.; Yin, D.; Jin, M.; Fang, J.; Dai, T.; Li, Y.; Li, Y.; Pu, Q.; Xie, G. Double-loop hairpin probe and doxorubicin-loaded gold nanoparticles for the ultrasensitive electrochemical sensing of microRNA. *Biosens. Bioelectron.* **2017**, *96*, 99–105. [CrossRef]
70. Yuan, Y.-H.; Chi, B.-Z.; Wen, S.-H.; Liang, R.-P.; Li, Z.-M.; Qiu, J.-D. Ratiometric electrochemical assay for sensitive detecting microRNA based on dual-amplification mechanism of duplex-specific nuclease and hybridization chain reaction. *Biosens. Bioelectron.* **2018**, *102*, 211–216. [CrossRef]
71. Zouari, M.; Campuzano, S.; Pingarrón, J.; Raouafi, N. Femtomolar direct voltammetric determination of circulating miRNAs in sera of cancer patients using an enzymeless biosensor. *Anal. Chim. Acta* **2020**, *1104*, 188–198. [CrossRef] [PubMed]
72. Yuan, Y.-H.; Wu, Y.-D.; Chi, B.-Z.; Wen, S.-H.; Liang, R.-P.; Qiu, J.-D. Simultaneously electrochemical detection of microRNAs based on multifunctional magnetic nanoparticles probe coupling with hybridization chain reaction. *Biosens. Bioelectron.* **2017**, *97*, 325–331. [CrossRef] [PubMed]
73. Mohammadniaeia, M.; Goa, A.; Chavan, S.G.; Koyappayila, A.; Kimb, S.-E.; Yoo, H.J.; Min, J.; Lee, M.-H. Relay-race RNA/barcode gold nanoflower hybrid for wide and sensitive detection of microRNA in total patient serum. *Biosens. Bioelectron.* **2019**, *141*, 111468. [CrossRef] [PubMed]
74. Zhang, J.; Hun, X. Electrochemical determination of miRNA-155 using molybdenum carbide nanosheets and colloidal gold modified electrode coupled with mismatched catalytic hairpin assembly strategy. *Microchem. J.* **2019**, *150*, 104095. [CrossRef]
75. Tian, L.; Qi, J.; Ma, X.; Wang, X.; Yao, C.; Song, W.; Wang, Y. A facile DNA strand displacement reaction sensing strategy of electrochemical biosensor based on N-carboxymethyl chitosan/molybdenum carbide nanocomposite for microRNA-21 detection. *Biosens. Bioelectron.* **2018**, *122*, 43–50. [CrossRef]
76. Miao, P.; Tang, Y.; Zhang, Q.; Bo, B.; Wang, J. Identification of Cellular MicroRNA Coupling Strand Displacement Polymerization and Nicking-Endonuclease-Based Cleavage. *ChemPlusChem* **2015**, *80*, 1712–1715. [CrossRef]
77. Miao, P.; Tang, Y.; Yin, J. MicroRNA detection based on analyte triggered nanoparticle localization on a tetrahedral DNA modified electrode followed by hybridization chain reaction dual amplification. *Chem. Commun.* **2015**, *51*, 15629–15632. [CrossRef]
78. Que, H.; Zhang, D.; Guoa, B.; Wanga, T.; Wua, H.; Hana, D.; Yan, Y. Label-free and ultrasensitive electrochemical biosensor for the detection of EBV-related DNA based on AgDNCs@DNA/AgNCs nanocomposites and lambda exonuclease-assisted target recycling. *Biosens. Bioelectron.* **2019**, *143*, 111610. [CrossRef]
79. Cheng, W.; Ma, J.; Cao, P.; Zhang, Y.; Xu, C.; Yi, Y.; Li, J. Enzyme-free electrochemical biosensor based on double signal amplification strategy for the ultra-sensitive detection of exosomal microRNAs in biological samples. *Talanta* **2020**, *219*, 121242. [CrossRef]
80. Hakimian, F.; Ghourchian, H. Ultrasensitive electrochemical biosensor for detection of microRNA-155 as a breast cancer risk factor. *Anal. Chim. Acta* **2020**, *1136*, 1–8. [CrossRef]
81. Deng, K.; Liu, X.; Li, C.; Huang, H. Sensitive electrochemical sensing platform for microRNAs detection based on shortened multi-walled carbon nanotubes with high-loaded thionin. *Biosens. Bioelectron.* **2018**, *117*, 168–174. [CrossRef] [PubMed]
82. Yu, N.; Wang, Z.; Wang, C.; Han, J.; Bu, H. Combining padlock exponential rolling circle amplification with $CoFe_2O_4$ magnetic nanoparticles for microRNA detection by nanoelectrocatalysis without a substrate. *Anal. Chim. Acta* **2017**, *962*, 24–31. [CrossRef] [PubMed]
83. Meng, T.; Jia, H.; An, S.; Wang, H.; Yang, X.; Zhang, Y. Pd nanoparticles-DNA layered nanoreticulation biosensor based on target-catalytic hairpin assembly for ultrasensitive and selective biosensing of microRNA-21. *Sens. Actuators B Chem.* **2020**, *323*, 128621. [CrossRef]

84. Tang, H.; Zhu, J.; Wang, D.; Li, Y. Dual-signal amplification strategy for miRNA sensing with high sensitivity and selectivity by use of single Au nanowire electrodes. *Biosens. Bioelectron.* **2019**, *131*, 88–94. [CrossRef] [PubMed]
85. Ge, L.; Wang, W.; Li, F. Electro-Grafted Electrode with Graphene-Oxide-Like DNA Affinity for Ratiometric Homogeneous Electrochemical Biosensing of MicroRNA. *Anal. Chem.* **2017**, *89*, 11560–11567. [CrossRef]
86. Li, B.; Liu, F.; Peng, Y.; Yin, H.; Fan, W.; Yin, H.; Ai, S.; Zhang, X.-S. Two-stage cyclic enzymatic amplification method for ultrasensitive electrochemical assay of microRNA-21 in the blood serum of gastric cancer patients. *Biosens. Bioelectron.* **2016**, *79*, 307–312. [CrossRef]
87. Shen, Z.; He, L.; Wang, W.; Tan, L.; Gan, N. Highly sensitive and simultaneous detection of microRNAs in serum using stir-bar assisted magnetic DNA nanospheres-encoded probes. *Biosens. Bioelectron.* **2019**, *148*, 111831. [CrossRef]
88. Fu, P.; Xing, S.; Xu, M.; Zhao, Y.; Zhao, C. Peptide nucleic acid-based electrochemical biosensor for simultaneous detection of multiple microRNAs from cancer cells with catalytic hairpin assembly amplification. *Sens. Actuators B Chem.* **2020**, *305*, 127545. [CrossRef]
89. Azzouzi, S.; Fredj, Z.; Turner, A.P.F.; Ben Ali, M.; Mak, W.C. Generic Neutravidin Biosensor for Simultaneous Multiplex Detection of MicroRNAs via Electrochemically Encoded Responsive Nanolabels. *ACS Sens.* **2019**, *4*, 326–334. [CrossRef]
90. Mohammadniaei, M.; Koyappayil, A.; Sun, Y.; Min, J.; Lee, M.-H. Gold nanoparticle/MXene for multiple and sensitive detection of oncomiRs based on synergetic signal amplification. *Biosens. Bioelectron.* **2020**, *159*, 112208. [CrossRef]
91. Kuah, E.; Toh, S.; Yee, J.; Ma, Q.; Gao, Z. Enzyme Mimics: Advances and Applications. *Chem. A Eur. J.* **2016**, *22*, 8404–8430. [CrossRef] [PubMed]
92. Kosman, J.; Juskowiak, B. Peroxidase-mimicking DNAzymes for biosensing applications: A review. *Anal. Chim. Acta* **2011**, *707*, 7–17. [CrossRef] [PubMed]
93. Wang, M.; Shen, B.; Yuan, R.; Cheng, W.; Xu, H.; Ding, S. An electrochemical biosensor for highly sensitive determination of microRNA based on enzymatic and molecular beacon mediated strand displacement amplification. *J. Electroanal. Chem.* **2015**, *756*, 147–152. [CrossRef]
94. Ma, W.; Situ, B.; Lv, W.; Li, B.; Yin, X.; Vadgama, P.; Zheng, L.; Wang, W. Electrochemical determination of microRNAs based on isothermal strand-displacement polymerase reaction coupled with multienzyme functionalized magnetic micro-carriers. *Biosens. Bioelectron.* **2016**, *80*, 344–351. [CrossRef] [PubMed]
95. Yang, J.; Tang, M.; Diao, W.; Cheng, W.; Zhang, Y.; Yan, Y. Electrochemical strategy for ultrasensitive detection of microRNA based on MNAzyme-mediated rolling circle amplification on a gold electrode. *Microchim. Acta* **2016**, *183*, 3061–3067. [CrossRef]
96. Wang, H.; Zuo, Z.; Ren, L.; Yuan, R.; Li, Q.; Ding, S.; Luo, R. Ultrasensitive electrochemical biosensing strategy for microRNA-21 detection based on homogeneous target-initiated transcription amplification. *J. Electroanal. Chem.* **2016**, *783*, 22–27. [CrossRef]
97. Xia, N.; Zhang, Y.; Wei, X.; Huang, Y.; Liu, L. An electrochemical microRNAs biosensor with the signal amplification of alkaline phosphatase and electrochemical–chemical–chemical redox cycling. *Anal. Chim. Acta* **2015**, *878*, 95–101. [CrossRef]
98. Shuai, H.-L.; Huang, K.-J.; Zhang, W.-J.; Cao, X.; Jia, M.-P. Sandwich-type microRNA biosensor based on magnesium oxide nanoflower and graphene oxide–gold nanoparticles hybrids coupling with enzyme signal amplification. *Sens. Actuators B Chem.* **2017**, *243*, 403–411. [CrossRef]
99. Mandli, J.; Mohammadi, H.; Amine, A. Electrochemical DNA sandwich biosensor based on enzyme amplified microRNA-21 detection and gold nanoparticles. *Bioelectrochemistry* **2017**, *116*, 17–23. [CrossRef]
100. Zouari, M.; Campuzano, S.; Pingarrón, J.M.; Raouafi, N.; Campuzano, S. Competitive RNA-RNA hybridization-based integrated nanostructured-disposable electrode for highly sensitive determination of miRNAs in cancer cells. *Biosens. Bioelectron.* **2017**, *91*, 40–45. [CrossRef]
101. Chen, Y.-X.; Zhang, W.-J.; Huang, K.-J.; Zheng, M.; Mao, Y.-C. An electrochemical microRNA sensing platform based on tungsten diselenide nanosheets and competitive RNA–RNA hybridization. *Analyst* **2017**, *142*, 4843–4851. [CrossRef] [PubMed]

102. Torrente-Rodríguez, R.M.; Montiel, V.R.-V.; Campuzano, S.; Farchado-Dinia, M.; Barderas, R.; Segundo-Acosta, P.S.; Montoya, J.J.; Pingarron, J.M. Fast Electrochemical miRNAs Determination in Cancer Cells and Tumor Tissues with Antibody-Functionalized Magnetic Microcarriers. *ACS Sens.* **2016**, *1*, 896–903. [CrossRef]
103. Zeng, D.; Wang, Z.; Meng, Z.; Wang, P.; San, L.; Wang, W.; Aldalbahi, A.; Lili, S.; Shen, J.; Mi, X. DNA Tetrahedral Nanostructure-Based Electrochemical miRNA Biosensor for Simultaneous Detection of Multiple miRNAs in Pancreatic Carcinoma. *ACS Appl. Mater. Interfaces* **2017**, *9*, 24118–24125. [CrossRef] [PubMed]
104. Zhai, Q.; He, Y.; Li, X.; Guo, J.; Li, S.; Yi, G. A simple and ultrasensitive electrochemical biosensor for detection of microRNA based on hybridization chain reaction amplification. *J. Electroanal. Chem.* **2015**, *758*, 20–25. [CrossRef]
105. Torrente-Rodríguez, R.; Campuzano, S.; Montiel, V.R.-V.; Montoya, J.J.; Pingarrón, J.M.; Campuzano, S. Sensitive electrochemical determination of miRNAs based on a sandwich assay onto magnetic microcarriers and hybridization chain reaction amplification. *Biosens. Bioelectron.* **2016**, *86*, 516–521. [CrossRef] [PubMed]
106. Liu, L.; Gao, Y.; Liu, H.; Xia, N. An ultrasensitive electrochemical miRNAs sensor based on miRNAs-initiated cleavage of DNA by duplex-specific nuclease and signal amplification of enzyme plus redox cycling reaction. *Sens. Actuators B Chem.* **2015**, *208*, 137–142. [CrossRef]
107. Shuai, H.-L.; Huang, K.-J.; Chen, Y.-X.; Fang, L.-X.; Jia, M.-P. Au nanoparticles/hollow molybdenum disulfide microcubes based biosensor for microRNA-21 detection coupled with duplex-specific nuclease and enzyme signal amplification. *Biosens. Bioelectron.* **2017**, *89*, 989–997. [CrossRef]
108. Wang, J.; Lu, J.; Dong, S.; Zhu, N.; Gyimah, E.; Wang, K.; Li, Y.; Zhang, Z. An ultrasensitive electrochemical biosensor for detection of microRNA-21 based on redox reaction of ascorbic acid/iodine and duplex-specific nuclease assisted target recycling. *Biosens. Bioelectron.* **2019**, *130*, 81–87. [CrossRef]
109. Chen, Y.-X.; Wu, X.; Huang, K.-J. A sandwich-type electrochemical biosensing platform for microRNA-21 detection using carbon sphere-MoS2 and catalyzed hairpin assembly for signal amplification. *Sens. Actuators B Chem.* **2018**, *270*, 179–186. [CrossRef]
110. Zhang, Y.; Yan, Y.; Chen, W.; Cheng, W.; Li, S.; Ding, X.; Li, D.; Wang, H.; Ju, H.; Ding, S. A simple electrochemical biosensor for highly sensitive and specific detection of microRNA based on mismatched catalytic hairpin assembly. *Biosens. Bioelectron.* **2015**, *68*, 343–349. [CrossRef]
111. Shuai, H.-L.; Huang, K.-J.; Xing, L.-L.; Chen, Y.-X. Ultrasensitive electrochemical sensing platform for microRNA based on tungsten oxide-graphene composites coupling with catalyzed hairpin assembly target recycling and enzyme signal amplification. *Biosens. Bioelectron.* **2016**, *86*, 337–345. [CrossRef] [PubMed]
112. Li, Q.; Zeng, F.; Lyu, N.; Liang, J. Highly sensitive and specific electrochemical biosensor for microRNA-21 detection by coupling catalytic hairpin assembly with rolling circle amplification. *Analyst* **2018**, *143*, 2304–2309. [CrossRef] [PubMed]
113. Zhang, H.; Fan, M.; Jiang, J.; Shen, Q.; Cai, C.; Shen, J. Sensitive electrochemical biosensor for MicroRNAs based on duplex-specific nuclease-assisted target recycling followed with gold nanoparticles and enzymatic signal amplification. *Anal. Chim. Acta* **2019**, *1064*, 33–39. [CrossRef] [PubMed]
114. Fang, C.S.; Kim, K.-S.; Yu, B.; Jon, S.; Kim, M.-S.; Yang, H. Ultrasensitive Electrochemical Detection of miRNA-21 Using a Zinc Finger Protein Specific to DNA–RNA Hybrids. *Anal. Chem.* **2017**, *89*, 2024–2031. [CrossRef]
115. Zouari, M.; Campuzano, S.; Pingarrón, J.M.; Raouafi, N. Amperometric Biosensing of miRNA-21 in Serum and Cancer Cells at Nanostructured Platforms Using Anti-DNA-RNA Hybrid Antibodies. *ACS Omega* **2018**, *3*, 8923–8931. [CrossRef]
116. Vargas, E.; Torrente-Rodríguez, R.; Montiel, V.R.-V.; Povedano, E.; Pedrero, M.; Montoya, J.J.; Campuzano, S.; Pingarrón, J.M. Magnetic Beads-Based Sensor with Tailored Sensitivity for Rapid and Single-Step Amperometric Determination of miRNAs. *Int. J. Mol. Sci.* **2017**, *18*, 2151. [CrossRef]
117. Zouari, M.; Campuzano, S.; Pingarrón, J.; Raouafi, N. Ultrasensitive determination of microribonucleic acids in cancer cells with nanostructured-disposable electrodes using the viral protein p19 for recognition of ribonucleic acid/microribonucleic acid homoduplexes. *Electrochim. Acta* **2018**, *262*, 39–47. [CrossRef]
118. Hu, T.; Zhang, L.; Wen, W.; Zhang, X.; Wang, S. Enzyme catalytic amplification of miRNA-155 detection with graphene quantum dot-based electrochemical biosensor. *Biosens. Bioelectron.* **2016**, *77*, 451–456. [CrossRef]

119. Zhang, H.; Wang, Q.; Yang, X.; Wang, K.; Li, Q.; Li, Z.; Gao, L.; Nie, W.; Zheng, Y. An isothermal electrochemical biosensor for the sensitive detection of microRNA based on a catalytic hairpin assembly and supersandwich amplification. *Analyst* **2017**, *142*, 389–396. [CrossRef]
120. Wang, H.; Jian, Y.; Kong, Q.; Liu, H.; Lan, F.; Liang, L.; Ge, S.; Yu, J. Ultrasensitive electrochemical paper-based biosensor for microRNA via strand displacement reaction and metal-organic frameworks. *Sens. Actuators B Chem.* **2018**, *257*, 561–569. [CrossRef]
121. Wang, Z.; Si, L.; Bao, J.; Dai, Z. A reusable microRNA sensor based on the electrocatalytic property of heteroduplex-templated copper nanoclusters. *Chem. Commun.* **2015**, *51*, 6305–6307. [CrossRef] [PubMed]
122. Zhang, K.; Dong, H.; Dai, W.; Meng, X.; Lu, H.; Wu, T.; Zhang, X. Fabricating Pt/Sn–In_2O_3 Nanoflower with Advanced Oxygen Reduction Reaction Performance for High-Sensitivity MicroRNA Electrochemical Detection. *Anal. Chem.* **2016**, *89*, 648–655. [CrossRef] [PubMed]
123. Guo, W.-J.; Wu, Z.; Yang, X.-Y.; Pang, D.-W.; Zhang, Z.-L. Ultrasensitive electrochemical detection of microRNA-21 with wide linear dynamic range based on dual signal amplification. *Biosens. Bioelectron.* **2019**, *131*, 267–273. [CrossRef] [PubMed]
124. Sun, X.; Wang, H.; Jian, Y.; Lan, F.; Zhang, L.; Liu, H.; Ge, S.; Yu, J. Ultrasensitive microfluidic paper-based electrochemical/visual biosensor based on spherical-like cerium dioxide catalyst for miR-21 detection. *Biosens. Bioelectron.* **2018**, *105*, 218–225. [CrossRef] [PubMed]
125. Lianga, Z.; Oua, D.; Sunab, D.; Tongc, Y.; Luo, H.-B.; Chen, Z. Ultrasensitive biosensor for microRNA-155 using synergistically catalytic nanoprobe coupled with improved cascade strand displacement reaction. *Biosens. Bioelectron.* **2019**, *146*, 111744. [CrossRef] [PubMed]
126. Wu, Y.; Sheng, K.; Liu, Y.; Yu, Q.; Ye, B. Enzyme spheres as novel tracing tags coupled with target-induced DNAzyme assembly for ultrasensitive electrochemical microRNA assay. *Anal. Chim. Acta* **2016**, *948*, 1–8. [CrossRef]
127. Zhou, L.; Wang, T.; Bai, Y.; Li, Y.; Qiu, J.; Yu, W.; Zhang, S. Dual-amplified strategy for ultrasensitive electrochemical biosensor based on click chemistry-mediated enzyme-assisted target recycling and functionalized fullerene nanoparticles in the detection of microRNA-141. *Biosens. Bioelectron.* **2020**, *150*, 111964. [CrossRef]
128. Lu, J.; Wang, J.; Hu, X.; Gyimah, E.; Yakubu, S.; Wang, K.; Wu, X.; Zhanga, Z. Electrochemical Biosensor Based on Tetrahedral DNA Nanostructures and G-Quadruplex–Hemin Conformation for the Ultrasensitive Detection of MicroRNA-21 in Serum. *Anal. Chem.* **2019**, *91*, 7353–7359. [CrossRef]
129. Liu, L.; Song, C.; Zhang, Z.; Yang, J.; Zhou, L.; Zhang, X.; Xie, G. Ultrasensitive electrochemical detection of microRNA-21 combining layered nanostructure of oxidized single-walled carbon nanotubes and nanodiamonds by hybridization chain reaction. *Biosens. Bioelectron.* **2015**, *70*, 351–357. [CrossRef]
130. Huang, Y.L.; Mo, S.; Gao, Z.F.; Chen, J.R.; Lei, J.L.; Luo, H.Q.; Li, N.B. Amperometric biosensor for microRNA based on the use of tetrahedral DNA nanostructure probes and guanine nanowire amplification. *Microchim. Acta* **2017**, *184*, 2597–2604. [CrossRef]
131. Cai, W.; Xie, S.; Tang, Y.; Chai, Y.; Yuan, R.; Zhang, J. A label-free electrochemical biosensor for microRNA detection based on catalytic hairpin assembly and in situ formation of molybdophosphate. *Talanta* **2017**, *163*, 65–71. [CrossRef] [PubMed]
132. Mohammadi, H.; Amine, A. Spectrophotometric and Electrochemical Determination of MicroRNA-155 Using Sandwich Hybridization Magnetic Beads. *Anal. Lett.* **2018**, *51*, 411–423. [CrossRef]
133. Jirakova, L.; Hrstka, R.; Campuzano, S.; Pingarrón, J.M.; Bartosik, M. Multiplexed Immunosensing Platform Coupled to Hybridization Chain Reaction for Electrochemical Determination of MicroRNAs in Clinical Samples. *Electroanalysis* **2018**, *31*, 293–302. [CrossRef]
134. Povedano, E.; Montiel, V.R.-V.; Gamella, M.; Serafín, V.; Pedrero, M.; Moranova, L.; Bartosik, M.; Montoya, J.J.; Yáñez-Sedeño, P.; Campuzano, S.; et al. A novel zinc finger protein–based amperometric biosensor for miRNA determination. *Anal. Bioanal. Chem.* **2020**, *412*, 5031–5041. [CrossRef]
135. Tian, L.; Qi, J.; Oderinde, O.; Yao, C.; Song, W.; Wang, Y. Planar intercalated copper (II) complex molecule as small molecule enzyme mimic combined with Fe_3O_4 nanozyme for bienzyme synergistic catalysis applied to the microRNA biosensor. *Biosens. Bioelectron.* **2018**, *110*, 110–117. [CrossRef]
136. Wang, J.; Hui, N.; Hui, N. Electrochemical functionalization of polypyrrole nanowires for the development of ultrasensitive biosensors for detecting microRNA. *Sens. Actuators B Chem.* **2019**, *281*, 478–485. [CrossRef]

137. Azimzadeh, M.; Rahaie, M.; Nasirizadeh, N.; Naderi-Manesh, H. Application of Oracet Blue in a novel and sensitive electrochemical biosensor for the detection of microRNA. *Anal. Methods* **2015**, *7*, 9495–9503. [CrossRef]
138. Tian, L.; Qian, K.; Qi, J.; Liu, Q.; Yao, C.; Song, W.; Wang, Y. Gold nanoparticles superlattices assembly for electrochemical biosensor detection of microRNA-21. *Biosens. Bioelectron.* **2018**, *99*, 564–570. [CrossRef]
139. Moccia, M.; Caratelli, V.; Cinti, S.; Pede, B.; Avitabile, C.; Saviano, M.; Imbriani, A.L.; Moscone, D.; Arduini, F. Paper-based electrochemical peptide nucleic acid (PNA) biosensor for detection of miRNA-492: A pancreatic ductal adenocarcinoma biomarker. *Biosens. Bioelectron.* **2020**, *165*, 112371. [CrossRef]
140. Zhang, C.; Li, D.; Li, D.; Wen, K.; Yang, X.; Zhu, Y. Rolling circle amplification-mediated in situ synthesis of palladium nanoparticles for the ultrasensitive electrochemical detection of microRNA. *Analyst* **2019**, *144*, 3817–3825. [CrossRef]
141. Ren, R.; Bi, Q.; Yuan, R.; Xiang, Y. An efficient, label-free and sensitive electrochemical microRNA sensor based on target-initiated catalytic hairpin assembly of trivalent DNAzyme junctions. *Sens. Actuators B Chem.* **2020**, *304*, 127068. [CrossRef]
142. Yang, C.; Shi, K.; Dou, B.; Xiang, Y.; Chai, Y.; Yuan, R. In Situ DNA-Templated Synthesis of Silver Nanoclusters for Ultrasensitive and Label-Free Electrochemical Detection of MicroRNA. *ACS Appl. Mater. Interfaces* **2015**, *7*, 1188–1193. [CrossRef] [PubMed]
143. Li, F.; Peng, J.; Zheng, Q.; Guo, X.; Tang, H.; Yao, S. Carbon Nanotube-Polyamidoamine Dendrimer Hybrid-Modified Electrodes for Highly Sensitive Electrochemical Detection of MicroRNA24. *Anal. Chem.* **2015**, *87*, 4806–4813. [CrossRef] [PubMed]
144. Bao, J.; Hou, C.; Zhao, Y.; Geng, X.; Samalo, M.; Yang, H.; Bian, M.; Huoa, D. An enzyme-free sensitive electrochemical microRNA-16 biosensor by applying a multiple signal amplification strategy based on Au/PPy–rGO nanocomposite as a substrate. *Talanta* **2019**, *196*, 329–336. [CrossRef] [PubMed]
145. Zhang, W.; Xu, H.; Zhao, X.; Tang, X.; Yang, S.; Yu, L.; Zhao, S.; Chang, K.; Chen, M. 3D DNA nanonet structure coupled with target-catalyzed hairpin assembly for dual-signal synergistically amplified electrochemical sensing of circulating microRNA. *Anal. Chim. Acta* **2020**, *1122*, 39–47. [CrossRef] [PubMed]
146. Liu, S.; Yang, Z.; Chang, Y.; Chai, Y.; Yuan, R. An enzyme-free electrochemical biosensor combining target recycling with Fe_3O_4/CeO_2@Au nanocatalysts for microRNA-21 detection. *Biosens. Bioelectron.* **2018**, *119*, 170–175. [CrossRef]
147. Huang, S.; Li, J.; Jin, X.; Liu, Y.; Huang, S. Ultrasensitive electrochemical microRNA-21 biosensor coupling with carboxylate-reduced graphene oxide-based signal-enhancing and duplex-specific nuclease-assisted target recycling. *Sens. Actuators B Chem.* **2019**, *297*, 126740. [CrossRef]
148. Guo, J.; Yuan, C.; Yan, Q.; Duan, Q.; Li, X.; Yi, G. An electrochemical biosensor for microRNA-196a detection based on cyclic enzymatic signal amplification and template-free DNA extension reaction with the adsorption of methylene blue. *Biosens. Bioelectron.* **2018**, *105*, 103–108. [CrossRef]
149. Su, S.; Wu, Y.; Zhu, D.; Chao, J.; Liu, X.; Wan, Y.; Su, Y.; Zuo, X.; Fan, C.; Wang, L. On-Electrode Synthesis of Shape-Controlled Hierarchical Flower-Like Gold Nanostructures for Efficient Interfacial DNA Assembly and Sensitive Electrochemical Sensing of MicroRNA. *Small* **2016**, *12*, 3794–3801. [CrossRef]
150. Yu, S.; Wang, Y.; Jiang, L.-P.; Bi, S.; Zhu, J. Cascade Amplification-Mediated In Situ Hot-Spot Assembly for MicroRNA Detection and Molecular Logic Gate Operations. *Anal. Chem.* **2018**, *90*, 4544–4551. [CrossRef]
151. Chen, X.; Yao, L.; Wang, Y.-C.; Chen, Q.; Deng, H.; Lin, Z.; Yang, H.-H. Novel electrochemical nanoswitch biosensor based on self-assembled pH-sensitive continuous circular DNA. *Biosens. Bioelectron.* **2019**, *131*, 274–279. [CrossRef] [PubMed]
152. Wang, S.; Lu, S.; Zhao, J.; Ye, J.; Huang, J.; Yang, X. An electric potential modulated cascade of catalyzed hairpin assembly and rolling chain amplification for microRNA detection. *Biosens. Bioelectron.* **2019**, *126*, 565–571. [CrossRef] [PubMed]
153. Wang, Y.-H.; Huang, K.-J.; Wu, X.; Ma, Y.-Y.; Song, D.-L.; Du, C.-Y.; Chang, S.-H. Ultrasensitive supersandwich-type biosensor for enzyme-free amplified microRNA detection based on N-doped graphene/Au nanoparticles and hemin/G-quadruplexes. *J. Mater. Chem. B* **2018**, *6*, 2134–2142. [CrossRef]
154. Asadzadeh-Firouzabadi, A.; Zare, H.R. Preparation and application of AgNPs/SWCNTs nanohybrid as an electroactive label for sensitive detection of miRNA related to lung cancer. *Sens. Actuators B Chem.* **2018**, *260*, 824–831. [CrossRef]

155. Wang, F.; Chu, Y.; Ai, Y.; Chen, L.; Gao, F. Graphene oxide with in-situ grown Prussian Blue as an electrochemical probe for microRNA-122. *Microchim. Acta* **2019**, *186*, 116. [CrossRef]
156. Liu, L.; Chang, Y.; Xia, N.; Peng, P.; Zhang, L.; Jiang, M.; Zhang, J.; Liu, L. Simple, sensitive and label–free electrochemical detection of microRNAs based on the in situ formation of silver nanoparticles aggregates for signal amplification. *Biosens. Bioelectron.* **2017**, *94*, 235–242. [CrossRef]
157. Azimzadeh, M.; Rahaie, M.; Nasirizadeh, N.; Ashtari, K.; Naderi-Manesh, H. An electrochemical nanobiosensor for plasma miRNA-155, based on graphene oxide and gold nanorod, for early detection of breast cancer. *Biosens. Bioelectron.* **2016**, *77*, 99–106. [CrossRef]
158. Cui, L.; Wang, M.; Sun, B.; Ai, S.; Wang, S.; Zhang, C.-Y. Substrate-free and label-free electrocatalysis-assisted biosensor for sensitive detection of microRNA in lung cancer cells. *Chem. Commun.* **2019**, *55*, 1172–1175. [CrossRef]
159. Bo, B.; Zhang, T.; Jiang, Y.; Cui, H.; Miao, P. Triple Signal Amplification Strategy for Ultrasensitive Determination of miRNA Based on Duplex Specific Nuclease and Bridge DNA–Gold Nanoparticles. *Anal. Chem.* **2018**, *90*, 2395–2400. [CrossRef]
160. Su, S.; Cao, W.; Liu, W.; Lu, Z.; Zhu, D.; Chao, J.; Weng, L.; Wang, L.; Fan, C.; Wang, L. Dual-mode electrochemical analysis of microRNA-21 using gold nanoparticle-decorated MoS2 nanosheet. *Biosens. Bioelectron.* **2017**, *94*, 552–559. [CrossRef]
161. Feng, K.; Liu, J.; Deng, L.; Yu, H.; Yang, M. Amperometric detection of microRNA based on DNA-controlled current of a molybdophosphate redox probe and amplification via hybridization chain reaction. *Microchim. Acta* **2017**, *185*, 28. [CrossRef] [PubMed]
162. Wang, Y.; Zhang, X.; Zhao, L.; Bao, T.; Wen, W.; Zhang, X.; Wang, S.-F. Integrated amplified aptasensor with in-situ precise preparation of copper nanoclusters for ultrasensitive electrochemical detection of microRNA 21. *Biosens. Bioelectron.* **2017**, *98*, 386–391. [CrossRef] [PubMed]
163. Smith, D.A.; Newbury, L.J.; Drago, G.; Bowen, T.; Redman, J.E. Electrochemical detection of urinary microRNAs via sulfonamide-bound antisense hybridisation. *Sens. Actuators B Chem.* **2017**, *253*, 335–341. [CrossRef] [PubMed]
164. Ebrahimi, A.; Nikokar, I.; Zokaei, M.; Bozorgzadeh, E. Design, development and evaluation of microRNA-199a-5p detecting electrochemical nanobiosensor with diagnostic application in Triple Negative Breast Cancer. *Talanta* **2018**, *189*, 592–598. [CrossRef] [PubMed]
165. Duan, F.; Guo, C.; Hu, M.; Song, Y.; Wang, M.; He, L.; Zhang, Z.; Pettinari, R.; Zhou, L. Construction of the 0D/2D heterojunction of $Ti_3C_2T_x$ MXene nanosheets and iron phthalocyanine quantum dots for the impedimetric aptasensing of microRNA-155. *Sens. Actuators B Chem.* **2020**, *310*, 127844. [CrossRef]
166. Yaman, Y.T.; Vural, O.A.; Bolat, G.; Abaci, S. One-pot synthesized gold nanoparticle-peptide nanotube modified disposable sensor for impedimetric recognition of miRNA 410. *Sens. Actuators B Chem.* **2020**, *320*, 128343. [CrossRef]
167. Yammouri, G.; Mandli, J.; Mohammadi, H.; Amine, A. Development of an electrochemical label-free biosensor for microRNA-125a detection using pencil graphite electrode modified with different carbon nanomaterials. *J. Electroanal. Chem.* **2017**, *806*, 75–81. [CrossRef]
168. Voccia, D.; Sosnowska, M.; Bettazzi, F.; Roscigno, G.; Fratini, E.; De Franciscis, V.; Condorelli, G.; Chitta, R.; D'Souza, F.; Kutner, W.; et al. Direct determination of small RNAs using a biotinylated polythiophene impedimetric genosensor. *Biosens. Bioelectron.* **2017**, *87*, 1012–1019. [CrossRef]
169. Mandli, J.; Amine, A. Impedimetric genosensor for miRNA-34a detection in cell lysates using polypyrrole. *J. Solid State Electrochem.* **2017**, *22*, 1007–1014. [CrossRef]
170. Meng, T.; Zhao, D.; Ye, H.; Feng, Y.; Wang, H.; Zhanga, Y. Construction of an ultrasensitive electrochemical sensing platform for microRNA-21 based on interface impedance spectroscopy. *J. Colloid Interface Sci.* **2020**, *578*, 164–170. [CrossRef]
171. Zhang, J.; Wu, D.-Z.; Cai, S.-X.; Chen, M.; Xia, Y.-K.; Wu, F.; Chen, J. An immobilization-free electrochemical impedance biosensor based on duplex-specific nuclease assisted target recycling for amplified detection of microRNA. *Biosens. Bioelectron.* **2016**, *75*, 452–457. [CrossRef] [PubMed]
172. Salimi, A.; Kavosi, B.; Navaee, A. Amine-functionalized graphene as an effective electrochemical platform toward easily miRNA hybridization detection. *Meas. J. Int. Meas. Confed.* **2019**, *143*, 191–198. [CrossRef]

173. Hu, F.; Zhang, W.; Zhang, J.; Zhang, Q.; Sheng, T.; Gu, Y. An electrochemical biosensor for sensitive detection of microRNAs based on target-recycled non-enzymatic amplification. *Sens. Actuators B Chem.* **2018**, *271*, 15–23. [CrossRef]
174. Bharti, A.; Agnihotri, N.; Prabhakar, N. A voltammetric hybridization assay for microRNA-21 using carboxylated graphene oxide decorated with gold-platinum bimetallic nanoparticles. *Microchim. Acta* **2019**, *186*, 185. [CrossRef] [PubMed]
175. Salahandish, R.; Ghaffarinejad, A.; Omidinia, E.; Zargartalebi, H.; Majidzadeh-A, K.; Naghib, S.M.; Sanati-Nezhad, A. Label-free ultrasensitive detection of breast cancer miRNA-21 biomarker employing electrochemical nano-genosensor based on sandwiched AgNPs in PANI and N-doped graphene. *Biosens. Bioelectron.* **2018**, *120*, 129–136. [CrossRef] [PubMed]
176. Boriachek, K.; Umer, M.; Islam, N.; Gopalan, V.; Lam, A.K.-Y.; Nguyen, N.-T.; Shiddiky, M.J. An amplification-free electrochemical detection of exosomal miRNA-21 in serum samples. *Analyst* **2018**, *143*, 1662–1669. [CrossRef]
177. Wan, Z.; Umer, M.; Lobino, M.; Thiel, D.; Nguyen, N.-T.; Trinchi, A.; Shiddiky, M.J.; Gao, Y.; Li, Q. Laser induced self-N-doped porous graphene as an electrochemical biosensor for femtomolar miRNA detection. *Carbon* **2020**, *163*, 385–394. [CrossRef]
178. Koo, K.M.; Carrascosa, L.G.; Shiddiky, M.J.A.; Trau, M. Poly(A) Extensions of miRNAs for Amplification-Free Electrochemical Detection on Screen-Printed Gold Electrodes. *Anal. Chem.* **2016**, *88*, 2000–2005. [CrossRef]
179. Kannan, P.; Maiyalagan, T.; Lin, B.; Lei, W.; Jie, C.; Guo, L.; Jiang, Z.; Mao, S.; Subramanian, P. Nickel-phosphate pompon flowers nanostructured network enables the sensitive detection of microRNA. *Talanta* **2020**, *209*, 120511. [CrossRef]
180. Gai, P.; Gu, C.; Li, H.; Sun, X.; Li, F. Ultrasensitive Ratiometric Homogeneous Electrochemical MicroRNA Biosensing via Target-Triggered Ru(III) Release and Redox Recycling. *Anal. Chem.* **2017**, *89*, 12293–12298. [CrossRef]
181. La, M.; Zhang, Y.; Gao, Y.; Li, M.; Liu, L.; Chang, Y. Impedimetric Detection of Micro RNAs by the SignalAmplification of Streptavidin Induced In Situ Formation ofBiotin Phenylalanine Nanoparticle Networks. *J. Electrochem. Soc.* **2020**, *167*. [CrossRef]
182. Azzouzi, S.; Mak, W.C.; Kor, K.; Turner, A.P.; Ben Ali, M.; Beni, V. An integrated dual functional recognition/amplification bio-label for the one-step impedimetric detection of Micro-RNA-21. *Biosens. Bioelectron.* **2017**, *92*, 154–161. [CrossRef] [PubMed]
183. Low, S.S.; Pan, Y.; Ji, D.; Li, Y.; Lu, Y.; He, Y.; Chen, Q.; Liu, Q. Smartphone-based portable electrochemical biosensing system for detection of circulating microRNA-21 in saliva as a proof-of-concept. *Sens. Actuators B Chem.* **2020**, *308*, 127718. [CrossRef]
184. Yin, H.; Wang, M.; Yang, Z.; Lu, L.; Yin, H.; Ai, S. Electrochemical biosensor for microRNA detection based on hybridization protection against nuclease S1 digestion. *J. Solid State Electrochem.* **2015**, *20*, 413–419. [CrossRef]
185. Jeong, B.; Kim, Y.J.; Jeong, J.-Y. Label-free electrochemical quantification of microRNA-375 in prostate cancer cells. *J. Electroanal. Chem.* **2019**, *846*, 113127. [CrossRef]
186. Li, J.; Wang, Y.; Deng, R.; Lin, L.; Liu, Y.; Li, J. Carbon nanotube enhanced label-free detection of microRNAs based on hairpin probe triggered solid-phase rolling-circle amplification. *Nanoscale* **2015**, *7*, 987–993. [CrossRef]
187. Akbarnia, A.; Zare, H.R.; Moshtaghioun, S.M.; Benvidi, A. Highly selective sensing and measurement of microRNA-541 based on its sequence-specific digestion by the restriction enzyme Hinf1. *Colloids Surf. B Biointerfaces* **2019**, *182*, 110360. [CrossRef]
188. Azab, S.M.; Elhakim, H.K.; Fekry, A.M. The strategy of nanoparticles and the flavone chrysin to quantify miRNA-let 7a in zepto-molar level: Its application as tumor marker. *J. Mol. Struct.* **2019**, *1196*, 647–652. [CrossRef]
189. Kangkamano, T.; Numnuam, A.; Limbut, W.; Kanatharana, P.; Vilaivan, T.; Thavarungkul, P. Pyrrolidinyl PNA polypyrrole/silver nanofoam electrode as a novel label-free electrochemical miRNA-21 biosensor. *Biosens. Bioelectron.* **2018**, *102*, 217–225. [CrossRef]
190. Yang, L.; Wang, H.; Lü, H.; Hui, N. Phytic acid functionalized antifouling conducting polymer hydrogel for electrochemical detection of microRNA. *Anal. Chim. Acta* **2020**, *1124*, 104–112. [CrossRef]

191. Zhu, D.; Liu, W.; Zhao, D.; Hao, Q.; Lianhui, W.; Huang, J.; Shi, J.; Chao, J.; Su, S.; Wang, L. Label-Free Electrochemical Sensing Platform for MicroRNA-21 Detection Using Thionine and Gold Nanoparticles Co-Functionalized MoS2 Nanosheet. *ACS Appl. Mater. Interfaces* **2017**, *9*, 35597–35603. [CrossRef] [PubMed]
192. Zouari, M.; Campuzano, S.; Pingarrón, J.M.; Raouafi, N. Determination of miRNAs in serum of cancer patients with a label- and enzyme-free voltammetric biosensor in a single 30-min step. *Microchim. Acta* **2020**, *187*, 1–11. [CrossRef] [PubMed]
193. Sabahi, A.; Salahandish, R.; Ghaffarinejad, A.; Omidinia, E. Electrochemical nano-genosensor for highly sensitive detection of miR-21 biomarker based on SWCNT-grafted dendritic Au nanostructure for early detection of prostate cancer. *Talanta* **2020**, *209*, 120595. [CrossRef] [PubMed]

biosensors

MDPI

Review

The Role of Peptides in the Design of Electrochemical Biosensors for Clinical Diagnostics

Patrick Severin Sfragano [1], Giulia Moro [2], Federico Polo [2] and Ilaria Palchetti [1,*]

[1] Department of Chemistry "Ugo Schiff", University of Florence, Via della Lastruccia 3, 50019 Sesto Fiorentino, Italy; patrickseverin.sfragano@unifi.it
[2] Department of Molecular Sciences and Nanosystems, Ca' Foscari University of Venice, Via Torino 155, 30172 Venice, Italy; giulia.moro@unive.it (G.M.); federico.polo@unive.it (F.P.)
* Correspondence: ilaria.palchetti@unifi.it

Abstract: Peptides represent a promising class of biorecognition elements that can be coupled to electrochemical transducers. The benefits lie mainly in their stability and selectivity toward a target analyte. Furthermore, they can be synthesized rather easily and modified with specific functional groups, thus making them suitable for the development of novel architectures for biosensing platforms, as well as alternative labelling tools. Peptides have also been proposed as antibiofouling agents. Indeed, biofouling caused by the accumulation of biomolecules on electrode surfaces is one of the major issues and challenges to be addressed in the practical application of electrochemical biosensors. In this review, we summarise trends from the last three years in the design and development of electrochemical biosensors using synthetic peptides. The different roles of peptides in the design of electrochemical biosensors are described. The main procedures of selection and synthesis are discussed. Selected applications in clinical diagnostics are also described.

Keywords: peptide; electrochemical biosensor; antifouling; protease; biomarker; bioreceptor

Citation: Sfragano, P.S.; Moro, G.; Polo, F.; Palchetti, I. The Role of Peptides in the Design of Electrochemical Biosensors for Clinical Diagnostics. *Biosensors* **2021**, *11*, 246. https://doi.org/10.3390/bios11080246

Received: 31 May 2021
Accepted: 19 July 2021
Published: 23 July 2021

1. Introduction

Peptides are sequences of amino acids of varying length and weight. Only 20 of the hundreds of known amino acids account for the vast majority of residues that make up human proteins [1]. The chemical structure of amino acids that occur in protein varies only in the R-group at the carbon in alpha position, Cα, and are referred to as α-amino acids [2]. Not all biologic amino acids are α-amino acids; β-amino acids (e.g., β-taurine), as well as γ-amino acids (e.g., γ-aminobutyric acid), also play important biochemical roles. α-amino acids are chiral, with the exception of glycine, and mainly occur in the L-form, even though small quantities of D-amino acids occur in biological fluids but without specific function. D-serine is an exception and serves as a neurotransmitter in cerebrospinal fluid. Isoleucine and threonine have a second asymmetric carbon that gives rise to stereoisomers. Furthermore, a number of rare amino acids are recovered from protein hydrolysates, in addition to the 20 protein-forming amino acids.

The chemical behaviour of the R group dictates the chemical behaviour of each α-amino acid, which can be categorized as charged, hydrophilic, or hydrophobic. The hydrophobic amino acids with aliphatic residues are alanine (A), isoleucine (I), leucine (L), methionine (M), and valine (V). Amino acids with aromatic residues such as phenylalanine (F), tryptophan (W), and tyrosine (Y) are also hydrophobic [3]. The aliphatic residues generally provide a hydrophobic environment whereas aromatic residues are usually involved in π–π stacking. The hydrophilic, polar residues participate in hydrogen bonding either via OH (serine (S) and threonine (T)) or $CONH_2$ groups (asparagine (N) and glutamine (Q)). The ionisable residues can be positively charged, (histidine (H), lysine (K), and arginine (R)) or negatively charged, such as in aspartic acid (D) and glutamic acid (E). Other natural amino acids are cysteine (C), glycine (G), and proline (P). Proline exhibits hydrophobic behaviour, whereas cysteine, with its thiol side chain, is an important source of sulfur in human metabolism.

Peptides adopt specific conformations depending on the position of each R-group in the amino acid sequence. The secondary structure of peptides (α- helices, β-sheets, and β-hairpins) is driven by noncovalent intermolecular interactions, such as hydrogen bonding, van der Waals forces, π-stacking, and hydrophobic and electrostatic interactions. The secondary structure of peptides can be modulated by introducing modifications in the amino acids, thus favouring interactions with other peptides or proteins. Amino acids can be considered as natural molecular building blocks that spontaneously arrange themselves to form highly organized structures with well-defined functional properties [2].

Recently, peptides have been proposed to be interesting and versatile tools for the design and development of biosensors [3–6]. Peptides can be easily obtained by chemical synthesis methods, avoiding the need for in-vivo, laborious procedures, as in the case of antibodies. Moreover, they are also biocompatible. Notably, research activity concerning peptide-based biosensors and bioassays is increasing, and, at the time of writing, around 3000 matches are found when searching for the keywords "peptide" AND "biosensor" in commonly employed search engines (SciFinder, CAS).

Electrochemical biosensors are powerful tools that allow for cost-effective, easy, and fast detection and/or monitoring of analytes in clinical diagnostics [7–12], and are often employed in the framework of point-of-care testing (PoCT). Peptides represent a promising class of affinity biorecognition elements that can be coupled to electrochemical transducers. The benefits lie mainly in their stability and selectivity toward a target analyte. Furthermore, they can be synthesized rather easily and modified with specific functional groups, thus making them suitable for the development of novel architectures for biosensing platforms, as well as alternative labelling tools. Also, peptides have been proposed as antibiofouling agents. Indeed, biofouling caused by the accumulation of biomolecules on electrode surfaces is one of the major issues and challenges to be addressed in the practical application of electrochemical biosensors.

Herein, we summarise trends from the last three years in the design and development of electrochemical biosensors using synthetic peptides. In comparison with other recent review papers mainly focused on protein detection [13] or on electrochemical methods in peptide-based assays [3], the different roles of peptides in the design of electrochemical biosensors are described here—from their use as antifouling agents to their role in the development of catalytic, as well as affinity, electrochemical biosensors. Moreover, the main procedures of selection and synthesis are discussed. Figure 1 shows a schematic summary of the various applications of peptides described throughout the review. Regarding detection, both label and label-free approaches are possible and different electrochemical detection methods are achievable using three main quantities: current (amperometric and voltammetric biosensors), potential, and impedance. Nonelectroactive peptides can be successfully combined with impedance/voltammetric transducers [14,15]. Furthermore, peptides can be easily labelled with redox-active probes, such as ferrocene (Fc) or methylene blue [16–18] for signal-on/signal-off detection. Selected applications in clinical diagnostics, in which these kinds of detection strategies are exploited, are discussed in the following sections.

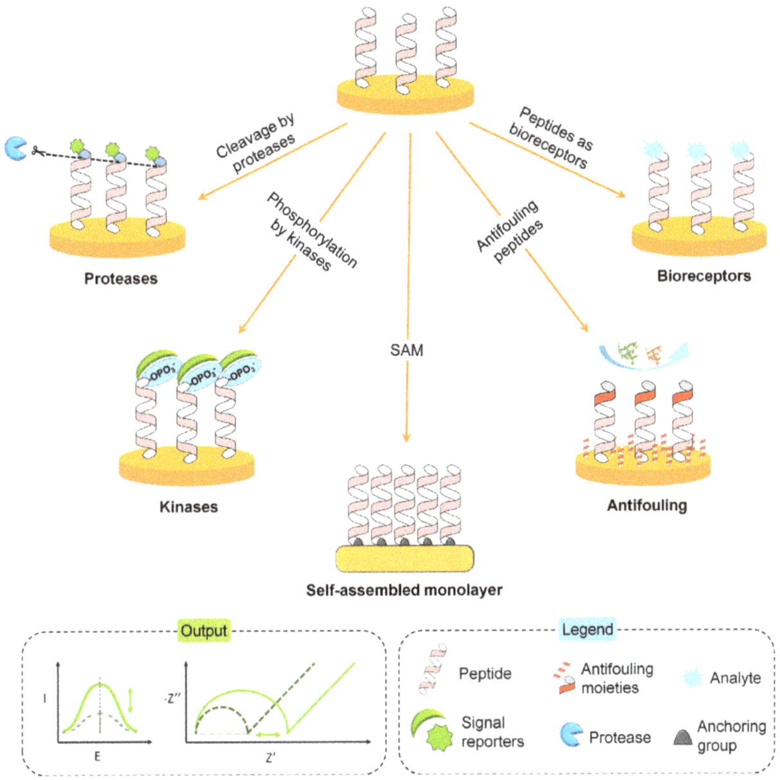

Figure 1. Schematic summary of the different roles of synthetic peptides in biosensors, as discussed in this review. Proteases can cause the cleavage of specific peptide sequences; kinases phosphorylate the hydroxyl groups in the peptide sequence; furthermore, peptides can form self-assembled monolayers and work as antifouling agents and biorecognition elements. The output can be an increase (signal-on) or a decrease (signal-off) of the electrochemical readout. Both label and label-free approaches are possible in biosensing. Picture not to scale.

2. Peptide Selection, Synthesis, and Characterisation

The design of successful peptide-based sensing platforms requires accurate selection, synthesis, and characterisation of the bioreceptor to optimize the surface coverage, while assuring and maximizing interaction with the target, and, to guarantee high-affinity, selective and reproducible recognition [19]. Ligand peptide selection can be challenging if one considers the commercial availability of hundreds of amino acid building blocks (naturally occurring and not) and the different folding of the final sequence (linear, cyclic, and bicyclic). Despite this high variability, the chemical synthesis of peptides can be easily implemented with great rapidity and high production rates. This aspect is of particular interest, as the availability of well-grounded and straightforward synthetic protocols allows several sequences to be tested in a short time, thus making these biomolecules highly competitive in pharmaceutical, as well as sensing, applications [20]. Therefore, genetically encoded peptide ligands with tailored properties can be generated by screening large combinatorial libraries using in-vitro display techniques [21]. Phage display was the first combinatorial technique used for the direct evolution of peptides, as described by Smith in 1985 [22]. The identification of high-affinity sequences is achieved by screening a wide library of random peptides that are displayed on the surface of the phage against the target of interest, such as a small molecule, a protein, etc. The displayed peptides, representing the phenotype, have a physical linkage with their encoding DNA or RNA sequences, the genotypes. After exposure to the target, only the binding peptides are sequenced via mass spectrometry-based methods to obtain the amino acid sequences [23]. To enhance binding affinity and to avoid nonspecific binding and blocking side-phenomena, phage display was further implemented in recent decades [24]. A similar selection mechanism also characterised other well-known combinatorial techniques described in the 1990s: from mRNA display [25] to ribosome display [26], bacteria display [27], and yeast display [28,29]. These experimental approaches can be integrated by computational ones from in-silico evolution and structural bioinformatics to atomistic simulations, as recently discussed by D'Annessa et al. [30]. Xiao et al. described the successful selection of peptides for biosensing applications using solely in-silico evolution [31]. This example underlines the wide variety of paths available for peptide selection. Regardless of the approach chosen for the selection, prior to proceeding with large-scale synthesis of the selected sequences, an in-depth characterisation of the peptide–target complex is required. The study of the binding kinetics and thermodynamics, along with the structural features of the peptide–target complex, is instrumental in evaluating the applicability of the selected peptide as a bioreceptor and, eventually, the identification of the most suitable design for the sensing platform. The design of the peptide–target characterisation protocol should take into account the final application of the peptide sequence (i.e., the biosensing platform) as the binding performance can vary depending on the physical and chemical properties of the surrounding environment, as recently discussed for other biorecognition elements [32]. Characterisation of the peptide–target complex is therefore fundamental to the evaluation of the peptide's applicability, the discrimination of a restricted pool of selected sequences, and, eventually, the consideration to improve biorecognition elements, for instance, by using peptides in conjugation with other biomolecules [33,34]. Once the peptide bioreceptor is characterised, it is possible to proceed with its synthesis following different approaches, such as solution-based [35] or solid-phase peptide synthesis (SPPS) [36], compatible with batch and continuous-flow reactors [37]. The possibility of carrying out peptide synthesis within partially or fully automated systems guarantees the ease and rapidity of synthesis and large-scale applicability of these biomolecules. The synthesis is coupled with a final purification step, usually performed via reversed-phase high-performance liquid chromatography (RP-HPLC) before checking the molecular mass by mass spectrometry.

3. Peptides as Self-Assembled Layers

Peptides can be immobilized at noble metal surfaces by spontaneous chemisorption processes forming ordered two-dimensional supermolecular systems known as self-assembled monolayers (SAMs). Covalent anchoring on gold surfaces is achieved mainly via gold–sulfur interaction using nonpeptide synthetic thiols or the natural thiol-containing amino acid cysteine [38–40]. Self-assembling peptides (SAPs) are tuneable building blocks compatible with numerous sensing strategies and nanosized biomaterials, as highlighted by the examples reported in the following sections. Heterogeneous SAMs can also be formed by mixing different biomolecules, in particular peptides and aptamers, allowing for the design of highly sensitive platforms [41]. An interface composed of a redox-tagged peptide, integrated with receptive aptamers, was developed to target C-reactive protein (CRP), a biomarker of systemic inflammation [42]. The study was further extended by designing peptides that could attach to antibodies instead of aptamers and achieve good sensitivity for clinically relevant levels of CRP [16]. By means of SPPS, both works produced and employed the Fc-tagged peptide sequence EAAC-NH_2, in which the cysteine residue was used to obtain covalent anchoring onto a Au electrode. The resulting SAM shows high surface density and a well-ordered structure.

Other known immobilization procedures can be used to develop peptide-based biosensors, namely physical adsorption (based on the noncovalent interaction between peptides and the transducer surface), the entrapment into a three-dimensional network of gel or polymers, as well as covalent chemical binding via functional moieties and selected reagents such as carbodiimide and hydroxysuccinimide derivatives [43].

4. Peptides as Antifouling Agents

Modification of the electrode surface may occur during electrochemical measurement in clinical specimens due to nonspecific binding and an accumulation of the products derived from electrochemical reactions or the components of the complex matrix. The nonspecific adsorption of proteins, cells, or micro-organisms on electrode surfaces is a major concern in biomedical applications, as well as the electrochemical oxidation of phenolic compounds that form radicals and therefore polymeric structures, which are insoluble and precipitate from the solution onto the electrode surface.

The layer of these modifiers impedes the direct contact of any electroactive compound with the electrode surface, thus hampering electron transfer and diminishing the electrochemical signal. This phenomenon is known as the fouling process [44,45] and it significantly affects the sensitivity and reproducibility of electrochemical biosensors. Several physicochemical causes are involved in the fouling process, which depend on the chemical/biochemical species involved and the nature of the electrode surface. These include electrostatic interactions and hydrophobic and intermolecular forces. Proteins, for instance, generally tend to adsorb onto hydrophobic interfaces rather than onto hydrophilic ones.

Antifouling procedures and treatments are therefore required to improve the reliability, stability, and performance of electrochemical biosensors, especially when clinical specimens are analysed. To date, approaches to enhance antifouling resistance can be classified as physical treatments, which alter the surface morphology, and chemical treatments, which immobilise selected reagent monolayers on the electrode surface. Whitesides and coworkers proposed four molecular-level characteristics for the evaluation of protein-resistant monolayers: (1) the presence of polar functional groups, i.e., hydrophilicity, (2) the presence of hydrogen bond acceptor groups, (3) the absence of hydrogen bond donor groups, and (4) the absence of net charge [46].

Thus, several bio-inert molecules have been developed or employed that effectively decrease the adsorption of protein or other biomolecules on electrode surfaces, including poly(ethyleneglycol)s, polyglycerols, zwitterionic polymers, and polysaccharides [47]. Among these molecules, the antifouling property of hydrophilic, nonionic molecules is due to hydrogen bonding-induced surface hydration. Furthermore, strongly ionic solvation can also generate surface hydration and thus form a tightly bound water layer, which provides a physical and energetic barrier to prevent protein adsorption and cell adhesion to surfaces [48]. Peptides are claimed to be interesting antifouling materials because, apart from their easy and cost-effective synthesis, they are composed of natural amino acids which are biocompatible zwitterionic molecules and possess high hydrogen bond-donor/acceptor abilities due to the carbonyl, amine, and hydroxyl groups in the peptide backbone and side chains.

A zwitterionic peptide composed of alternating negatively charged glutamic acid (E) and positively charged lysine (K) residues which exhibits antifouling abilities and a well-defined secondary structure for closer packing of the monolayer due to a proline (P) linker peptide (PPPP) was designed by Nowinski et al. [49]. These peptide sequences have been proposed in many different SAPs, obtaining hierarchical assemblies characterized by: an interfacial region that operates as a biomolecular recognition layer or as an enhancer of the target signal [50], an antifouling region that stabilises the SAM via intermolecular interactions, and a surface anchoring portion [49], mainly using a cysteine (C) residue.

An inverted Y-shaped peptide was recently used for COVID-19 nucleic acid electrochemical detection in complex biological media [51]. The peptide consists of one antifouling main chain (KEPPPPKEKEKEKEK-biotin) in the upper part, in which the four proline residues (PPPP) assist in the formation of a stable secondary structure, and two anchor-antifouling side chains (CKEKEKEKE) in the lower part. Two (C) residues at the ends of the two side chains were used as the surface anchor to immobilise the peptides onto the electrode surface. Hierarchical peptide brushes composed of the zwitterionic antifouling peptides (CPPPPEKEKEKEK) and short-chain peptides (CPPPPEKEKEK), with the possibility of tethering more water molecules than other structures, have been proposed for the electrochemical determination of alpha-fetoprotein in serum by using an aptamer as a selective bioreceptor [52].

Many examples of multifunctional all-in-one SAPs combining anchoring, antifouling, and recognizing functions are reported in the literature [3,41,53–58]. For instance, a Y-shaped peptide (CPPPPEK (HWRGWVA)EKEKE) with both recognizing and antifouling branches was designed and attached to the electrode surface via a gold–sulfur bond to construct a biosensor for IgG determination in human serum. One of the two zwitterionic branches of this Y-shaped peptide was designed with a (EKEKEKE) sequence for antifouling, and the other one with a (HWEGWVA) sequence for recognizing the IgG [59].

Other peptide sequences with antifouling properties have recently been designed and used in the development of electrochemical sensors [60–63].

5. Peptides as Substrate and Signal Development Agents in Catalytic Biosensors

Enzymes represent valid biomarkers to assess the status or the progression of a variety of diseases and health conditions. Indeed, the catalytic activity of an enzyme can be used for its detection when a specific substrate is present. In peptide-based biosensors, such enzymatic substrate can be a (synthetic) peptide sequence; instead of capturing the target analyte, the peptide is used to transform the catalytic activity of the enzyme into a detectable electrochemical signal. The most important enzymes that are currently detected using peptide-based biosensors are proteases and kinases.

Proteases have potential diagnostic relevance due to their ability to hydrolyse specific peptide bonds, causing proteolysis. The proteolytic activity of proteases induces the cleavage of the peptide sequence used as substrate; in order to convert this event into a measurable signal, such peptides are usually conjugated with a signal reporter, such as a redox probe [64]. The cleavage of this labelled sequence portion provides either an increase (signal-on mechanism) or a decrease (signal-off mechanism) of the electrochemical output. In this respect, it has been shown that signal-on sensors are less susceptible to false positives [65,66]. The redox reporter can be located at the N-terminus or at the C-terminus of the amino acid sequence. In general, the choice of its location is determined by the synthetic process used (SPPS, etc.), the structural characteristics of the sequence, and the design of the sensing platform. The most common redox labels are Fc, horseradish peroxidase (HRP), and methylene blue, together with signal-enhancing nanocomposites based on reduced graphene oxide (rGO) or (noble) metals such as gold, silver, and copper. Moreover, the insertion of a flexible spacer (i.e., polyethylene glycol (PEG)) within the redox reporter seems to enhance the redox signal, promote enzyme accessibility, and confer flexibility to the probe. In this regard, Bradley and coworkers presented a systematic study evaluating the effect of different PEG-based spacers on the performances of peptide-based biosensors, highlighting their pivotal role [67].

Label-free approaches, in which a change of the system's impedance is correlated to the concentration of the analyte, are also employed, although less frequently.

One of the most investigated proteases is a family of endopeptidases, namely matrix metalloproteinases (MMPs), which have an important clinical application (when upregulated) in the identification of various pathological and physiological conditions such as neurodegenerative and cardiovascular disorders, diabetes, sepsis, arthritis, angiogenesis, and others. Moreover, as matrix-degrading enzymes, MMPs can attack and degrade various extracellular protein components of cell membranes and the extracellular matrix, and hence play a significant role in the progression, invasion, and metastasis of tumours [68]. The expression of MMPs is thus considered a good parameter to monitor the occurrence and prognosis of neoplasia. Cleavage-based electrochemical biosensors that use peptides as substrate for the proteolytic activity of MMPs constitute a booming research field due to their advantages: low cost, high selectivity, and applicability in PoCT.

Among MMPs, MMP-2 is one of the most investigated using the abovementioned biosensors, usually employing the peptide sequence PLGVR as the proteolytic target operated by MMP-2. However, other MMPs, such as MMP-7 [69] and MMP-14 [70], are also attractive clinical-related biomarkers.

Often, the current intensity measured by these protease-based platforms is quite low. One of the main challenges of modern biosensor technology is to achieve ultrasensitivity so as to detect analytes present at extremely low concentrations. Therefore, some form of signal amplification is highly desirable. Nanomaterials are widely used to enhance the performances of biosensors; for instance, by increasing the electrochemically active surface area and improving mass transport while leading to better electrocatalytic activity and fast heterogeneous electron transfer kinetics [71]. An interesting example is the modification of the electrode surface with carbon nanotubes (CNTs) and electrochemically synthesized Au nanoparticles (AuNPs), which led to the sensitive monitoring of the activity of MMP-7 in a label-free approach [72]. The electrode surface was further functionalized with a peptide (JR2EC) that presented two binding sites for MMP-7. Its MMP-mediated hydrolysis was monitored by means of differential pulse voltammetry (DPV), achieving a limit of detection (LOD) of 6 pg/mL. The sensor was successfully tested in human serum and synthetic urine.

Nanozymes also represent an attractive alternative for the attainment of remarkable signal amplification along with stability, easy development at low cost, and resistance to acids and alkalis [73,74]. Inspired by these characteristics, Xi et al. [75] fabricated an H_2O_2-free peptide-based biosensor for the detection of MMP-2 using a Au@Pt bimetallic nanozyme as a signal amplification label. A peptide including the sequence PLGVR allowed detection of the protease. DPV measurement showed good linear correlation of the current intensity against MMP-2 concentration, achieving a LOD of 0.18 ng/mL.

Other signal amplification strategies have been used to enhance the biosensor's performance and to detect MMP-2. An appealing case is the anodic stripping of silver nanoparticles (AgNPs) on the electrode surface. In particular, a first peptide presenting a proteolytic motif sequence for the specific cleavage by MMP-2 was immobilised onto the surface of a Au electrode through a Au–S chemical bond, thus forming a SAM [76]. A complex composed of a second peptide and AgNPs was then captured by the peptides in the SAM by means of host–guest interactions. In the absence of MMP-2, AgNPs produce a drastic output in square wave voltammetry (SWV). On the other hand, when MMP-2 is present, the first peptide in the SAM is cleaved, releasing the second peptide functionalized with AgNPs from the electrode surface, resulting in a weaker current response (Figure 2a). A LOD of 0.12 pg/mL has been estimated.

Aside from methods that use nanomaterials, various forms of amplified biodetection signals are obtainable. Radical polymerizations reactions, such as reversible addition-fragmentation chain-transfer (RAFT) polymerization and atom transfer radical polymerization (ATRP), are interesting implementations in biosensing platforms. Kim and Sikes recently wrote an exhaustive review that presents the principles of these reactions, comparing them in terms of performance and ease of application [77].

Hu and coworkers [65] managed to immobilise a recognition peptide via a Au–S bond on Au electrodes (Figure 2b). This peptide acted as proteolytic substrate to assess the MMP-2′s activity in a signal-on strategy. The grafting of ferrocenyl (Fc) polymers through electrochemically mediated RAFT (eRAFT) polymerization was responsible for the efficient accumulation of a vast quantity of Fc redox reporters on the electrode surface, lowering the LOD to 0.27 pg/mL under optimal conditions. Good performance was also demonstrated in complex serum samples and in the presence of interferents for the evaluation of selectivity. The authors also presented a similar method based on RAFT polymerization for the signal-amplified determination of thrombin activity, a serine protease routinely checked for in the diagnosis of coagulation disorders [78].

Working again with MMP-2 as analyte, Wang et al. instead used the electrochemically mediated ATRP (eATRP) reaction in a signal amplification strategy with ferrocenylmethyl methacrylate monomers to obtain a chain-growth polymer of Fc as an electroactive probe [79]. A specific peptide used as a recognition substrate is cleaved in the presence of MMP-2, hence lowering the peak current of Fc measured with SWV. A LOD of 0.53 fM was obtained under optimal conditions. A potential application in human serum was also verified by running experiments with spiked human serum, which were diluted 1000-fold, with recoveries ranging from 97% to 112%.

Applying a very similar eATRP-based approach, Hu et al. targeted a different protease, namely the prostate-specific antigen (PSA), down to femtomolar concentrations [80]. As one of the most studied biomarkers for prostate carcinoma, PSA, a glycoprotein with endopeptidase activity, is always widely discussed in clinical research [81]. A quick view at the number of cases and victims of prostate cancer per year enlightens the importance of early diagnosis, given that the vast majority of patients rarely show symptoms before the latest stages of the disease [82]. In recent years, several peptide-based biosensors for the highly sensitive detection of PSA have been developed, harnessing different detection and amplification techniques, and exploiting the cleavage activity of the protease. As for MMPs, nanocomposites are widely used materials to enhance the sensitivity of the PSA detection mechanism. Meng et al., for instance, proposed the combination of graphene oxide and AgNPs on a Au electrode (Figure 2c) [83]. The use of DNAzymes (i.e., G-quadruplets/hemin, which possesses peroxidase-like activity) may also provide a dramatic boost to the sensor's sensitivity. A few interesting applications of hemin/G-quadruplex DNAzymes coupled to peptides as recognition substrates for PSA detection have been reported in the recent literature [66,84].

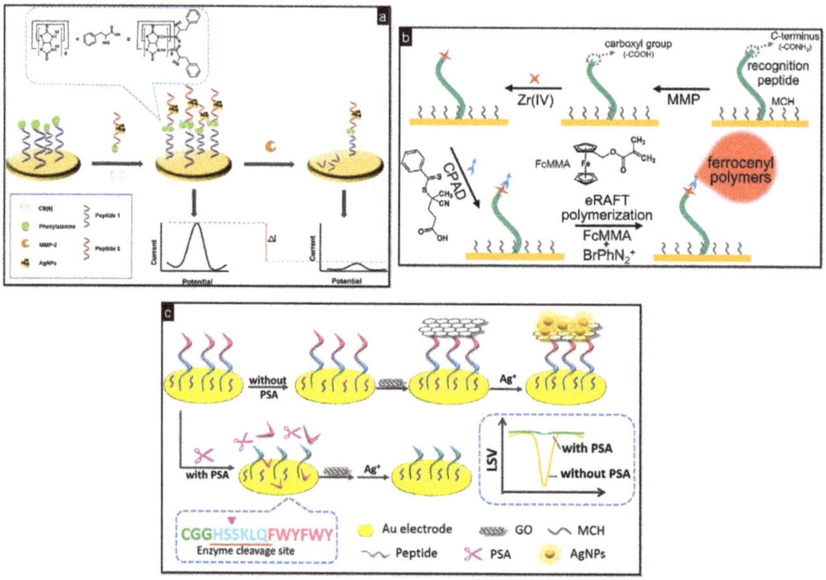

Figure 2. Schematic illustrations of different protease-based catalytic biosensors: (**a**) signal-amplified detection of MMP-2 through anodic stripping of AgNPs, using CB [8] as macrocyclic receptor to bind two aromatic amino acid residues via host–guest interactions, reprinted with permission from [76]; (**b**) signal-on MMP's activity detection using a carboxyl group-free recognition peptide as proteolytic substrate, immobilised via Au–S self-assembly. Grafting of Fc polymers through eRAFT polymerization of ferrocenylmethyl methacrylate (FcMMA), reprinted with permission from [65]; (**c**) GO/AgNPs nanocomposite for the determination of PSA on Au electrode by means of linear sweep voltammetry (LSV), reprinted with permission from [83].

Proteases represent markers for a variety of other applications. For instance, proteases produced from bacteria can be used to identify the presence of bacteria. Indeed, specific (synthetic) peptide sequences may find application as recognition receptors in the quantitative/qualitative detection and monitoring of different bacteria. Thus, peptide-based biosensors may constitute a cost-effective and rapid system for protection against pathogenic bacteria. With this in mind, Eissa and Zourob [85] worked on the multiplexed detection of *Listeria monocytogenes* (LOD of 9 CFU/mL) and *Staphylococcus aureus* (LOD of 3 CFU/mL) by exploiting the proteolytic activities of proteases produced from these two bacteria to hydrolyse a synthetic peptide sequence used as substrate. Magnetic nanoparticles were used to immobilise the peptide, harnessing the streptavidin–biotin interaction. An increased reduction in the peak current of $[Fe(CN)_6]^{3-/4-}$ was found in SWV when, due to the cleavage of the peptide sequence operated by the specific enzyme for each bacteria, the peptide/magnetic nanobeads were pulled away from the surface of AuNPs-modified screen-printed carbon electrodes (SPCEs). Selectivity experiments were also carried out.

Often, magnetic beads (MBs) offer a simple and practical solution for sample treatment and management. MBs are usually made of a thin polymer shell coupled to a dispersion of magnetic materials, presenting superparamagnetic properties. In the presence of a magnetic field, they exhibit magnetic properties; this effect ceases totally when the magnetic field is removed. These characteristics make MBs very useful for many different applications [86], including purification processes in bioanalytics; instead of centrifugation, filtration, or precipitation procedures, a simple magnet is sufficient. MB-assisted electrochemical biosensors pave the way for fast and handy protocols by decreasing electrode biofouling [87,88]. The immobilisation of peptide sequences on MBs merges the advantages of the abovementioned biosensors with peptide-based platforms. The attachment of a short peptide sequence labelled with biotin and fluorescein isothiocyanate (FITC) onto neutravidin-modified MBs recently allowed for the detection of an important protease in human cell lysates that finds clinical applications: trypsin, which is considered a biomarker for multiple forms of cancer when upregulated [89]. Together with other serine proteases, it activates other proteases (i.e., the abovementioned MMPs), thus inducing a proteolytic cascade, resulting in a decisive phase of tumour progression. Upon peptide digestion by trypsin, the modified MBs were enzymatically labelled with Fab fragments from anti-FITC antibodies conjugated with horseradish peroxidase (HRP). After being magnetically captured on the surface of unmodified SPCE, amperometric detection was conducted, which relies on the hydroquinone (HQ)/HRP/H_2O_2 system. Trypsin was successfully detected in cell lysates from pancreatic cancer, cervix carcinoma, and kidney cells, discriminating between pancreatic and nonpancreatic cancer cells.

An alternative to nanostructured macroscopic electrodes could be microelectrodes [90]. Pt-based microelectrodes of 25 μm diameter were recently applied by Mount's group for the detection of trypsin in a peptide-based biosensor, demonstrating their applicability for the determination of clinically relevant concentrations of proteases [17].

As mentioned in the introduction of this paragraph, kinases are the second most important group of enzymes analysed with these catalytic peptide-based biosensors. In the case of kinase activity, detection is based on the determination of the phosphorylation process of the peptide used as substrate. In particular, kinases use adenosine 5′-triphosphate (ATP) as a phosphate group donor to catalyse the (reversible) phosphorylation of the hydroxyl groups of specific amino acid residues (i.e., serine, tyrosine, and threonine) in the peptide/protein sequence. This event is usually followed by conjugation with a signal reporter. Indeed, this kind of approach requires a more complex design compared with that of cleavage-based sensors for proteases. Likely due to this reason, and to the best of our knowledge, very few papers have been published in recent years on the detection of kinase activity. Cyclic adenosine monophosphate (cAMP)-dependent protein kinase and, more commonly, protein kinase A (PKA) indicate, when oversecreted, several pathological conditions including Alzheimer's disease, cancer, diabetes, cardiovascular diseases, and others. A noteworthy example of its detection is the use of the aforementioned RAFT polymerization process to augment sensitivity, employing the peptide sequence LRRASLGGGGC as the recognition substrate [91,92].

Table 1 summarises various characteristics of the biosensors reported in the prior section, including remarks, performance, and whether or not an analysis on real samples was performed.

Table 1. Catalytic peptide-based biosensors for the detection of various proteases and kinases. GCE = glassy carbon electrode; NHS = normal human serum; SA = sodium alginate; EIS = electrochemical impedance spectroscopy; PEI = polyethyleneimine; PtNTs = platinum nanotubes; CFU = colony-forming unit; HNE = human neutrophil elastase.

Target	Remarks	Target Peptide Sequence	Electrode	LOD	Real Samples	Ref.
MMP-2	Grafting of ferrocenyl polymers through eRAFT polymerization. Signal-on sensor. Fc as redox reporter.	PLGVR	Au electrode	0.27 pg/mL	/	[65]
MMP-2	Signal amplification via Au@Pt (nanorods) bimetallic nanozyme. H_2O_2-free peptide biosensor.	PLGVR	GCE	0.18 ng/mL	100-fold diluted human serum	[75]
MMP-2	Signal amplification via eATRP reaction and Fc polymers as electroactive probe. Measurements in SWV: Fc signal is decreased when the peptide used as recognition substrate is cleaved by MMP-2.	CGAPLGVRGA	Au electrode	0.53 fM	1000-fold diluted NHS	[79]
MMP-2	Signal amplification by anodic stripping of AgNPs. A first peptide is anchored onto the Au electrode and second-peptide-templated AgNPs are used to generate the signal. MMP-2 cleaves the first peptide, lowering the signal.	PLGVR	Au electrode	0.12 pg/mL	Human serum	[76]
MMP-7	JR2EC peptide as substrate. DPV analysis. Label-free approach: current increases linearly at higher concentrations of MMP-7 due to the cleavage of the peptide, which gives an electron transfer hindering effect (less surface area available).	/	CNTs/AuNPs/Au electrode	6 pg/mL	Spiked undiluted synthetic urine and 100-fold diluted human serum	[72]
MMP-7	Dual-reaction enhanced sensitivity. Amperometric detection. PdNPs catalytic probes combined with Au-rGO/methylene blue-SA nanocomposite.	KKKRPLALWRSCCC	GCE	3.1 fg/mL	Spiked healthy human serum	[69]
MMP-14	MMP-14-mediated cleavage of a Fc-carrying peptide placed on a Au electrode.	CPLPLRSWGLK	Au electrode	0.1 ng/L	Breast cancer cell lines type MCF-7	[70]
PSA	Signal amplification via eATRP reaction and Fc polymers as electroactive probe.	CSGGSSHSSKLQKK	Au electrode	3.2 fM	NHS	[80]
PSA	Signal-on biosensor based on peptide-conjugated hemin/G-quadruplex DNAzyme and rosebud-like $MoSe_2$@rGO nanocomposite.	HSSKLQ	GCE	0.3 fg/mL	Clinical serum samples	[66]
PSA	Aggregation of silver ions and formation of AgNPs on a GO-modified Au electrode. If PSA is cleaved, the immobilisation of graphene oxide and the formation of AgNPs will not occur, hence leading to a subsequently decreased electrochemical response.	CGGHSSKLQFWYFWY	Au electrode	0.33 pg/mL	Spiked healthy human serum	[83]

Table 1. *Cont.*

Target	Remarks	Target Peptide Sequence	Electrode	LOD	Real Samples	Ref.
PSA	Peptide-hemin/G-quadruplex conjugate. GCE modified with PEI-rGO@PtNTs nanocomposites. In the presence of PSA, the peptide-DNAzyme conjugate is cleaved, reducing the electrochemical signal.	CAAAHHHHHHHSSKLQ	GCE	2 fg/mL	Spiked 100-fold diluted human serum	[84]
Proteases from *L. monocytogenes* and *S. aureus*	Magnetic beads/peptide immobilised on an array of AuNPs-modified SPCE. Increased SWV reduction peak of ferro/ferricyanide when the cleaved magnetic beads/peptide were pulled away from the electrode surface.	*S. aureus*: ETKVEENEAIQK; *L. monocytogenes*: NMLSEVERE	AuNPs-modified SPCE	3 and 9 CFU/mL for *S. aureus* and *L. monocytogenes*, respectively	/	[85]
Trypsin	Amperometric detection of trypsin activity using the HQ/HRP/H_2O_2 system, and a peptide-sequence immobilised onto neutravidin-modified magnetic beads, dually labelled with biotin and fluorescein isothiocyanate.	FRR	SPCE	7 nM	HEK293T, HeLa, BxPC3 and PANC-1 cell lysates	[89]
Trypsin	Evaluation of Pt-based microelectrodes in a peptide-based biosensor for the detection of trypsin, envisaging a possible implantable application.	FRR	Pt microelectrode	2.9 nM	/	[17]
Trypsin	$NiCo_2O_4$ nanosheets and g-C_3N_4 nanocomposite for signal amplification.	CAGRAAADAD	GCE	10^{-10} mg/mL	10-fold diluted healthy human serum	[71]
Thrombin	RAFT polymerization as signal amplification. Recruitment of a large quantity of Fc tags on the electrode surface.	CGLVPRGS	Au electrode	2.7 µU/mL	Spiked NHS	[78]
HNE	HNE-mediated peptide cleavage leads to the release of a redox-labelled probe fragment, resulting in a measurable decrease of the electrochemical output via SWV. Immobilisation of a methylene blue-labelled peptide sequence.	APEEIMRRQ	Polycrystalline Au electrode	4 nM	Human blood	[64]
PKA	RAFT polymerization as signal amplification. Recruitment of a large quantity of Fc electroactive probes to each phosphorylated site.	LRRASLGGGGC	Au electrode	1.05 mU/mL	HepG2 cell lysates	[91]
PKA	eRAFT polymerization as signal amplification. Recruitment of a large quantity of Fc electroactive probes to each phosphorylated site.	LRRASLGGGGC	Au electrode	1.02 mU/mL	/	[92]

6. Peptides as Bioreceptors in Affinity Biosensors

Cancer diagnosis is a vast clinical field, constantly enriched with novel biomarkers enabling discrimination between healthy and ill subjects, as well as between precancerous conditions and early stages of the disease. Many of these biomarkers are specific to certain types of tumours [93], while others may help to individuate the onset of different cancer-related processes and carcinogenesis. The anterior gradient proteins (AGR), for instance, are a family of proteins overexpressed in various human cancers. Ostatná et al. studied extensively the anterior gradient-2 (AGR2) oncoprotein with label-free current chronopotentiometry stripping (CPS) analysis, which allowed for the discrimination between specific and nonspecific interactions of AGR2 with a peptide aptamer [94]. Another promising tumour-related biomarker is poly(ADP-ribose) polymerase-1 (PARP-1). Wang et al. proposed an interesting method of labelling the peptide probe that was not based on unspecific electrostatic interactions [95]. In particular, they used peptide-templated copper nanoparticles (CuNPs) as a probe and harnessed specific covalent-like interactions between the guanidine groups of the probe and the acidic phosphate groups of PARP-1 (Figure 3a). This method allowed them to avoid unspecific interactions and achieve a low LOD of 0.004 U. Other interesting uses of metal nanoparticles such as AgNPs as labels can be found in the recent cancer-related literature [96].

Globally, colorectal cancer is the third most common type of cancer with an incidence of 10% of all cases [97]. Early diagnosis can truly constitute a life-saving step with this tumour. However, the gold standard technique for early detection, colonoscopy, is often despised by the vast majority of patients. That is why other less-invasive approaches are highly desirable and have already been utilized. Attractive analyses, for instance, are the determination of carcinoembryonic antigen (CEA) levels [98] and cytosensing of circulating tumour cells [99]. However, some of these methods often cannot discriminate between precancerous adenomas and carcinomas. An interesting exception was recently published concerning the development of an electrochemical affinity biosensor that uses synthetic peptides, designed using in silico modelling [100]. Such peptides were covalently immobilised on a Au electrode using benzoquinone through a surface chemistry approach. The detection of the leucine-rich α-2-glycoprotein-1 (LRG1) biomarker made possible the identification of the adenoma to carcinoma transition in 100-fold diluted human serum.

Interactions between proteins and metallic ions play a pivotal role and are very frequent at the biological and biochemical levels, defining structures and functions of proteins in the organism. Therefore, it is easy to imagine that peptides may share this kind of interaction with metallic ions, thus representing good recognition elements in peptide-based metallic ion sensing platforms [101]. With this in mind, Zhang and coworkers recently studied colorectal cancer-related oxidative stress under inflammatory conditions by investigating protein function and detecting proteins and their metal ion cofactors using peptide probes [102]. The cellular response to oxidative stress, indeed, is highly linked to the translocation of proteins and metal ions, as well as oxidative modifications of their functions and interactions.

Besides cancer, neurodegenerative disorders are among the most serious and debilitating diseases, responsible for heavy social and economic burdens. The two most prevalent are Alzheimer's disease (AD) and Parkinson's disease [103]. AD is strongly related to the aggregation of amyloid-β (Aβ) in the form of insoluble plaques in the brain, causing memory loss and dementia. The determination of Aβ in biological fluids such as blood, plasma, serum, and (above all) cerebrospinal fluid can give vital information for the (early) diagnosis of AD. For this reason, several peptide-based methods that aim at the detection of this biomarker have emerged over the years, for instance, by analysing Aβ using nanostructured platforms [104] or collecting platelets via peripheral blood sampling [105]. In a recent publication, this was accomplished by capturing the Aβ oligomer in a sandwich formed of two peptides, one as the capture probe, immobilised on a Au electrode, and the other, functionalized with Fc, as the label [106]. This latter peptide, after binding to the biomarker, was able to self-assemble on the surface of the electrode, generating an interesting form of signal amplification due to the large number of Fc moieties accumulated (Figure 3b).

Peptide-based biosensors have also been employed in the detection of biomarkers for other conditions and pathophysiological processes [107], including rheumatoid [108,109] and juvenile idiopathic [15] arthritis and acute kidney injury [110]. Furthermore, some peptide sequences for the affinity recognition of proteases have been selected. An efficient strategy to convert the binding event into a measurable electrochemical output is the conjugation of the peptide with a redox probe. For example, concerning the MMPs previously introduced, an uncommon approach was followed by Ma et al. for the detection of MMP-14: comparing a label-based method to a label-free one in an affinity biosensor instead of employing the previously mentioned catalytic approach [111]. In particular, a specific peptide that recognises the hemopexin domain PEX-14 of the protease, namely peptide ISC, was used either unlabelled or tagged with a Fc redox reporter. Both versions were immobilised on Au electrodes. However, the label-free architecture exhibited a signal-on trend, in which the EIS semicircle radius increased together with the concentration of MMP-14, whereas the Fc-labelled architecture showed a signal-off behaviour in DPV. The latter architecture performed slightly better, achieving a LOD of 0.3 pg/mL, compared with the LOD of 0.03 ng/mL obtained by the former one. Subsequently, a similar example was published by the same group using different peptides [112].

Apart from direct self-assembly, peptides demonstrate great compatibility with alkanethiol SAM, allowing for the design of peptide-based platforms on gold by covalent immobilisation of the recognition layer. This is the case for the sensing platform reported by Kim et al. [113] for the determination of nonstructural 1 protein, a biomarker of dengue virus. This simple architecture allows for the detection of the analyte via SWV and ESI in the presence of a redox probe with a LOD of 1.49 μg/mL. A similar sensing platform was designed for monitoring human norovirus in various food samples [114]. Here, eight different peptides were screened and compared after immobilisation at portable gold screen-printed electrodes via thiol SAM. The resulting portable impedimetric sensor allowed for discrimination among the sequences and selection of the one with better performance in terms of LOD. This was further applied as a bioreceptor in another electrochemical sensor based on tungsten disulfide nanoflowers decorated with gold nanoparticles [115]. The nanohybrid material functionalized with the peptide was incubated with oyster samples spiked with the analyte (Figure 3c). After sizing the norovirus, the biohybrid composite was separated from the sample solution, rinsed, and immobilised at carbon screen-printed electrodes with the help of Nafion ionomer. This strategy prevents the adsorption of interfering agents and is suggested when working with complex matrices, such as oyster samples.

Matsubara et al. [116] developed a tunable peptide-based biosensing platform for the determination of the antiviral nucleoprotein antibodies of Avian influenza, anti-hemagglutinin (HA), and several virus variants (from H1N1 and H3N2 to H5N3, H7N1, and H9N2), as illustrated in Figure 3d. The success of this double-analyte sensing relies on its biorecognition layer made of dendrimers bearing pentapeptides sequences able to recognize the receptor-binding site of all HA variants. In this example, the low steric hindrance of the peptide branches is instrumental to the recognition of both analytes, while the possibility to directly immobilise the dendrimers at boron-doped diamond (BDD) electrode surfaces assures high control and reproducibility of the modification itself. After characterisation with voltammetric techniques, the analytical protocol was defined using EIS as the detection technique. Apart from viruses, peptide-based sensors were also designed to monitor bacteria and toxins such as *Escherichia coli* (*E. coli*), *Staphylococcus aureus* (*S. aureus*), and *Salmonella typhimurium* (*S. typhi*) [117] or endotoxin [118].

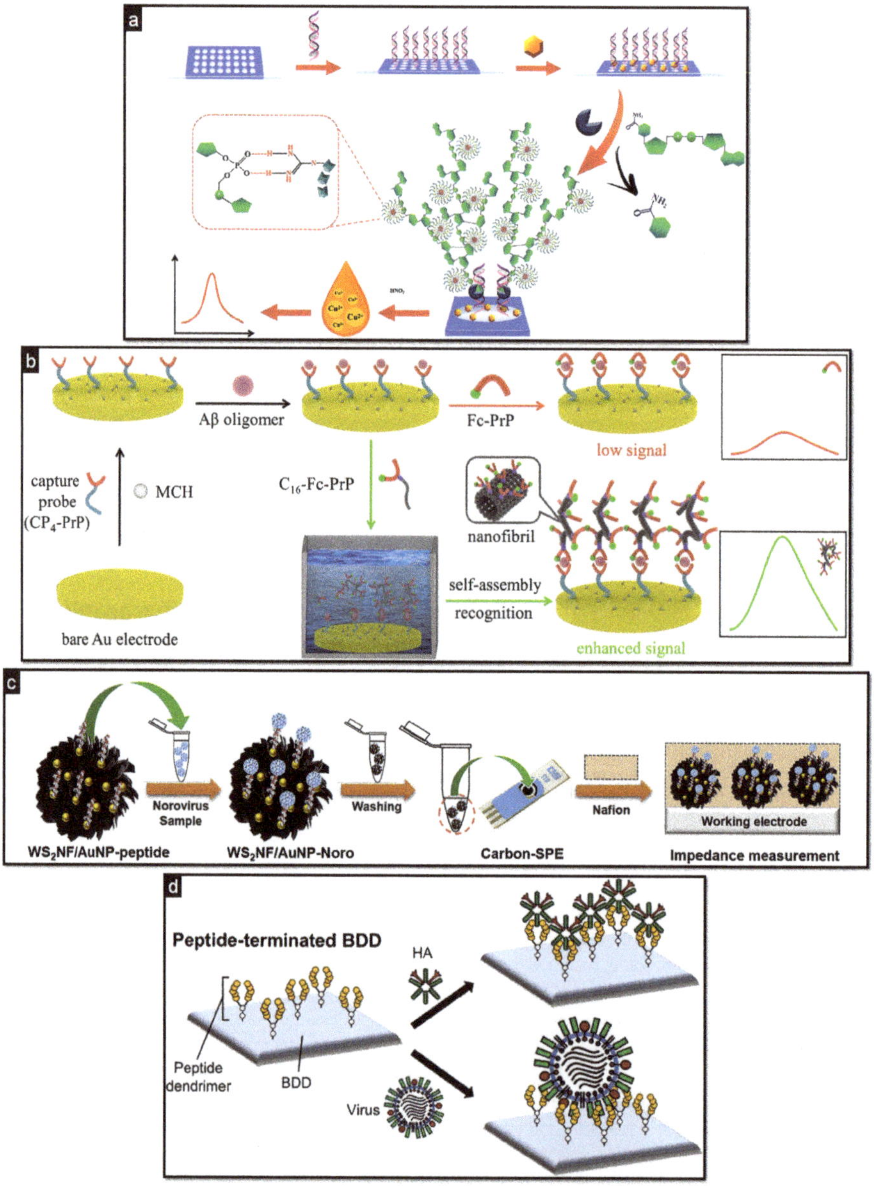

Figure 3. Schematic representation of some examples of peptide-based affinity platforms: (**a**) peptide-templated CuNPs as a probe for the detection of PARP-1, recognising and labelling PAR (PARP-1 catalysed form) by covalent-like interactions between guanidine groups and phosphate groups of PAR; quantitative determination via trace-level stripping voltammetry, reprinted with permission from [95]; (**b**) signal amplification strategy based on in situ peptide self-assembly for the detection, through SWV, of Aβ oligomer by designing a sandwich with a prion protein residue (PrP) that worked as a capture and Fc-conjugated signalling probe, reprinted with permission from [106]; (**c**) design of the label-free detection scheme based on peptide-functionalised WS_2NF/AuNPs for norovirus through EIS analysis, reprinted with permission from [115] (**d**) HA and avian influenza virus immobilisation at BDD electrodes in a Fc-labelled approach, reprinted with permission from [116] Copyright (2020) American Chemical Society.

7. Conclusions and Outlook

The synthetic nature, stability, and high yield of production of peptides are all very interesting properties for their use in different fields of science, especially in clinical diagnostics. An additional advantage is that different detection schemes are possible by using peptides; they can be used as substrates of proteases and kinases, which are enzymes considered to be important biomarkers of many different diseases. Furthermore, on the basis of their secondary structures, peptides can be used as affinity molecules for the specific binding of different analytes. Due to their physicochemical properties, peptides have also been proposed as antifouling molecules. Many examples of all-in-one multifunctional molecules with antifouling and biorecognition properties on the same peptide have also been proposed and reviewed in this manuscript. Despite these interesting properties, several issues remain—mainly, the total number of peptide sequences enabling recognition discovered until now is still significantly lower than that of antibodies.

In addition, peptides have been proposed as structural materials [2] and many examples are reported in the literature. Due to their tunable physicochemical properties, peptides are able to fold in compact structural motifs, shaping nanosized architectures in fibres, micelles, tubes, monolayers, bilayers, and strips that can have many different applications, including in vivo diagnostics.

The advantages of peptides versus antibodies in biosensing are evident in terms of their cost efficiency, high yield, and easier chemical synthesis. By contrast, it is hard to compare nucleic acids, including nucleic acid aptamers, and peptides. Peptides possess a variety of functional groups not present in nucleic acids (including nucleic acid aptamers) that can both enhance interactions, and thus affinity, with the target analyte and explain their functional and structural properties. Moreover, peptides have a different acid-base behaviour than nucleic acids. Thus, a comparison of these classes of interesting molecules in biosensing is not a trivial matter. Different considerations have to be kept in mind when making this comparison, such as selection or production procedures, which can lead to different evaluations. Therefore, it is not easy to predict which molecule is the best for a particular application. However, from the perspective of a researcher, it is important to have many different structural and functional molecules in order to better solve different bioanalytical issues and to increase the selectivity or multiplexing properties of the developed biosensors.

Author Contributions: Conceptualization, I.P.; writing—original draft preparation, P.S.S., G.M. and I.P.; writing—review and editing, I.P. and F.P. All authors have read and agreed to the published version of the manuscript.

Funding: This research was funded by Regione Toscana Bando Salute 2018, (Research project CUP n. D78D20000870002) and by Fondazione CR Firenze ID 2018.0944 and ID 2020.1662 (P.S. fellowship).

Acknowledgments: The authors acknowledge Alessandro Angelini for the technical support.

Conflicts of Interest: The authors declare no conflict of interest. The funders had no role in the design of the study; in the collection, analyses, or interpretation of data; in the writing of the manuscript, or in the decision to publish the results.

References

1. Rifai, N. *Tietz Fundamentals of Clinical Chemistry and Molecular Diagnostics—E-Book*; Elsevier Health Sciences: Amsterdam, The Netherlands, 2018; ISBN 9780323549738.
2. Ulijn, R.V.; Smith, A.M. Designing Peptide Based Nanomaterials. *Chem. Soc. Rev.* **2008**, *37*, 664. [CrossRef]
3. Puiu, M.; Bala, C. Peptide-Based Biosensors: From Self-Assembled Interfaces to Molecular Probes in Electrochemical Assays. *Bioelectrochemistry* **2018**, *120*, 66–75. [CrossRef]
4. Mascini, M.; Palchetti, I.; Tombelli, S. Nucleic Acid and Peptide Aptamers: Fundamentals and Bioanalytical Aspects. *Angew. Chem. Int. Ed.* **2012**, *51*, 1316–1332. [CrossRef] [PubMed]
5. Kerman, K.; Song, H.; Duncan, J.S.; Litchfield, D.W.; Kraatz, H.-B. Peptide Biosensors for the Electrochemical Measurement of Protein Kinase Activity. *Anal. Chem.* **2008**, *80*, 9395–9401. [CrossRef]

6. Puiu, M.; Bala, C. Building Switchable Peptide-Architectures on Gold/Composite Surfaces: New Perspectives in Electrochemical Bioassays. *Curr. Opin. Electrochem.* **2018**, *12*, 13–20. [CrossRef]
7. Sfragano, P.S.; Pillozzi, S.; Palchetti, I. Electrochemical and PEC Platforms for MiRNA and Other Epigenetic Markers of Cancer Diseases: Recent Updates. *Electrochem. Commun.* **2021**, *124*, 106929. [CrossRef]
8. Sfragano, P.S.; Laschi, S.; Palchetti, I. Sustainable Printed Electrochemical Platforms for Greener Analytics. *Front. Chem.* **2020**, *8*, 1–7. [CrossRef] [PubMed]
9. Bettazzi, F.; Palchetti, I. Nanotoxicity Assessment: A Challenging Application for Cutting Edge Electroanalytical Tools. *Anal. Chim. Acta* **2019**, *1072*, 61–74. [CrossRef] [PubMed]
10. Xia, L.; Liang, B.; Li, L.; Tang, X.; Palchetti, I.; Mascini, M.; Liu, A. Direct Energy Conversion from Xylose Using Xylose Dehydrogenase Surface Displayed Bacteria Based Enzymatic Biofuel Cell. *Biosens. Bioelectron.* **2013**, *44*. [CrossRef]
11. Palchetti, I.; Laschi, S.; Marrazza, G.; Mascini, M. Electrochemical Imaging of Localized Sandwich DNA Hybridization Using Scanning Electrochemical Microscopy. *Anal. Chem.* **2007**, *79*, 7206–7213. [CrossRef]
12. Liang, B.; Li, L.; Tang, X.; Lang, Q.; Wang, H.; Li, F.; Shi, J.; Shen, W.; Palchetti, I.; Mascini, M.; et al. Microbial Surface Display of Glucose Dehydrogenase for Amperometric Glucose Biosensor. *Biosens. Bioelectron.* **2013**, *45*. [CrossRef]
13. Vanova, V.; Mitrevska, K.; Milosavljevic, V.; Hynek, D.; Richtera, L.; Adam, V. Peptide-Based Electrochemical Biosensors Utilized for Protein Detection. *Biosens. Bioelectron.* **2021**, *180*, 113087. [CrossRef]
14. Lim, J.M.; Ryu, M.Y.; Yun, J.W.; Park, T.J.; Park, J.P. Electrochemical Peptide Sensor for Diagnosing Adenoma-Carcinoma Transition in Colon Cancer. *Biosens. Bioelectron.* **2017**, *98*, 330–337. [CrossRef] [PubMed]
15. Rodovalho, V.R.; Araujo, G.R.; Vaz, E.R.; Ueira-Vieira, C.; Goulart, L.R.; Madurro, J.M.; Brito-Madurro, A.G. Peptide-Based Electrochemical Biosensor for Juvenile Idiopathic Arthritis Detection. *Biosens. Bioelectron.* **2018**, *100*, 577–582. [CrossRef]
16. Piccoli, J.P.; Soares, A.C.; Oliveira, O.N.; Cilli, E.M. Nanostructured Functional Peptide Films and Their Application in C-Reactive Protein Immunosensors. *Bioelectrochemistry* **2021**, *138*, 107692. [CrossRef] [PubMed]
17. Ucar, A.; González-Fernández, E.; Staderini, M.; Avlonitis, N.; Murray, A.F.; Bradley, M.; Mount, A.R. Miniaturisation of a Peptide-Based Electrochemical Protease Activity Sensor Using Platinum Microelectrodes. *Analyst* **2020**, *145*, 975–982. [CrossRef] [PubMed]
18. Puiu, M.; Idili, A.; Moscone, D.; Ricci, F.; Bala, C. A Modular Electrochemical Peptide-Based Sensor for Antibody Detection. *Chem. Commun.* **2014**, *50*, 8962. [CrossRef]
19. Morales, M.A.; Halpern, J.M. Guide to Selecting a Biorecognition Element for Biosensors. *Bioconjug. Chem.* **2018**, *29*, 3231–3239. [CrossRef]
20. Bodanszky, M. In Search of New Methods in Peptide Synthesis. A Review of the Last Three Decades. *Int. J. Pept. Protein Res.* **2009**, *25*, 449–474. [CrossRef]
21. Ullman, C.G.; Frigotto, L.; Cooley, R.N. In Vitro Methods for Peptide Display and Their Applications. *Brief. Funct. Genom.* **2011**, *10*, 125–134. [CrossRef]
22. Smith, G. Filamentous Fusion Phage: Novel Expression Vectors That Display Cloned Antigens on the Virion Surface. *Science* **1985**, *228*, 1315–1317. [CrossRef]
23. Tang, L. Next-Generation Peptide Sequencing. *Nat. Methods* **2018**, *15*, 997. [CrossRef] [PubMed]
24. Yun, S.; Lee, S.; Park, J.P.; Choo, J.; Lee, E.K. Modification of Phage Display Technique for Improved Screening of High-Affinity Binding Peptides. *J. Biotechnol.* **2019**, *289*, 88–92. [CrossRef]
25. Roberts, R.W.; Szostak, J.W. RNA-Peptide Fusions for the in Vitro Selection of Peptides and Proteins. *Proc. Natl. Acad. Sci. USA* **1997**, *94*, 12297–12302. [CrossRef]
26. Hanes, J.; Pluckthun, A. In Vitro Selection and Evolution of Functional Proteins by Using Ribosome Display. *Proc. Natl. Acad. Sci. USA* **1997**, *94*, 4937–4942. [CrossRef] [PubMed]
27. Francisco, J.A.; Campbell, R.; Iverson, B.L.; Georgiou, G. Production and Fluorescence-Activated Cell Sorting of Escherichia Coli Expressing a Functional Antibody Fragment on the External Surface. *Proc. Natl. Acad. Sci. USA* **1993**, *90*, 10444–10448. [CrossRef]
28. Boder, E.T.; Wittrup, K.D. Yeast Surface Display for Screening Combinatorial Polypeptide Libraries. *Nat. Biotechnol.* **1997**, *15*, 553–557. [CrossRef] [PubMed]
29. Linciano, S.; Pluda, S.; Bacchin, A.; Angelini, A. Molecular Evolution of Peptides by Yeast Surface Display Technology. *Medchemcomm* **2019**, *10*, 1569–1580. [CrossRef] [PubMed]
30. D'Annessa, I.; Di Leva, F.S.; La Teana, A.; Novellino, E.; Limongelli, V.; Di Marino, D. Bioinformatics and Biosimulations as Toolbox for Peptides and Peptidomimetics Design: Where Are We? *Front. Mol. Biosci.* **2020**, *7*. [CrossRef]
31. Xiao, X.; Kuang, Z.; Slocik, J.M.; Tadepalli, S.; Brothers, M.; Kim, S.; Mirau, P.A.; Butkus, C.; Farmer, B.L.; Singamaneni, S.; et al. Advancing Peptide-Based Biorecognition Elements for Biosensors Using in-Silico Evolution. *ACS Sens.* **2018**, *3*, 1024–1031. [CrossRef]
32. Daems, E.; Moro, G.; Campos, R.; De Wael, K. Mapping the Gaps in Chemical Analysis for the Characterisation of Aptamer-Target Interactions. *Trends Anal. Chem.* **2021**, *142*, 116311. [CrossRef]
33. Pusuluri, A.; Krishnan, V.; Lensch, V.; Sarode, A.; Bunyan, E.; Vogus, D.R.; Menegatti, S.; Soh, H.T.; Mitragotri, S. Treating Tumors at Low Drug Doses Using an Aptamer–Peptide Synergistic Drug Conjugate. *Angew. Chem. Int. Ed.* **2019**, *58*, 1437–1441. [CrossRef] [PubMed]

34. Lee, K.; Yoo, Y.K.; Chae, M.-S.; Hwang, K.S.; Lee, J.; Kim, H.; Hur, D.; Lee, J.H. Highly Selective Reduced Graphene Oxide (RGO) Sensor Based on a Peptide Aptamer Receptor for Detecting Explosives. *Sci. Rep.* **2019**, *9*, 10297. [CrossRef]
35. Ponnamperuma, C.; Peterson, E. Peptide Synthesis from Amino Acids in Aqueous Solution. *Science* **1965**, *147*, 1572–1574. [CrossRef] [PubMed]
36. Palomo, J.M. Solid-Phase Peptide Synthesis: An Overview Focused on the Preparation of Biologically Relevant Peptides. *RSC Adv.* **2014**, *4*, 32658–32672. [CrossRef]
37. Gordon, C.P. The Renascence of Continuous-Flow Peptide Synthesi—An Abridged Account of Solid and Solution-Based Approaches. *Org. Biomol. Chem.* **2018**, *16*, 180–196. [CrossRef]
38. Rosenberg, R.A.; Rozhkova, E.A.; Novosad, V. Investigations into Spin- and Unpolarized Secondary Electron-Induced Reactions in Self-Assembled Monolayers of Cysteine. *Langmuir* **2021**, *37*, 2985–2992. [CrossRef]
39. Secchi, V.; Franchi, S.; Santi, M.; Dettin, M.; Zamuner, A.; Iucci, G.; Battocchio, C. Self-Assembling Behavior of Cysteine-Modified Oligopeptides: An XPS and NEXAFS Study. *J. Phys. Chem. C* **2018**, *122*, 6236–6239. [CrossRef]
40. Piccoli, J.P.; Santos, A.; Santos-Filho, N.A.; Lorenzón, E.N.; Cilli, E.M.; Bueno, P.R. The Self-Assembly of Redox Active Peptides: Synthesis and Electrochemical Capacitive Behavior. *Biopolymers* **2016**, 357–367. [CrossRef]
41. Wang, Y.; Cui, M.; Jiao, M.; Luo, X. Antifouling and Ultrasensitive Biosensing Interface Based on Self-Assembled Peptide and Aptamer on Macroporous Gold for Electrochemical Detection of Immunoglobulin E in Serum. *Anal. Bioanal. Chem.* **2018**, *410*, 5871–5878. [CrossRef] [PubMed]
42. Piccoli, J.; Hein, R.; El-Sagheer, A.H.; Brown, T.; Cilli, E.M.; Bueno, P.R.; Davis, J.J. Redox Capacitive Assaying of C-Reactive Protein at a Peptide Supported Aptamer Interface. *Anal. Chem.* **2018**, *90*, 3005–3008. [CrossRef]
43. Reynoso, E.C.; Torres, E.; Bettazzi, F.; Palchetti, I. Trends and Perspectives in Immunosensors for Determination of Currently-Used Pesticides: The Case of Glyphosate, Organophosphates, and Neonicotinoids. *Biosensors* **2019**, *9*, 20. [CrossRef] [PubMed]
44. Lin, P.-H.; Li, B.-R. Antifouling Strategies in Advanced Electrochemical Sensors and Biosensors. *Analyst* **2020**, *145*, 1110–1120. [CrossRef] [PubMed]
45. Campuzano, S.; Pedrero, M.; Yáñez-Sedeño, P.; Pingarrón, J. Antifouling (Bio)Materials for Electrochemical (Bio)Sensing. *Int. J. Mol. Sci.* **2019**, *20*, 423. [CrossRef]
46. Ostuni, E.; Chapman, R.G.; Holmlin, R.E.; Takayama, S.; Whitesides, G.M. A Survey of Structure−Property Relationships of Surfaces That Resist the Adsorption of Protein. *Langmuir* **2001**, *17*, 5605–5620. [CrossRef]
47. Wei, Q.; Becherer, T.; Angioletti-Uberti, S.; Dzubiella, J.; Wischke, C.; Neffe, A.T.; Lendlein, A.; Ballauff, M.; Haag, R. Protein Interactions with Polymer Coatings and Biomaterials. *Angew. Chem. Int. Ed.* **2014**, *53*, 8004–8031. [CrossRef]
48. Ye, H.; Wang, L.; Huang, R.; Su, R.; Liu, B.; Qi, W.; He, Z. Superior Antifouling Performance of a Zwitterionic Peptide Compared to an Amphiphilic, Non-Ionic Peptide. *ACS Appl. Mater. Interfaces* **2015**, *7*, 22448–22457. [CrossRef]
49. Nowinski, A.K.; Sun, F.; White, A.D.; Keefe, A.J.; Jiang, S. Sequence, Structure, and Function of Peptide Self-Assembled Monolayers. *J. Am. Chem. Soc.* **2012**, *134*, 6000–6005. [CrossRef] [PubMed]
50. Yawitz, T.M.; Patterson, K.S.; Onkst, B.X.; Youmbi, F.; Clark, R.A. Cytochrome c Electrochemistry on Peptide Self-Assembled Monolayers. *J. Electroanal. Chem.* **2018**, *828*, 59–62. [CrossRef]
51. Song, Z.; Ma, Y.; Chen, M.; Ambrosi, A.; Ding, C.; Luo, X. Electrochemical Biosensor with Enhanced Antifouling Capability for COVID-19 Nucleic Acid Detection in Complex Biological Media. *Anal. Chem.* **2021**, *93*, 5963–5971. [CrossRef]
52. Liu, N.; Fan, X.; Hou, H.; Gao, F.; Luo, X. Electrochemical Sensing Interfaces Based on Hierarchically Architectured Zwitterionic Peptides for Ultralow Fouling Detection of Alpha Fetoprotein in Serum. *Anal. Chim. Acta* **2021**, *1146*, 17–23. [CrossRef]
53. Liu, N.; Ma, Y.; Han, R.; Lv, S.; Wang, P.; Luo, X. Antifouling Biosensors for Reliable Protein Quantification in Serum Based on Designed All-in-One Branched Peptides. *Chem. Commun.* **2021**, *57*, 777–780. [CrossRef] [PubMed]
54. Wang, D.; Wang, J.; Song, Z.; Hui, N. Highly Selective and Antifouling Electrochemical Biosensors for Sensitive MicroRNA Assaying Based on Conducting Polymer Polyaniline Functionalized with Zwitterionic Peptide. *Anal. Bioanal. Chem.* **2021**, *413*, 543–553. [CrossRef] [PubMed]
55. Wang, G.; Han, R.; Li, Q.; Han, Y.; Luo, X. Electrochemical Biosensors Capable of Detecting Biomarkers in Human Serum with Unique Long-Term Antifouling Abilities Based on Designed Multifunctional Peptides. *Anal. Chem.* **2020**, *92*, 7186–7193. [CrossRef] [PubMed]
56. Song, Z.; Chen, M.; Ding, C.; Luo, X. Designed Three-in-One Peptides with Anchoring, Antifouling, and Recognizing Capabilities for Highly Sensitive and Low-Fouling Electrochemical Sensing in Complex Biological Media. *Anal. Chem.* **2020**, *92*, 5795–5802. [CrossRef]
57. Liu, N.; Hui, N.; Davis, J.J.; Luo, X. Low Fouling Protein Detection in Complex Biological Media Supported by a Designed Multifunctional Peptide. *ACS Sens.* **2018**, *3*, 1210–1216. [CrossRef] [PubMed]
58. Huang, S.; Tang, R.; Zhang, T.; Zhao, J.; Jiang, Z.; Wang, Q. Anti-Fouling Poly Adenine Coating Combined with Highly Specific CD20 Epitope Mimetic Peptide for Rituximab Detection in Clinical Patients' Plasma. *Biosens. Bioelectron.* **2021**, *171*, 112678. [CrossRef] [PubMed]
59. Chen, M.; Song, Z.; Han, R.; Li, Y.; Luo, X. Low Fouling Electrochemical Biosensors Based on Designed Y-Shaped Peptides with Antifouling and Recognizing Branches for the Detection of IgG in Human Serum. *Biosens. Bioelectron.* **2021**, *178*, 113016. [CrossRef]

60. Liu, N.; Song, J.; Lu, Y.; Davis, J.J.; Gao, F.; Luo, X. Electrochemical Aptasensor for Ultralow Fouling Cancer Cell Quantification in Complex Biological Media Based on Designed Branched Peptides. *Anal. Chem.* **2019**, *91*, 8334–8340. [CrossRef]
61. Ding, C.; Wang, X.; Luo, X. Dual-Mode Electrochemical Assay of Prostate-Specific Antigen Based on Antifouling Peptides Functionalized with Electrochemical Probes and Internal References. *Anal. Chem.* **2019**, *91*, 15846–15852. [CrossRef]
62. Xu, Y.; Wang, X.; Ding, C.; Luo, X. Ratiometric Antifouling Electrochemical Biosensors Based on Multifunctional Peptides and MXene Loaded with Au Nanoparticles and Methylene Blue. *ACS Appl. Mater. Interfaces* **2021**, *13*, 20388–20396. [CrossRef]
63. Wang, S.; Ma, Y.; Wang, Y.; Jiao, M.; Luo, X.; Cui, M. One-Step Electrodeposition of Poly(m-Aminobenzoic Acid) Membrane Decorated with Peptide for Antifouling Biosensing of Immunoglobulin, E. *Colloids Surf. B Biointerfaces* **2020**, *186*, 110706. [CrossRef]
64. González-Fernández, E.; Staderini, M.; Yussof, A.; Scholefield, E.; Murray, A.F.; Mount, A.R.; Bradley, M. Electrochemical Sensing of Human Neutrophil Elastase and Polymorphonuclear Neutrophil Activity. *Biosens. Bioelectron.* **2018**, *119*, 209–214. [CrossRef] [PubMed]
65. Hu, Q.; Su, L.; Mao, Y.; Gan, S.; Bao, Y.; Qin, D.; Wang, W.; Zhang, Y.; Niu, L. Electrochemically Induced Grafting of Ferrocenyl Polymers for Ultrasensitive Cleavage-Based Interrogation of Matrix Metalloproteinase Activity. *Biosens. Bioelectron.* **2021**, *178*, 113010. [CrossRef]
66. Ye, Z.; Li, G.; Xu, L.; Yu, Q.; Yue, X.; Wu, Y.; Ye, B. Peptide-Conjugated Hemin/G-Quadruplex as a Versatile Probe for "Signal-on" Electrochemical Peptide Biosensor. *Talanta* **2020**, *209*, 120611. [CrossRef] [PubMed]
67. González-Fernández, E.; Staderini, M.; Avlonitis, N.; Murray, A.F.; Mount, A.R.; Bradley, M. Effect of Spacer Length on the Performance of Peptide-Based Electrochemical Biosensors for Protease Detection. *Sens. Actuators B Chem.* **2018**, *255*, 3040–3046. [CrossRef]
68. Cox, T.R. The Matrix in Cancer. *Nat. Rev. Cancer* **2021**, *21*, 217–238. [CrossRef] [PubMed]
69. Zheng, Y.; Ma, Z. Dual-Reaction Triggered Sensitivity Amplification for Ultrasensitive Peptide-Cleavage Based Electrochemical Detection of Matrix Metalloproteinase-7. *Biosens. Bioelectron.* **2018**, *108*, 46–52. [CrossRef]
70. Sun, L.; Chen, Y.; Chen, F.; Ma, F. Peptide-Based Electrochemical Biosensor for Matrix Metalloproteinase-14 and Protein-Overexpressing Cancer Cells Based on Analyte-Induced Cleavage of Peptide. *Microchem. J.* **2020**, *157*, 105103. [CrossRef]
71. Lin, Y.; Shen, R.; Liu, N.; Yi, H.; Dai, H.; Lin, J. A Highly Sensitive Peptide-Based Biosensor Using $NiCo_2O_4$ Nanosheets and g-C_3N_4 Nanocomposite to Construct Amplified Strategy for Trypsin Detection. *Anal. Chim. Acta* **2018**, *1035*, 175–183. [CrossRef]
72. Palomar, Q.; Xu, X.X.; Selegård, R.; Aili, D.; Zhang, Z. Peptide Decorated Gold Nanoparticle/Carbon Nanotube Electrochemical Sensor for Ultrasensitive Detection of Matrix Metalloproteinase-7. *Sens. Actuators B Chem.* **2020**, *325*, 128789. [CrossRef]
73. Campuzano, S.; Pedrero, M.; Yáñez-Sedeño, P.; Pingarrón, J.M. Nanozymes in Electrochemical Affinity Biosensing. *Microchim. Acta* **2020**, *187*, 1–16. [CrossRef]
74. Mahmudunnabi, R.G.; Farhana, F.Z.; Kashaninejad, N.; Firoz, S.H.; Shim, Y.B.; Shiddiky, M.J.A. Nanozyme-Based Electrochemical Biosensors for Disease Biomarker Detection. *Analyst* **2020**, *145*, 4398–4420. [CrossRef]
75. Xi, X.; Wen, M.; Song, S.; Zhu, J.; Wen, W.; Zhang, X.; Wang, S. A H2O2-Free Electrochemical Peptide Biosensor Based on Au@Pt Bimetallic Nanorods for Highly Sensitive Sensing of Matrix Metalloproteinase 2. *Chem. Commun.* **2020**, *56*, 6039–6042. [CrossRef] [PubMed]
76. Cheng, W.; Ma, J.; Kong, D.; Zhang, Z.; Khan, A.; Yi, C.; Hu, K.; Yi, Y.; Li, J. One Step Electrochemical Detection for Matrix Metalloproteinase 2 Based on Anodic Stripping of Silver Nanoparticles Mediated by Host-Guest Interactions. *Sens. Actuators B Chem.* **2021**, *330*, 129379. [CrossRef]
77. Kim, S.; Sikes, H.D. Radical Polymerization Reactions for Amplified Biodetection Signals. *Polym. Chem.* **2020**, *11*, 1424–1444. [CrossRef]
78. Hu, Q.; Bao, Y.; Gan, S.; Zhang, Y.; Han, D.; Niu, L. Amplified Electrochemical Biosensing of Thrombin Activity by RAFT Polymerization. *Anal. Chem.* **2020**, *92*, 3470–3476. [CrossRef] [PubMed]
79. Wang, Q.; Liu, J.; Yu, S.; Sun, H.; Wang, L.; Li, L.; Kong, J.; Zhang, X. A Highly Sensitive Assay for Matrix Metalloproteinase 2 via Signal Amplification Strategy of EATRP. *Microchem. J.* **2021**, *164*, 106015. [CrossRef]
80. Hu, Q.; Gan, S.; Bao, Y.; Zhang, Y.; Han, D.; Niu, L. Electrochemically Controlled ATRP for Cleavage-Based Electrochemical Detection of the Prostate-Specific Antigen at Femtomolar Level Concentrations. *Anal. Chem.* **2020**, *92*, 15982–15988. [CrossRef] [PubMed]
81. Chang, Y.; Wang, M.; Wang, L.; Xia, N. Recent Progress in Electrochemical Biosensors for Detection of Prostate-Specific Antigen. *Int. J. Electrochem. Sci.* **2018**, *13*, 4071–4084. [CrossRef]
82. Dowlatshahi, S.; Abdekhodaie, M.J. Electrochemical Prostate-Specific Antigen Biosensors Based on Electroconductive Nanomaterials and Polymers. *Clin. Chim. Acta* **2021**, *516*, 111–135. [CrossRef] [PubMed]
83. Meng, F.; Sun, H.; Huang, Y.; Tang, Y.; Chen, Q.; Miao, P. Peptide Cleavage-Based Electrochemical Biosensor Coupling Graphene Oxide and Silver Nanoparticles. *Anal. Chim. Acta* **2019**, *1047*, 45–51. [CrossRef] [PubMed]
84. Yu, Q.; Wu, Y.; Liu, Z.; Lei, S.; Li, G.; Ye, B. Novel Electrochemical Biosensor Based on Cationic Peptide Modified Hemin/G-Quadruples Enhanced Peroxidase-like Activity. *Biosens. Bioelectron.* **2018**, *107*, 178–183. [CrossRef]
85. Eissa, S.; Zourob, M. Ultrasensitive Peptide-Based Multiplexed Electrochemical Biosensor for the Simultaneous Detection of *Listeria monocytogenes* and *Staphylococcus aureus*. *Microchim. Acta* **2020**, *187*, 1–11. [CrossRef]

86. Armanetti, P.; Flori, A.; Àvigo, C.; Conti, L.; Valtancoli, B.; Petroni, D.; Doumett, S.; Cappiello, L.; Ravagli, C.; Baldi, G.; et al. Spectroscopic and Photoacoustic Characterization of Encapsulated Iron Oxide Super-Paramagnetic Nanoparticles as a New Multiplatform Contrast Agent. *Spectrochim. Acta Part A Mol. Biomol. Spectrosc.* **2018**, *199*, 248–253. [CrossRef]
87. Baydemir, G.; Bettazzi, F.; Palchetti, I.; Voccia, D. Strategies for the Development of an Electrochemical Bioassay for TNF-Alpha Detection by Using a Non-Immunoglobulin Bioreceptor. *Talanta* **2016**, *151*, 141–147. [CrossRef]
88. Bettazzi, F.; Enayati, L.; Sánchez, I.C.; Motaghed, R.; Mascini, M.; Palchetti, I. Electrochemical Bioassay for the Detection of TNF-α Using Magnetic Beads and Disposable Screen-Printed Array of Electrodes. *Bioanalysis* **2013**, *5*, 11–19. [CrossRef]
89. Muñoz-San Martín, C.; Pedrero, M.; Gamella, M.; Montero-Calle, A.; Barderas, R.; Campuzano, S.; Pingarrón, J.M. A Novel Peptide-Based Electrochemical Biosensor for the Determination of a Metastasis-Linked Protease in Pancreatic Cancer Cells. *Anal. Bioanal. Chem.* **2020**, *412*, 6177–6188. [CrossRef] [PubMed]
90. Forster, R.J. Microelectrodes: New Dimensions in Electrochemistry. *Chem. Soc. Rev.* **1994**, *23*, 289. [CrossRef]
91. Hu, Q.; Kong, J.; Han, D.; Bao, Y.; Zhang, X.; Zhang, Y.; Niu, L. Ultrasensitive Peptide-Based Electrochemical Detection of Protein Kinase Activity Amplified by RAFT Polymerization. *Talanta* **2020**, *206*, 120173. [CrossRef]
92. Hu, Q.; Kong, J.; Han, D.; Zhang, Y.; Bao, Y.; Zhang, X.; Niu, L. Electrochemically Controlled RAFT Polymerization for Highly Sensitive Electrochemical Biosensing of Protein Kinase Activity. *Anal. Chem.* **2019**, *91*, 1936–1943. [CrossRef] [PubMed]
93. Sun, Z.; Wang, L.; Wu, S.; Pan, Y.; Dong, Y.; Zhu, S.; Yang, J.; Yin, Y.; Li, G. An Electrochemical Biosensor Designed by Using Zr-Based Metal–Organic Frameworks for the Detection of Glioblastoma-Derived Exosomes with Practical Application. *Anal. Chem.* **2020**, *92*, 3819–3826. [CrossRef]
94. Ostatná, V.; Kasalová, V.; Sommerová, L.; Hrstka, R. Electrochemical Sensing of Interaction of Anterior Gradient-2 Protein with Peptides at a Charged Interface. *Electrochim. Acta* **2018**, *269*, 70–75. [CrossRef]
95. Wang, Z.; Xu, E.; Wang, C.; Wei, W.; Liu, Y.; Liu, S. High Specificity and Efficiency Electrochemical Detection of Poly(ADP-Ribose) Polymerase-1 Activity Based on Versatile Peptide-Templated Copper Nanoparticles and Detection Array. *Anal. Chim. Acta* **2019**, *1091*, 95–102. [CrossRef] [PubMed]
96. Tang, Y.; Dai, Y.; Huang, X.; Li, L.; Han, B.; Cao, Y.; Zhao, J. Self-Assembling Peptide-Based Multifunctional Nanofibers for Electrochemical Identification of Breast Cancer Stem-like Cells. *Anal. Chem.* **2019**, *91*, 7531–7537. [CrossRef]
97. Global Cancer Observatory (GLOBOCAN). Available online: https://gco.iarc.fr/today/online-analysis-pie?v=2020&mode=cancer&mode_population=conti-nents&population=900&populations=900&key=total&sex=0&cancer=39&type=0&statistic=5&prevalence=0&population_group=0&ages_group%5B%5D=0&ages_group%5B%5D=17&nb_items=7&grou (accessed on 28 May 2021).
98. Wu, Y.; Li, G.; Zou, L.; Lei, S.; Yu, Q.; Ye, B. Highly Active DNAzyme-Peptide Hybrid Structure Coupled Porous Palladium for High-Performance Electrochemical Aptasensing Platform. *Sens. Actuators B Chem.* **2018**, *259*, 372–379. [CrossRef]
99. Yaman, Y.T.; Akbal, Ö.; Bolat, G.; Bozdogan, B.; Denkbas, E.B.; Abaci, S. Peptide Nanoparticles (PNPs) Modified Disposable Platform for Sensitive Electrochemical Cytosensing of DLD-1 Cancer Cells. *Biosens. Bioelectron.* **2018**, *104*, 50–57. [CrossRef]
100. Cho, C.H.; Kim, J.H.; Kim, J.; Yun, J.W.; Park, T.J.; Park, J.P. Re-Engineering of Peptides with High Binding Affinity to Develop an Advanced Electrochemical Sensor for Colon Cancer Diagnosis. *Anal. Chim. Acta* **2021**, *1146*, 131–139. [CrossRef]
101. Georgieva, S.; Todorov, P.; Peneva, P.; Varbanov, M.; Gartsiyanova, K. VV-Hemorphin-5 Analogue for Trace Copper Determination in Water Samples. *J. Iran. Chem. Soc.* **2020**, *17*, 2885–2894. [CrossRef]
102. Zhang, K.; Zhou, L.; Zhang, T.; Fan, Z.; Xie, M.; Ding, Y.; Li, H. Peptide Based Biosensing of Protein Functional Control Indicates Novel Mechanism of Cancerous Development under Oxidative Stress. *Sens. Actuators B Chem.* **2021**, *329*, 129121. [CrossRef]
103. Lee, M.H.; Liu, K.T.; Thomas, J.L.; Su, Z.L.; O'Hare, D.; Van Wuellen, T.; Chamarro, J.M.; Bolognin, S.; Luo, S.C.; Schwamborn, J.C.; et al. Peptide-Imprinted Poly(Hydroxymethyl 3,4-Ethylenedioxythiophene) Nanotubes for Detection of α Synuclein in Human Brain Organoids. *ACS Appl. Nano Mater.* **2020**, *3*, 8027–8036. [CrossRef]
104. Negahdary, M.; Heli, H. An Electrochemical Peptide-Based Biosensor for the Alzheimer Biomarker Amyloid-β(1–42) Using a Microporous Gold Nanostructure. *Microchim. Acta* **2019**, *186*, 1–8. [CrossRef]
105. Zhang, K.; Yang, Q.; Fan, Z.; Zhao, J.; Li, H. Platelet-Driven Formation of Interface Peptide Nano-Network Biosensor Enabling a Non-Invasive Means for Early Detection of Alzheimer's Disease. *Biosens. Bioelectron.* **2019**, *145*, 111701. [CrossRef] [PubMed]
106. Huang, Y.; Zhang, B.; Yuan, L.; Liu, L. A Signal Amplification Strategy Based on Peptide Self-Assembly for the Identification of Amyloid-β Oligomer. *Sens. Actuators B Chem.* **2021**, *335*, 129697. [CrossRef]
107. He, Y.; Zhou, L.; Deng, L.; Feng, Z.; Cao, Z.; Yin, Y. An Electrochemical Impedimetric Sensing Platform Based on a Peptide Aptamer Identified by High-Throughput Molecular Docking for Sensitive l-Arginine Detection. *Bioelectrochemistry* **2021**, *137*, 107634. [CrossRef] [PubMed]
108. Chinnadayyala, S.R.; Cho, S. Electrochemical Immunosensor for the Early Detection of Rheumatoid Arthritis Biomarker: Anti-Cyclic Citrullinated Peptide Antibody in Human Serum Based on Avidin-Biotin System. *Sensors* **2021**, *21*, 124. [CrossRef]
109. Guerrero, S.; Sánchez-Tirado, E.; Martínez-García, G.; González-Cortés, A.; Yáñez-Sedeño, P.; Pingarrón, J.M. Electrochemical Biosensor for the Simultaneous Determination of Rheumatoid Factor and Anti-Cyclic Citrullinated Peptide Antibodies in Human Serum. *Analyst* **2020**, *145*, 4680–4687. [CrossRef]
110. Cho, C.H.; Kim, J.H.; Song, D.-K.; Park, T.J.; Park, J.P. An Affinity Peptide-Incorporated Electrochemical Biosensor for the Detection of Neutrophil Gelatinase-Associated Lipocalin. *Biosens. Bioelectron.* **2019**, *142*, 111482. [CrossRef]

111. Ma, F.; Zhu, Y.; Chen, Y.; Liu, J.; Zeng, X. Labeled and Non-Label Electrochemical Peptide Inhibitor-Based Biosensing Platform for Determination of Hemopexin Domain of Matrix Metalloproteinase-14. *Talanta* **2019**, *194*, 548–553. [CrossRef]
112. Ma, F.; Yan, J.; Sun, L.; Chen, Y. Electrochemical Impedance Spectroscopy for Quantization of Matrix Metalloproteinase-14 Based on Peptides Inhibiting Its Homodimerization and Heterodimerization. *Talanta* **2019**, *205*, 120142. [CrossRef]
113. Kim, J.H.; Cho, C.H.; Ryu, M.Y.; Kim, J.-G.; Lee, S.-J.; Park, T.J.; Park, J.P. Development of Peptide Biosensor for the Detection of Dengue Fever Biomarker, Nonstructural 1. *PLoS ONE* **2019**, *14*, e0222144. [CrossRef]
114. Baek, S.H.; Kim, M.W.; Park, C.Y.; Choi, C.-S.; Kailasa, S.K.; Park, J.P.; Park, T.J. Development of a Rapid and Sensitive Electrochemical Biosensor for Detection of Human Norovirus via Novel Specific Binding Peptides. *Biosens. Bioelectron.* **2019**, *123*, 223–229. [CrossRef]
115. Baek, S.H.; Park, C.Y.; Nguyen, T.P.; Kim, M.W.; Park, J.P.; Choi, C.; Kim, S.Y.; Kailasa, S.K.; Park, T.J. Novel Peptides Functionalized Gold Nanoparticles Decorated Tungsten Disulfide Nanoflowers as the Electrochemical Sensing Platforms for the Norovirus in an Oyster. *Food Control.* **2020**, *114*, 107225. [CrossRef]
116. Matsubara, T.; Ujie, M.; Yamamoto, T.; Einaga, Y.; Daidoji, T.; Nakaya, T.; Sato, T. Avian Influenza Virus Detection by Optimized Peptide Termination on a Boron-Doped Diamond Electrode. *ACS Sens.* **2020**, *5*, 431–439. [CrossRef] [PubMed]
117. Wilson, D.; Materón, E.M.; Ibáñez-Redín, G.; Faria, R.C.; Correa, D.S.; Oliveira, O.N. Electrical Detection of Pathogenic Bacteria in Food Samples Using Information Visualization Methods with a Sensor Based on Magnetic Nanoparticles Functionalized with Antimicrobial Peptides. *Talanta* **2019**, *194*, 611–618. [CrossRef]
118. Yu, N.; Zhang, X.; Gao, Y.; You, H.; Zhang, J.; Miao, P. Highly Sensitive Endotoxin Assay Combining Peptide/Graphene Oxide and DNA-Modified Gold Nanoparticles. *ACS Omega* **2019**, *4*, 14312–14316. [CrossRef] [PubMed]

biosensors

MDPI

Review

State of the Art on the SARS-CoV-2 Toolkit for Antigen Detection: One Year Later

Laura Fabiani [1], Veronica Caratelli [1], Luca Fiore [1], Viviana Scognamiglio [2], Amina Antonacci [2], Silvia Fillo [3], Riccardo De Santis [3], Anella Monte [3], Manfredo Bortone [3], Danila Moscone [1], Florigio Lista [3] and Fabiana Arduini [1,4,*]

1 Department of Chemical Science and Technologies, University of Rome "Tor Vergata", Via della Ricerca Scientifica, 00133 Rome, Italy; laura.fabiani@uniroma2.it (L.F.); veronica.caratelli@uniroma2.it (V.C.); luca.fiore@uniroma2.it (L.F.); moscone@uniroma2.it (D.M.)
2 Institute of Crystallography (IC-CNR), Department of Chemical Sciences and Materials Technologies, Via Salaria km 29.300, 00015 Monterotondo, Italy; viviana.scognamiglio@ic.cnr.it (V.S.); amina.antonacci@ic.cnr.it (A.A.)
3 Scientific Department, Army Medical Center, Via Santo Stefano Rotondo 4, 00184 Rome, Italy; silviafillo@gmail.com (S.F.); riccardo.desantis@gmail.com (R.D.S.); nellymonte88@gmail.com (A.M.); fabiana_arduini@yahoo.it (M.B.); romano.lista@gmail.com (F.L.)
4 SENSE4MED, via Renato Rascel 30, 00128 Rome, Italy
* Correspondence: fabiana.arduini@uniroma2.it

Abstract: The recent global events of COVID-19 in 2020 have alerted the world to the risk of viruses and their impacts on human health, including their impacts in the social and economic sectors. Rapid tests are urgently required to enable antigen detection and thus to facilitate rapid and simple evaluations of contagious individuals, with the overriding goal to delimitate spread of the virus among the population. Many efforts have been achieved in recent months through the realization of novel diagnostic tools for rapid, affordable, and accurate analysis, thereby enabling prompt responses to the pandemic infection. This review reports the latest results on electrochemical and optical biosensors realized for the specific detection of SARS-CoV-2 antigens, thus providing an overview of the available diagnostics tested and marketed for SARS-CoV-2 antigens as well as their pros and cons.

Keywords: SARS-CoV-2 detection; nasopharyngeal swab; saliva; serum; droplets

Citation: Fabiani, L.; Caratelli, V.; Fiore, L.; Scognamiglio, V.; Antonacci, A.; Fillo, S.; De Santis, R.; Monte, A.; Bortone, M.; Moscone, D.; et al. State of the Art on the SARS-CoV-2 Toolkit for Antigen Detection: One Year Later. *Biosensors* **2021**, *11*, 310. https://doi.org/10.3390/bios11090310

Received: 30 June 2021
Accepted: 18 August 2021
Published: 31 August 2021

1. Introduction

Since the early 1900s, diverse pathogenic viruses have been identified to cause severe diseases worldwide, including Rift Valley fever (1931), Crimean Congo hemorrhagic fever (1944), Zika virus (1947), Chikungunya (1952), Marburg (1967), Lassa fever (1969), Ebola virus (1976), human immunodeficiency virus (1980), Nipah (1998), severe acute respiratory syndrome (SARS, 2003), influenza A virus (2009), and Middle East respiratory syndrome coronavirus (MERS, 2012), among others (Figure 1A) [1]. In 2020, severe acute respiratory syndrome-coronavirus (SARS-CoV-2) caused an outbreak of the respiratory disease named COVID-19, which has had a significant impact on human health and in all economic sectors [2], leading to the most serious socioeconomic crisis since World War II [3].

Initially, the diagnosis of COVID-19 was usually carried out in the hospital by medical imaging through high-cost instrumentation and skilled personnel, including the use of computed tomography, radiograph X-rays, ultrasound, echocardiograms, and magnetic resonance imaging (Figure 1B) [4]. However, considering the wide spread of COVID-19, the availability of a cost-effective and laboratory-free detection method would help to prevent outbreaks of the virus and lessen its associated mortality.

In general, SARS-CoV-2 detection systems are divided into three general categories: (i) RNA-based diagnostics, (ii) antigen-based diagnostics, and (iii) antibody-based diagnostics (Figure 1C) [5].

To establish a unique approach in the application of the available diagnostics, the European Commission (EU) released "Guidelines on COVID-19 for in vitro diagnostic tests and their performance (2020/C 122 I/01)". The aim of this publication was to outline the regulatory context of the in vitro diagnostic devices used in EU countries and provide an overview of the different procedures and purposes of these tests. In detail, the tests available today for COVID-19 fall broadly into two categories: (i) tests based on evaluating the contagiousness of SARS-CoV-2 through the detection of viral genetic material (Polymerase Chain Reaction) and viral components, such as proteins on the virus surface (antigen tests); and (ii) tests that estimate exposure to the virus based on the immune response of the human body to the infection. However, the EU also highlighted that diagnostics for immune response have been not able to provide "a definite answer on the presence or absence of the SARS-CoV-2 virus and thus they are not suitable to assess if the tested individual may be contagious for others. Nevertheless, antibody tests could prove essential for performing large-scale sero-epidemiological population surveys for assessing, e.g., the immune status of workers and as one of the elements for guiding de-escalation strategies when the pandemic is under control" [6].

For this reason, rapid tests are urgently required for antigen detection to easily and quickly evaluate contagious individuals and thus delimitate spread of the virus among the population. To this end, on 30 January 2020, the EC promptly launched a Call for Projects entitled "SC1-PHECORONAVIRUS-2020: Advancing knowledge for the clinical and public health response to the [COVID-19] epidemic", featuring 18 Projects with a budget of EUR 48.5 million and involving 151 research groups across Europe and beyond, for research activities devoted to counteracting the COVID-19 emergency [7]. Four main pillars have been proposed based on: (i) infection monitoring systems, (ii) point-of-care diagnostic tests, (iii) new treatments, and (iv) the development of new vaccines. Among them, the requirement for novel rapid diagnostics "will concentrate on enabling front-line health workers to make the diagnosis more quickly and more accurately, which will, in turn, reduce the risk of further spread of the virus", according to the EC.

The following projects have been awarded support for the development of novel diagnostics:

- CoNVat: Combating 2019-nCoV: Advanced Nanobiosensing platforms for POC global diagnostics and surveillance to develop a point-of-care device using optical biosensor technology for rapid diagnosis and monitoring of the new coronavirus directly in the patient's sample (four partners: ES(2), FR, and IT) [8].
- CORONADX: Three rapid diagnostic tests (point-of-care) for COVID-19 Coronavirus, improving epidemic preparedness, public health, and socioeconomic benefits to deliver three complementary diagnostic tools, including one point-of-care diagnostic that can be used with minimal training (eight partners: AT, CN(2), DK(2), IT(2), and SE) [9].
- HG nCoV19 test: Development and validation of a rapid molecular diagnostic test for nCoV19 to develop and validate a novel rapid molecular diagnostic test for coronavirus (four partners: CN, IE, IT, and UK) [10].

It is evident that the high potential of diagnostics could help improve knowledge on virus diffusion, as well as diminish the danger of further spread, considering the continuous emergence and re-emergence of viral infections, as highlighted by Cheng et al. [11]. As the authors asserted, "The findings that horseshoe bats are the natural reservoir for SARS-CoV-like virus and that civet are the amplification host highlight the importance of wildlife and biosecurity in farms and wet markets, which can serve as the source and amplification centers for emerging infections".

Therefore, early-stage detection of viral infection could help to circumvent further infection from highly contagious viruses and prevent viral disease morbidity and premature death among the worldwide population. To highlight the relevance of biosensors as smart analytical tools, several authors reviewed the advantages and disadvantages of the many biosensing configurations realized for the detection of viruses [12–14]. Eden Morales-Narváez and Can Dincer discussed the potential of using biosensing tools beyond PCR-based systems, reporting that "researchers around the world are pushing hard to develop different methods and devices, allowing an easy, rapid, affordable and highly sensitive and selective quantification of nucleic acids in low resource settings (such as doctors' practices, or directly at home)" [15]. This review, to our knowledge, was the first on the topic of biosensors and COVID-19, and its impact as a widely cited paper was recently recognized by Clarivate Web of Science (May 2021). Afterward, other reviews were published, highlighting how nanotechnology [13–15] plays a crucial role in the design of reliable and miniaturized devices.

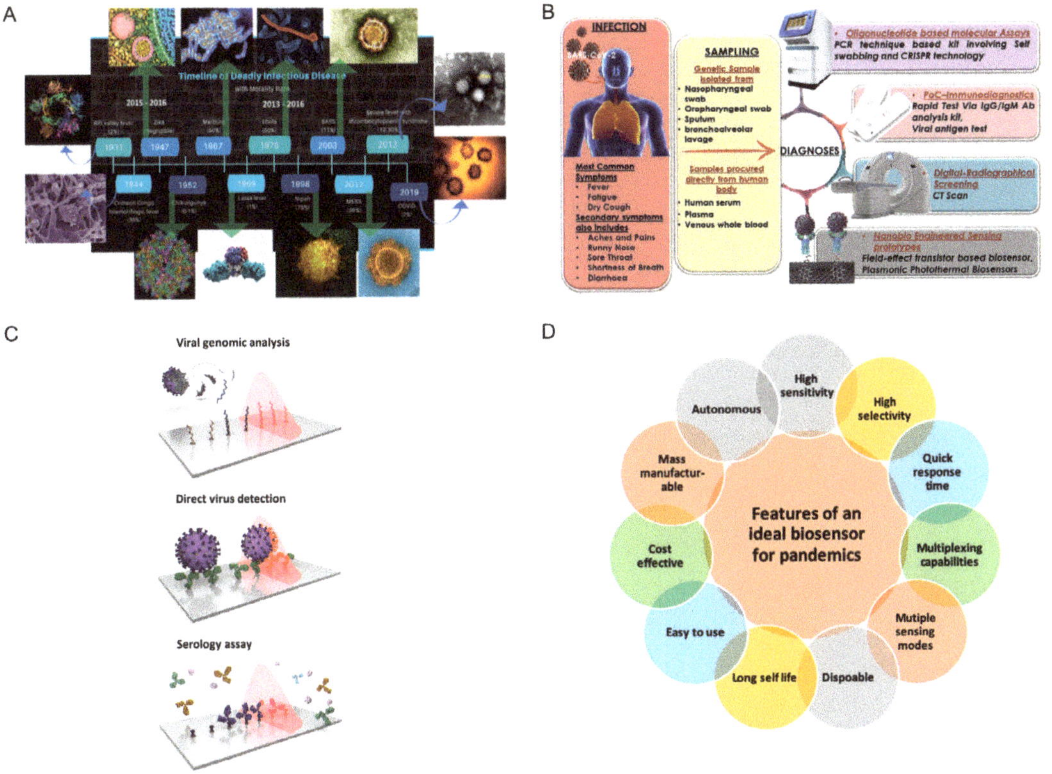

Figure 1. (**A**) Timeline of virus-based diseases. Reprinted with permission from [1], 2021 Elsevier. (**B**) different diagnostic methods for COVID-19. Reprinted with permission from [4], 2020 Elsevier. (**C**) different strategies for biosensing tool development in the COVID-19 outbreak. Reprinted with permission from [5], 2020 American Chemical Society and (**D**) features of an ideal biosensor for pandemics. Reprinted with permission from [16], 2020 American Chemical Society.

The lessons learned during the first year of the COVID-19 pandemic guided the design of innovative toolkits with strong potential to be exploited for wide screening under low resource settings. As outlined by Bhalla et al. [16], an ideal biosensor for effective use in pandemics should be single-use and offer a long shelf life, ease of use, cost-effectiveness, mass-manufacturing ability, autonomy, high sensitivity, high selectivity, rapidity, multiplexing capabilities, and multiple sensing modes (Figure 1D). The convergence of interdisciplinary technologies represents an immediate solution for the main bottlenecks constraining biosensor prototypes to achieve real applications with the desirable features. Such technologies include: (i) nanomaterial technology to improve the analytical figures of merit; (ii) microfluidics to enhance biosensor performance in terms of sustainability (by decreasing the use of reagents and waste volume), automation, and suitability for in-field analysis; (iii) smartphone-assisted technology to support the realization of easy-to-use and portable systems, thus boosting data transmission and management in a timely fashion; and (iv) wearable tools to help collect previously inaccessible physical and biochemical signals, including those from epidermal tattoos, contact lenses, textiles, face masks, wristbands, and patches [17].

This review provides an overview of the biosensors for SARS-CoV-2 antigens available in the literature and tested on real matrices, such as nasopharynx swabs, saliva, serum, and droplets, approximately one year after the start of the COVID-19 outbreak. Indeed, beyond the development of biosensors for RNA sequences and antibodies, the detection of antigens such as the SARS-CoV-2 spike (S) protein and SARS-CoV-2 nucleocapsid (N) protein by biosensing tools has attracted significant attention. The pros and cons for the detection of S and N proteins are also highlighted to develop a feasible strategy for fabricating an ideal biosensor for the specific detection of SARS-CoV-2, thereby overcoming the limitation of commercially available lateral-flow immunosensors (Figure 2 and Table 1), which encompass the use of invasive nasopharyngeal swabs as the sampling system, which offers lower sensitivity.

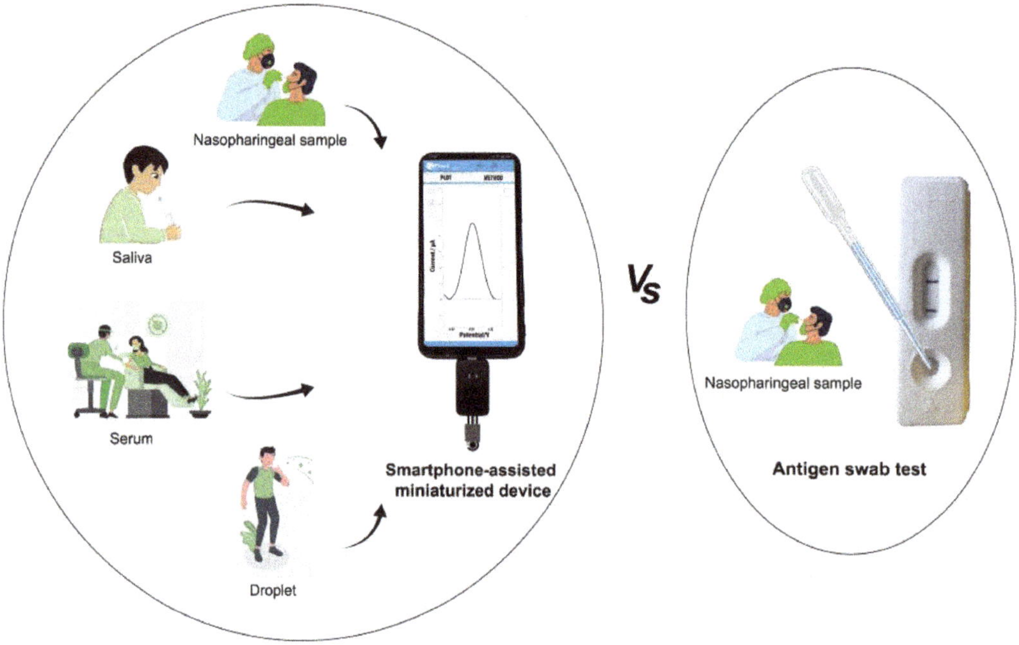

Figure 2. Different matrices used for the development of antigen biosensors at an academic level vs. commercially available antigen kits.

Table 1. Commercially available antigen kits.

Antigen Swab Test	Sensitivity %	Specificity %	Limit of Detection ($TCID_{50}$/mL)	Analysis Time (Min)	Ref.
STRONGSTEP	96	99	2.50×10^2	15	[18]
BIOCREDIT	90	90	Not reported	5–8	[19]
REALY TECH	90	100	1.25×10^3	10–20	[20]
VIVADIAG	83	100	1.35×10^3	15	[21]
ZKDENTAL	87	100	Not reported	15	[22]
MOLAB	99	98	1.15×10^2	15	[23]
JOYSBIO	89	99	1.60×10^2	15	[24]
CLUNGENE	91	100	$5 \times 10^{2.67}$	15	[25]

2. SARS-CoV-2 Antigen Detection Using Nasopharyngeal Swab

The first biosensor described in the literature for detecting the SARS-CoV-2 antigen was developed by the Seo et al. [26]. The method involves using the developed biosensor to measure S protein in nasopharyngeal swab specimens (Figure 3A).

The S protein was selected because it is a superficial glycoprotein of SARS-CoV-2 with an affinity for human angiotensin-converting enzyme 2 (hACE2), which is used as a receptor to infect human cells [27,28]. Nasopharyngeal swab specimens were selected because they offer the highest-yield samples for diagnostic testing, even though the collection of such samples, while generally considered safe, is invasive [29]. In detail, the Seo research group developed a graphene-based field-effect transistor immunosensor by immobilizing the SARS-CoV-2 spike antibody through the 1-pyrenebutyric acid N-hydroxysuccinimide ester, enabling detection of the S protein with a detection limit of 1 fg/mL in a standard solution. This field-effect transistor-based immunosensor was tested in nasopharyngeal swab specimens from COVID-19 patients and a cultured virus, observing detection limits equal to 100 fg/mL and 1.6×10^1 pfu/mL, respectively. This article opened global research avenues for the development of immunosensor-based sensors for the S protein, demonstrating the suitability of the immunosensing system for the rapid detection of patients affected by COVID-19. Besides the S protein, the N protein of the coronavirus is often used as a marker in diagnostic assays. Other authors also highlighted the usefulness of the N antigen of SARS-CoV-2 for reliable diagnosis [30,31].

Shao et al. used the same field-effect transistor approach by employing high-purity semiconducting single-walled carbon nanotubes functionalized with specific antibodies for the detection of both S and N proteins. The detection of S and N proteins was carried out by adding 10 μL of a nasopharyngeal swab sample for 2 min [32]. After this incubation time, the device was washed three times with water, and the measurement performed. The two types of field-effect transistor immunosensors demonstrated a LOD of 0.55 fg/mL for the S protein and 0.016 fg/mL, respectively, for the N protein in a standard solution. To evaluate the feasibility in real samples, a total of 28 PCR-positive samples and 10 negative nasopharyngeal swab samples were tested, finding a 17.8% false-negative rate. The low detection achieved for both proteins alongside the technique's application in clinical samples demonstrated the feasibility of immuno-based field-effect transistors for the rapid detection of SARS-CoV-2 in nasopharyngeal swab specimens. Furthermore, Chaimayo et al. proposed a rapid SARS-CoV-2 antigen detection test, the Standard™ Q COVID-19 Ag kit, which was able to detect SARS-CoV-2 in nasopharyngeal and throat swabs collected from 454 suspected COVID-19 cases. This Standard Q COVID-19 Ag test provides a rapid chromatographic immunoassay for the detection of N protein characterized by two precoated lines on the result window: a control (C) line coated with a mouse monoclonal anti-chicken Igγ antibody and a test (T) line coated with a mouse monoclonal antibody against N protein. The antigen–antibody color particles migrate via a complex process involving capillary force and are captured by the mouse monoclonal anti-SARS-CoV-2 antibody coated on the test (T) region. The colored test (T) line's intensity depends on the amount of SARS-CoV-2 N antigen present in the sample. This rapid Standard™ Q COVID-19 Ag kit showed comparable sensitivity (98.33%; 95% CI, 91.06–99.96%) and specificity (98.73%; 95% CI, 97.06–99.59%) to a real-time RT-PCR assay, demonstrating its potential use as a screening assay, especially in high prevalence areas [33].

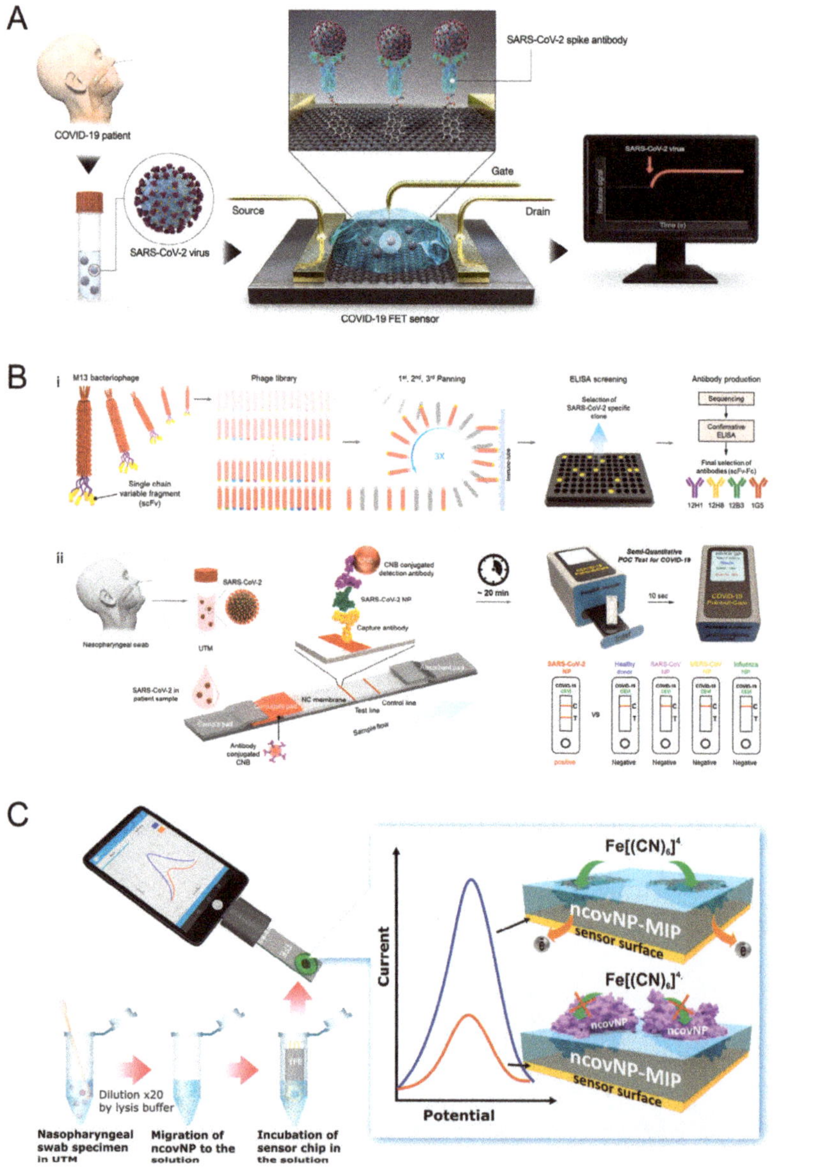

Figure 3. SARS-CoV-2 antigen detection in a nasopharyngeal swab. (**A**) S protein detection with a field-effect transistor-based immunosensor. Reprinted with permission from [26], 2020 American Chemical Society; (**B**) lateral-flow assay fabricated using the scFv-Fc antibody for N protein detection. Reprinted with permission from [34], 2021 Elsevier; (**C**) molecularly imprinted polymer-based electrochemical sensor for the detection of N protein. Reprinted with permission from [35], 2021 Elsevier.

Although commercially available antibodies are used as the main approach for detecting SARS-CoV-2 antigens, Kim et al. developed single-chain variable fragment (scFv)-crystallizable (Fc) fusion proteins (scFv-Fcs) for the detection of N protein with improved specificity [34]. To screen scFv binders that specifically interact with the SARS-CoV-2 N protein, the authors carried out a phage-display screening using a chicken-naïve scFv antibody library, followed by the isolation of positive clones and the elimination of scFv binders from MERS-CoV and SARS-CoV-2. After producing the specific antibodies, an analysis was carried out using four unique clones, 12H1, 12H8, 12B3, and 1G5, all characterized by different complementary–determining region sequences for heavy and light chains. The sensitivity was evaluated by binding experiments using the SARS-CoV-2 N protein, finding K_D values equal to 18.3, 1.31, 8.47, and 2.86 nM, respectively. The lateral-flow assay was designed by introducing the scFv-Fc antibody on the test line and anti-human IgG antibodies on the control line, while the conjugate pad was loaded with each scFv-Fc antibody–cellulose nanobead conjugate. The analytical performance of the developed device was tested using 100 μL of N protein or cultured virus in a lysis buffer, with 20 min as the analysis time. Then, the LOD was evaluated and found to be 2, 5, and 10 ng when using 12H8–12H1, 12H8–12B3, and 12H8-1G5, respectively (Figure 3B). When tested with the cultured virus, a LOD equal to 2.5×10^4 pfu was observed, as well as no cross-reactivity with the N proteins belonging to SARS-CoV-2, MERS-CoV, influenza virus, or the negative control on the nasal swab specimens.

To overcome the limitations of antibody production involving animal use, Raziq et al. developed a molecularly imprinted polymer-based electrochemical sensor for detecting the SARS-CoV-2 N protein (Figure 3C) [35]. The MIP sensor was prepared by modifying Micrux gold-based thin-film electrodes with a film generated from poly-m-phenylenediamine as a suitable functional monomer. Differential pulse voltammetry was used with ferro/ferricyanide as a redox probe for detecting N protein up to 111 fM, with LOD and LOQ values equal to 15 and 50 fM (0.7–2.2 pg/mL), respectively. To evaluate the matrix effect, the MIP sensor was tested in negative specimens by adding known concentrations of the N protein, with slightly higher values observed for the LOD and LOQ (27 fM and 90 fM, respectively). When tested with positive samples, good agreement was found between RT-PCR and the MIP sensor, demonstrating the feasibility of the developed MIP sensor.

3. SARS-CoV-2 Antigen Detection in Saliva

As highlighted above, nasopharyngeal swabs provide the main collection specimens, despite the procedure resulting in potential discomfort and requiring skilled healthcare personnel. Although underestimated in the first phase of the pandemic event as a specimen, saliva contains a detectable concentration of the virus and can be safely collected without the need for trained staff. To et al. reported that the salivary viral load was highest during the first week after symptom onset and subsequently declined over time [36]. Teo et al. collected saliva, nasopharyngeal swabs, and self-administered nasal swabs from 200 patients with acute respiratory infections and tested the samples via RT-PCR [37]. In total, 62.0%, 44.5%, and 37.7% of the saliva, nasopharyngeal, and self-administered nasal swabs gave positive results, highlighting that saliva represents a sensitive and suitable sample type for COVID-19 diagnosis.

For SARS-CoV-2 detection in saliva, we recently developed an electrochemical printed chip for the highly sensitive and accurate detection of SARS-CoV-2 in saliva. Since sensitivity and accuracy are key issues, we designed this immunosensor by employing: (i) magnetic beads as support for the immunological chain due to their ability to detect virus pre-concentration, thereby improving sensitivity; (ii) electrochemical detection, which is well-known as a sensitive and cost-effective detection method that uses a hand-held device; and (iii) carbon black as a nanomaterial to modify screen-printed sensors, thereby improving sensitivity in detecting the enzymatic by-product 1-naphtol and representing a cheap nanomaterial (around EUR 1 for 1 Kg). Furthermore, this device was conceived as an easy-to-use system. Thus, all the reagents needed for immunological chain creation can be added in a single step in untreated saliva, and during the incubation period of 30 min, stirring can be avoided (Figure 4A) [38]. To detect both N and S proteins, the antibodies for each antigen were selected and immobilized on magnetic beads. The two immunosensors developed were tested in untreated saliva, obtaining a detection limit equal to 19 ng/mL and 8 ng/mL, respectively, for S and N proteins. The effectiveness of these sensors was assessed using virus cultured in a biosafety-level-3 laboratory and in clinical samples from saliva for comparison against data obtained from nasopharyngeal swab specimens tested using Real-Time PCR. The immunosensor for S protein demonstrated higher sensitivity than the assay for N protein, with the former being able to measure 6.5 PFU/mL due to the high amount of S protein in SARS-CoV-2. Furthermore, when tested with saliva specimens, both immunosensors for N and S proteins were able, in almost all cases, to identify COVID-19 patient samples, even in the case of high CT values from Real-Time PCR (low viral load), demonstrating the high sensitivity of this cost-effective and miniaturized device.

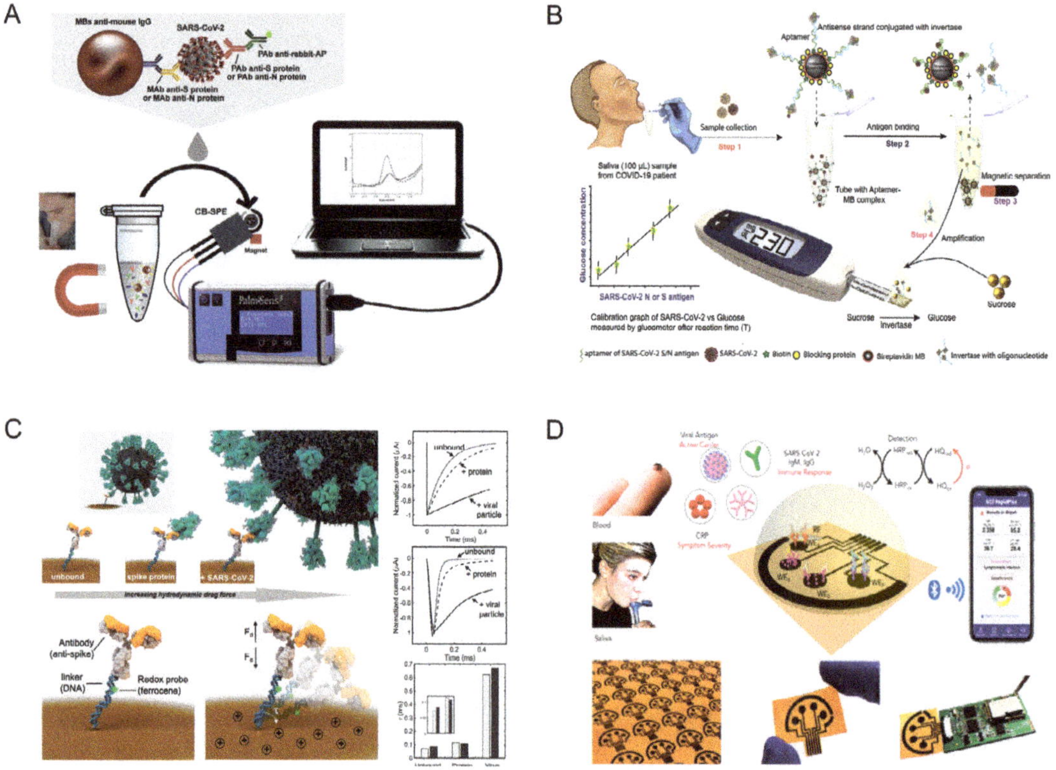

Figure 4. SARS-CoV-2 antigen detection in saliva: (**A**) magnetic beads combined with a nanomaterial-based-printed electrode for the development of two immunosensors for the detection of S and N proteins. Reprinted with permission from [38], 2021 Elsevier; (**B**) magnetic beads for the development of a cheap aptamer assay for the detection of S and N protein antigens, exploiting an off-the-shelf glucometer. Reprinted with permission from [39], 2021 Elsevier; (**C**) a reagent-free electrochemical immunosensor for directly reading out viral particles in 5 min. Reprinted with permission from [40], 2020 American Chemical Society; (**D**) an electrochemical biosensing system for the detection of N protein, IgM and IgG antibodies, and inflammatory biomarker C-reactive protein using the same hand-held device. Reprinted with permission from [41], 2020 Elsevier.

Subsequently, Hall's group used magnetic beads to develop a cheap (USD 3.20/test) aptamer assay for the detection of SARS-CoV-2 antigens using an off-the-shelf glucometer. In this study, a SARS-CoV-2 N- or S-protein-specific biotinylated aptamer was conjugated to a streptavidin-coated magnetic bead and pre-hybridized with a complementary antisense oligonucleotide strand covalently bonded to the invertase enzyme (Figure 4B) [39]. The analytical system is based on measuring the viral antigen's interactions with the aptamer by quantifying invertase-antisense oligo release. The aptamer-antigen complex on magnetic beads was removed with a magnet, and the remaining aptamer-antisense-invertase complex was collected and incubated with sucrose, which was then converted to glucose and measured using the glucometer. To verify the effectiveness of the S and N aptamer-antisense-invertase system in detecting authentic virus and the native proteins produced during SARS-CoV-2 infection, the authors created viral stocks of SARS-CoV-2 in a biosafety-level-3 laboratory, demonstrating that the aptamer-antisense-invertase systems can recognize their native targets when produced by replicating authentic SARS-CoV-2. Subsequently, this aptasensor was challenged in saliva samples, showing a detection limit in saliva equal to 5.27 and 6.31 pM for N and S proteins, respectively. Finally, the authors tested the developed assays to discriminate SARS-CoV-2-infected and healthy individuals using validated saliva samples, with 100% positive percent agreement and 100% negative agreement with the RT-qPCR data performed on the same samples analyzed, demonstrating high accuracy and speed combined with cost-effectiveness.

Kelly et al. developed a faster reagent-free electrochemical immunosensor able to directly read out viral particles in 5 min using a sensor-modified electrode chip, without the addition of any reagents [40]. The sensor was built from an analyte-recognizing antibody attached to a rigid, negatively charged linker of DNA labeled with a ferrocene redox probe to produce the electrochemical signal. In this system, the application of a positive potential attracts the negatively charged DNA-labeled linker to the surface, thus producing a current. Because the drag force is affected by the size of the bound analyte, in the presence of the S protein (and better in the case of the virus), the response is changed. This sensing tool was successfully tested with saliva samples inactivated by heating at 65 °C for 30 min, and the results were found to be comparable with gold-standard RT-PCR approaches, demonstrating the effectiveness of this smart device (Figure 4C).

Gao et al. [41] developed a highly innovative electrochemical biosensing system called SARS-CoV-2 RapidPlex, which is characterized by multiple abilities, portability, and wireless connection for the detection of N protein, IgM and IgG antibodies, and inflammatory biomarker C-reactive protein using the same hand-held device (Figure 4D). This sensing tool is composed of mass-producible laser-engraved four-channel graphene arrays combined with a PCB system for wireless data transmission to a mobile user interface. For selective detection, the platform was chemically modified with captured antigens and antibodies to detect the target analytes. To assess the effectiveness of the device, N protein, IgM and IgG antibodies, and inflammatory biomarker C-reactive protein were analyzed in commercial saliva samples from RT-PCR COVID-19-confirmed patients (n = 5) and healthy subjects (n = 3). Using this device, the analysis required saliva-sample dilution in a phosphate buffer, followed by incubation for 10 min at room temperature, a washing step with the PBS buffer, and addition of the necessary reagents for 5 min. The results demonstrated the suitability of this smart device for multiplexing detection in saliva and serum samples, paving the way toward a highly innovative Telemedicine Platform for COVID-19 management.

4. SARS-CoV-2 Antigen Detection in Serum

The effectiveness of serum as a specimen for the detection of SARS-CoV-2 antigens has been also evaluated. For instance, Li et al. analyzed fifty cases of SARS-CoV-2 nucleic acid-positive and SARS-CoV-2 antibody-negative patients, observing an N protein positivity rate of 76%, suggesting that the serum measurement of SARS-CoV-2 N protein can have high diagnostic value for infected patients before the antibody appears, thus shortening the window of serological diagnosis [42]. Li and Lillehoj [43] developed a microfluidic device for high sensitivity measurements of SARS-CoV-2 N protein in undiluted and 5× diluted serum (Figure 5A). The printed electrochemical sensor was embedded in a microfluidic device able to minimize sample (25 μL) and reagent (80 μL) consumption and simplify handling of the sample. The sample was previously mixed with dually-labeled magnetic nanobeads (the beads were coated with a detection antibody and enzyme to improve signal amplification) and then dispensed into the chip using a capillary tube and plunger. Subsequently, the microfluidic chip was placed onto a magnet for 1 min to pre-concentrate the magnetic beads. Then, an incubation time of 50 min, in the case of whole serum samples, or 25 min, in the case of diluted serum samples, was selected. Subsequently, a buffer solution was flushed through the chip for 4 min at 100 μL/min, followed by the addition of an enzymatic substrate for 1 min at 100 μL/min for electrochemical measurements. The reported LOD of this immunosensor for SARS-CoV-2 N protein in the whole serum and 5× diluted serum was 50 and 10 pg/mL, respectively. To evaluate the effectiveness of the developed microfluidic device, the device was tested using serum samples obtained from seven COVID-19 patients and four healthy patients, observing a very low current (<1 μA) in the case of healthy people and a current in the range of 5–17 μA for COVID-19 patients, demonstrating results consistent with the PCR method.

5. SARS-CoV-2 Antigen Detection in Droplets

The mucosalivary droplets formed during breathing, speaking, coughing, and sneezing are the principal avenue by which people are infected. As described by Bourouiba [44], mucosalivary droplets are primarily composed of a multiphase turbulent gas cloud, which is unable to evaporate for a much longer time than isolated droplets. Mucosalivary droplets are thus characterized by a longer lifetime (by a factor of up to 1000), increasing the time of possible transmission from seconds to minutes. This behavior, unfortunately, increases the ease of infection among people that come into contact with such droplets in the absence of correctly worn masks.

A recent novel approach for evaluating an individual's infection considers a mask not only as a protection system able to cut the diffusion of droplets [45] but also as a sampling and detection system. Several groups have sought to develop smart masks able to provide information on COVID-19 infection. For instance, Marrocco et al. developed a sensing face mask integrated with a radio frequency identification (RFID) tag for humidity sensing to monitor the wetness of the mask [46].

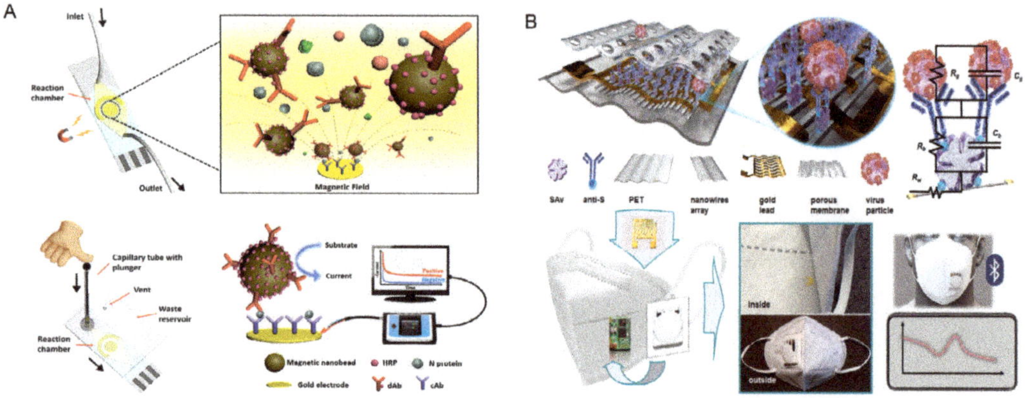

Figure 5. SARS-CoV-2 antigen detection in serum and droplets. (**A**) Microfluidic device for the high-sensitivity measurement of N protein in undiluted and 5× diluted serum. Reprinted with permission from [43], 2021 American Chemical Society; (**B**) immunosensor for the detection of SARS-CoV-2 in droplets by exploiting the surface of the face mask to collect and enrich the respiratory droplets. Reprinted with permission from [47], 2021 Elsevier.

The only completed sensor embedded in a face mask for antigen detection was reported by Xue et al. [47]. These authors were the first to develop an immunosensor for the detection of SARS-CoV-2 in droplets by exploiting the surface of the face mask to collect and enrich the respiratory droplets (Figure 5B). This intelligent mask includes an impedimetric label-free immunosensor, a miniaturized impedance circuit including an A/D converter, an operational amplifier, and a wireless transmission unit. The authors developed the immunosensor to immobilize the antibodies for S protein on nanowires doped with biotin groups and thus achieve immobilization through streptavidin–biotin interactions. The nanowire array was designed with parallel patterns on the substrates and vertically connected via gold interdigitated electrodes. The width and spacing of the nanowires were set at 75 nm to increase their sensitivity for the detection of SARS-CoV-2 in aerosols, taking into account that high-density nanowire arrays allow for higher collision frequency between the immobilized antibodies and virus present in the droplets. The developed sensing system was able to detect the S protein and whole virus in simulated human breath, with a detection limit as low as 7 pfu/mL from an atomized sample of a coronavirus aerosol mimic and a measurement time of only 5 min.

6. Biosensors in the Literature vs. Commercialized Toolkits

As reported in the literature [16], ideal biosensors for deployment in pandemics should be simple to use. The ability to carry out measurements simply and effectively refers to both the detection of the target analyte and the sample treatment. Among commercially available kits for antigen detection, analytical tools are characterized by the collection of nasopharyngeal swabs, followed by simple suspension in a viral/universal transport medium and the addition of some drops on the strips. The response usually occurs in few minutes, with a range from 5 to 20 min (Table 1).

In commercial kits, unmeasured SARS-CoV-2 is largely caused by the uncorrected sampling of nasopharyngeal swab specimens. As reported by Lippi et al. for RT-PCR analyses based on nasopharyngeal swabs [48], this type of specimen sampling is characterized by preanalytical issues, such as: identification problems; inadequate procedures for the collection, handling, transport, and storage of the swabs; the collection of inappropriate or inadequate materials (in terms of quality or volume); and manual errors. Some analytical problems may also jeopardize diagnostic accuracy, including testing outside the diagnostic window, active viral recombination, the use of inadequately validated assays, insufficient harmonization, instrument malfunctions, and other specific technical issues. Moreover, this type of sampling is invasive, and its sensitivity is not sufficient to diagnose COVID-19 when a low load virus is present, which means high CT values.

The most significant advantage of the biosensors in the literature is their ability to work with other types of specimens—especially saliva, which is not invasive and does not require any sample treatment, as highlighted in Table 2. Indeed, both nasopharyngeal swabs and serum require complex sampling and/or sample treatments. In the case of serum, a laboratory-set-up treatment is required, which precludes the application of biosensors developed on-site [43]. To boost the applicability of saliva-based biosensors, which are less invasive and still highly sensitive, and enable them to reach market, several challenges remain to be addressed, including scalable manufacturing and storage stability, which are primary issues for any successful commercially available point-of-care device.

Table 2. Sample treatment of biosensors in the literature.

Sample Matrix	Treatment	Ref.
Nasopharyngeal swab	Nasopharyngeal swabs were suspended in a universal transport medium	[26]
Nasopharyngeal swab	Nasopharyngeal swabs were suspended in a viral transport medium	[32]
Nasopharyngeal and throat swabs	Nasopharyngeal and throat swabs were mixed in a viral transport medium	[33]
Nasopharyngeal swab	Not reported	[34]
Nasopharyngeal swab	Nasopharyngeal specimens were vortexed in a universal transport medium	[35]
Saliva	No treatment	[38]
Saliva	No treatment	[39]
Saliva	No treatment	[40]
Saliva	No treatment	[41]
Serum	Whole and 5× diluted	[43]
Droplets	No treatment	[47]

7. Conclusions

From the start of the present pandemic, all disciplines have made efforts to deliver useful tools to assist in the management of the outbreak. For on-site antigen detection, the industrial sector has combined established sampling techniques using nasopharyngeal swabs with customized lateral-flow systems and replaced previously used antibodies with other analytes and antibodies for S protein or N protein detection, with minimal variation in industrial-scale fabrication. Different companies have commercialized these types of devices. However, even when widely characterized by sufficient selectivity and sensitivity, these devices are not able to diagnose the infection at its start, at which point patients are characterized by a low viral load. To address this issue, researchers have begun to develop more sensitive devices by exploiting nanomaterial technology, microfluidics, and smartphone-assisted systems (Table 3). Nanomaterials, such as graphene and carbon black, have been used to increase the sensitivity of biosensors, and microfluidics combined with printed electrodes have facilitated the simple management of samples. Moreover, the presence of miniaturized potentiostats (e.g., Sensit Smart, PalmSens instrument) embedded in smartphones will help foster the synergic combination of biosensing tools with the Internet of Things. Indeed, the convergence of interdisciplinary technologies presents an immediate solution for the main bottlenecks that constrain biosensor prototypes from achieving real applications, matching the suitable features for effective use of a biosensor in pandemics, including long shelf life, ease of use, cost-effectiveness, mass manufacturing, autonomy, high sensitivity, high selectivity, rapidity, multiplexing capabilities, multiple sensing modes, and single-use [16].

Table 3. Analytical features of biosensors for the detection of N and S proteins reported in the literature.

Analyte	Type of Biosensor	Type of Transduction	Matrix Analyzed	Linear Range (LR)/Detection Limit (LOD)	Time of Analysis	Ref.
S protein/virus	Graphene-based field-effect transistor immunosensor	FET	Nasopharyngeal swab	S protein LR: 0.1–100 pg/mL LOD: 100 fg/mL Virus: LR: 1.6×10^1–1.6×10^4 pfu/mL LOD: 1.6×10^1 pfu/mL	<1 min	[18]
S/N protein	Single-walled carbon nanotube-based field-effect transistor immunosensor	FET	Nasopharyngeal swab	S protein LR: 5.5 fg/mL–5.5 pg/mL LOD: 0.55 fg/mL N protein LR: 16 fg/mL–16 pg/mL LOD: 0.016 fg/mL	<5 min	[24]
N protein	Lateral-flow immunoassay	Colorimetric (visual) detection	Nasopharyngeal swab	sensitivity 98.33%	15–30 min	[25]
N protein/virus	Lateral-flow immunoassay based on scFv-Fc fusion proteins	Colorimetric detection	Nasopharyngeal swab	N protein LOD: 2 ng Virus LOD: 2.5×10^4 pfu	20 min	[26]
N protein	Molecularly imprinted polymer-based electrochemical sensor	Differential Pulse Voltammetry	Nasopharyngeal swab	LOD: 27 fM in clinical samples	15 min	[27]
S/N protein and virus	Magnetic bead-based immunosensor combined with carbon black-modified screen-printed electrode	Differential Pulse Voltammetry	Saliva	S protein LOD: 19 ng/mL in saliva N protein LOD: 8 ng/mL in saliva Virus: 6.5 pfu/mL concentration tested using S protein immunosensor and 6.5×10^3 pfu/mL concentration tested using N protein immunosensor	30 min	[30]
S/N protein	Magnetic bead-based sensor using a biotinylated aptamer-oligo-invertase complex	Glucometer	Saliva	N protein LOD: 5.27 pM in saliva S protein LOD: 6.31 pM in saliva	60 min	[31]

Table 3. *Cont.*

Analyte	Type of Biosensor	Type of Transduction	Matrix Analyzed	Linear Range (LR)/Detection Limit (LOD)	Time of Analysis	Ref.
S protein/virus	A reagent-free electrochemical Sensor modified with an antibody attached to DNA linker functionalized with a ferrocene redox probe	Chronoamperometry	Saliva	S protein LOD: 1 pg/mL Virus LOD: 4000 copies per mL	5 min/ 10 min	[32]
N protein	An electrochemical immunosensing platform using laser-engraved graphene electrodes and a wireless transmission unit	Chronoamperometry	Saliva	LR: Up to 5000 pg/mL	1 min	[33]
N protein	Microfluidic immunosensor based on screen-printed gold electrode combined with magnetic nanobeads	Chronoamperometry	Serum	Whole serum LOD: 50 pg/mL 5× Diluted serum LOD: 10 pg/mL	Whole serum: 50 min 5× diluted serum: 25 min	[35]
S protein/virus	Nanowire-based immunosensor combined with a miniaturized impedance circuit and a wireless transmission unit	Electrochemical impedance spectroscopy	Droplets	S protein in aerosol concentration tested: 1, 10 ng/mL Virus aerosol LOD: 7 pfu/mL corresponding to an air concentration of 0.35 pfu/L	S protein aerosol: 10 min Virus aerosol: 5 min	[39]

However, several main drawbacks still need to be overcome, as highlighted by Eden Morales-Narváez and Can Dincer [12]. Previous recommendations include the need for: (i) investments in diagnostic tools; (ii) collaborative networks within the biosecurity sector; (iii) autonomy for each country to manufacture its own biosensing technologies and protection equipment; (iv) the development of new diagnostic tools to meet government requirements; (v) widely establishing the necessary features of biosensors; (vi) the connection of biosensors with the Internet of Things; and (vii) training of the population for self-sampling and testing.

Taking into account the results achieved to date as well as the recommendations for the successful use of biosensors in virus detection, we are confident that this pandemic event will positively affect biosensing research activity. Biosensors with all the features required for reliable applications should be developed with the overriding goal of producing devices not only confined in articles but also able to be used among the population; this point was highlighted by Mao et al. [49] when discussing "the feasibility of an integrated point-of-care biosensor system with mobile health for wastewater-based epidemiology (iBMW) for early warning of COVID-19, screening and diagnosis of potential infectors, and improving health care and public health". Thus, beyond scientific publications, the delivery of useful toolkits in collaboration with companies should be one of the main goals for the scientific community, in order to avoid the monitoring issues observed in the COVID-19 pandemic during a future unexpected outbreak.

Author Contributions: Conceptualization, F.A., writing—original draft preparation, F.A., V.S., A.A., L.F. (Laura Fabiani), V.C., L.F. (Luca Fiore); writing—review and editing, F.A., D.M., S.F., R.D.S., F.L., M.B., A.M. All authors have read and agreed to the published version of the manuscript.

Funding: This research received no external funding.

Institutional Review Board Statement: Not applicable.

Informed Consent Statement: Not applicable.

Data Availability Statement: Not applicable.

Conflicts of Interest: The authors declare no conflict of interest.

References

1. Jain, S.; Nehra, M.; Kumar, R.; Dilbaghi, N.; Hu, T.; Kumar, S.; Kaushik, A.; Li, C.Z. Internet of Medical Things (IoMT)-integrated biosensors for point-of-care testing of infectious diseases. *Biosens. Bioelectron.* **2021**, *179*, 113074. [CrossRef]
2. Everyone Included: Social Impact of COVID-19 | DISD. Available online: https://www.un.org/development/desa/dspd/everyone-included-covid-19.html/ (accessed on 28 June 2021).
3. The Territorial Impact of COVID-19: Managing the Crisis Across Levels of Government. Available online: https://www.oecd.org/coronavirus/policy-responses/the-territorial-impact-of-covid-19-managing-the-crisis-across-levels-of-government-d3e314e1/ (accessed on 28 June 2021).
4. Mahapatra, S.; Chandra, P. Clinically practiced and commercially viable nanobio engineered analytical methods for COVID-19 diagnosis. *Biosens. Bioelectron.* **2020**, *165*, 112361. [CrossRef]
5. Soler, M.; Estevez, M.C.; Cardenosa-Rubio, M.; Astua, A.; Lechuga, L.M. How nanophotonic label-free biosensors can contribute to rapid and massive diagnostics of respiratory virus infections: COVID-19 Case. *ACS Sens.* **2020**, *5*, 2663–2678. [CrossRef]
6. Guidelines on COVID-19 In Vitro Diagnostic Tests and Their Performance (2020/C 122I/01). Available online: https://eur-lex.europa.eu/legal-content/EN/TXT/?uri=CELEX:52020XC0415(04) (accessed on 1 June 2021).
7. European Research Area Corona Platform. Available online: https://ec.europa.eu/info/sites/info/files/research_and_innovation/research_by_area/documents/ec_rtd_cv-projects.pdf (accessed on 1 June 2021).
8. Combating 2019-nCoV: Advanced Nanobiosensing Platforms for POC Global Diagnostics and Surveillance. Available online: https://cordis.europa.eu/project/id/101003544 (accessed on 1 June 2021).
9. Three Rapid Diagnostic Tests (Point-of-Care) for COVID-19 CoronaThree Rapid Diagnostic Tests (Point-of-Care) for Coronavirus, Improving Epidemic Preparedness, Public Health and Socio-Economic Benefits. Available online: https://cordis.europa.eu/project/id/101003562 (accessed on 1 June 2021).
10. Development and Validation of Rapid Molecular Diagnostic Test for nCoV19. Available online: https://cordis.europa.eu/project/id/101003713 (accessed on 1 June 2021).
11. Cheng, V.C.C.; Lau, S.K.P.; Woo, P.C.Y.; Yuen, K.Y. Severe acute respiratory syndrome coronavirus as an agent of emerging and reemerging Infection. *Clin. Microbiol. Rev.* **2007**, *20*, 660–694. [CrossRef] [PubMed]
12. Morales-Narváez, E.; Dincer, C. The impact of biosensing in a pandemic outbreak: COVID-19. *Biosens. Bioelectron.* **2020**, *163*, 112274. [CrossRef] [PubMed]
13. Chan, W.C.W. Nano Research for COVID-19. *ACS Nano* **2020**, *14*, 3719–3720. [CrossRef]
14. Chung, Y.H.; Beiss, V.; Fiering, S.N.; Steinmetz, N.F. COVID-19 Vaccine frontrunners and their nanotechnology design. *ACS Nano* **2020**, *14*, 12522–12537. [CrossRef] [PubMed]
15. Chauhan, G.; Madou, M.J.; Kalra, S.; Chopra, V.; Ghosh, D.; Martinez-Chapa, S.O. Nanotechnology for COVID-19: Therapeutics and vaccine research. *ACS Nano* **2020**, *14*, 7760–7782. [CrossRef]
16. Bhalla, N.; Pan, Y.; Yang, Z.; Payam, A.F. Opportunities and challenges for biosensors and nanoscale analytical tools for pandemics: COVID-19. *ACS Nano* **2020**, *14*, 7783–7807. [CrossRef]
17. Ates, H.C.; Yetisen, A.K.; Güder, F.; Dincer, C. Wearable devices for the detection of COVID-19. *Nat. Electron.* **2021**, *4*, 13–14. [CrossRef]
18. Strongstep SARS-CoV-2 Antigen Rapid Test. Available online: https://www.finddx.org/product/strongstep-sars-cov-2-antigen-rapid-test/ (accessed on 30 August 2021).

19. Biocredit COVID-19 Ag Test. Available online: https://www.biovendor.com/biocredit-covid-19-ag-detection-kit?utm_source=google&utm_medium=organic (accessed on 30 August 2021).
20. Realy Tech Novel Coronavirus (SARS-Cov-2) Antigen Rapid Test (Swab). Available online: https://feldundstall.at/wp-content/uploads/2020/12/%e6%9c%80%e6%96%b0Realy-COVID-Antigen-kit112.pdf (accessed on 30 August 2021).
21. VivaDiag Pro SARS-CoV-2 Ag Rapid Test. Available online: https://vivacare.gr/wp-content/uploads/2020/10/VivaDiag-SARS-CoV-2-Ag-Rapid-Test-Package-Insert%EF%BC%88sealed-pouch.pdf (accessed on 30 August 2021).
22. Healgen Coronavirus Antigen Rapid Test Kit. Available online: https://theppeonlineshop.co.uk/pdfs/Healgen-Test-Data-Sheet.pdf (accessed on 30 August 2021).
23. Molab Corona Antigen Test + Prefilled Buffer. Available online: https://www.quadratech.co.uk/product/molab-covid-19-rapid-antigen-test-kit/ (accessed on 30 August 2021).
24. Joysbio COVID-19 Antigen Rapid Test Kit. Available online: https://en.joysbio.com/covid-19-antigen-rapid-test-kit/ (accessed on 28 June 2021).
25. Antigen Rapid Test Cassette Clungene. Available online: https://www.mmbiotech.it/wp-content/uploads/2021/03/Bugiardino-CLUNGENE-for-COVID-19-Antigen-Rapid-Test-Cassette-EN-109155103-version-3.0.pdf (accessed on 28 June 2021).
26. Seo, G.; Lee, G.; Kim, M.J.; Baek, S.H.; Choi, M.; Ku, K.B.; Lee, C.S.; Jun, S.; Park, D.; Kim, H.G.; et al. Rapid detection of COVID-19 causative virus (SARS-CoV-2) in human nasopharyngeal swab specimens using field-effect transistor-based biosensor. *ACS Nano* **2020**, *14*, 5135–5142. [CrossRef]
27. Verdecchia, P.; Cavallini, C.; Spanevello, A.; Angeli, F. The pivotal link between ACE2 deficiency and SARS-CoV-2 infection. *Eur. J. Intern. Med.* **2020**, *76*, 14–20. [CrossRef] [PubMed]
28. Xia, S.; Liu, M.; Wang, C.; Xu, W.; Lan, Q.; Feng, S.; Qi, F.; Bao, L.; Du, L.; Liu, S.; et al. Inhibition of SARS-CoV-2 (previously 2019-NCoV) infection by a highly potent pan-coronavirus fusion inhibitor targeting its spike protein that harbors a high capacity to mediate membrane fusion. *Cell Res.* **2020**, *30*, 343–355. [CrossRef] [PubMed]
29. Föh, B.; Borsche, M.; Balck, A.; Taube, S.; Rupp, J.; Klein, C.; Katalinic, A. Complications of nasal and pharyngeal swabs: A relevant challenge of the COVID-19 pandemic? *Eur. Respir. J.* **2021**, *57*, 2004004. [CrossRef]
30. Fehr, A.R.; Perlman, S. Coronaviruses: An Overview of Their Replication and Pathogenesis. In *Coronaviruses*; Maier, H.J., Bickerton, E., Britton, P., Eds.; Springer: New York, NY, USA, 2015; Volume 1282, pp. 1–23. ISBN 9781493924370.
31. Di, B.; Hao, W.; Gao, Y.; Wang, M.; Wang, Y.; Qiu, L.; Wen, K.; Zhou, D.; Wu, X.; Lu, E.; et al. Monoclonal antibody-based antigen capture enzyme-linked immunosorbent assay reveals high sensitivity of the nucleocapsid protein in acute-phase sera of severe acute respiratory syndrome patients. *Clin. Diagn. Lab. Immunol.* **2005**, *12*, 135–140. [CrossRef]
32. Shao, W.; Shurin, M.R.; Wheeler, S.E.; He, X.; Star, A. Rapid detection of SARS-CoV-2 antigens using high-purity semiconducting single-walled carbon nanotube-based field-effect transistors. *ACS Appl. Mater. Interfaces* **2021**, *13*, 10321–10327. [CrossRef]
33. Chaimayo, C.; Kaewnaphan, B.; Tanlieng, N.; Athipanyasilp, N.; Sirijatuphat, R.; Chayakulkeeree, M.; Angkasekwinai, N.; Sutthent, R.; Puangpunngam, N.; Tharmviboonsri, T.; et al. Rapid SARS-CoV-2 antigen detection assay in comparison with real-time RT-PCR assay for laboratory diagnosis of COVID-19 in Thailand. *Virol. J.* **2020**, *17*, 1–7. [CrossRef] [PubMed]
34. Kim, H.-Y.; Lee, J.-H.; Kim, M.J.; Park, S.C.; Choi, M.; Lee, W.; Ku, K.B.; Kim, B.T.; Changkyun Park, E.; Kim, H.G.; et al. Development of a SARS-CoV-2-specific biosensor for antigen detection using scFv-Fc fusion proteins. *Biosens. Bioelectron.* **2021**, *175*, 112868. [CrossRef]
35. Raziq, A.; Kidakova, A.; Boroznjak, R.; Reut, J.; Öpik, A.; Syritski, V. Development of a portable MIP-based electrochemical sensor for detection of SARS-CoV-2 antigen. *Biosens. Bioelectron.* **2021**, *178*, 113029. [CrossRef]
36. To, K.K.-W.; Tsang, O.T.-Y.; Leung, W.-S.; Tam, A.R.; Wu, T.-C.; Lung, D.C.; Yip, C.C.-Y.; Cai, J.-P.; Chan, J.M.-C.; Chik, T.S.-H.; et al. Temporal profiles of viral load in posterior oropharyngeal saliva samples and serum antibody responses during infection by SARS-CoV-2: An observational cohort study. *Lancet Infect. Dis.* **2020**, *20*, 565–574. [CrossRef]
37. Teo, A.K.J.; Choudhury, Y.; Tan, I.B.; Cher, C.Y.; Chew, S.H.; Wan, Z.Y.; Cheng, L.T.E.; Oon, L.L.E.; Tan, M.H.; Chan, K.S.; et al. Saliva is more sensitive than nasopharyngeal or nasal swabs for diagnosis of asymptomatic and mild COVID-19 infection. *Sci. Rep.* **2021**, *11*, 3134. [CrossRef]
38. Fabiani, L.; Saroglia, M.; Galatà, G.; De Santis, R.; Fillo, S.; Luca, V.; Faggioni, G.; D'Amore, N.; Regalbuto, E.; Salvatori, P.; et al. Magnetic beads combined with carbon black-based screen-printed electrodes for COVID-19: A Reliable and miniaturized electrochemical immunosensor for SARS-CoV-2 detection in saliva. *Biosens. Bioelectron.* **2021**, *171*, 112686. [CrossRef]
39. Singh, N.K.; Ray, P.; Carlin, A.F.; Magallanes, C.; Morgan, S.C.; Laurent, L.C.; Aronoff-Spencer, E.S.; Hall, D.A. Hitting the diagnostic sweet spot: Point-of-care SARS-CoV-2 salivary antigen testing with an off-the-shelf Glucometer. *Biosens. Bioelectron.* **2021**, *180*, 113111. [CrossRef] [PubMed]
40. Yousefi, H.; Mahmud, A.; Chang, D.; Das, J.; Gomis, S.; Chen, J.B.; Wang, H.; Been, T.; Yip, L.; Coomes, E.; et al. Detection of SARS-CoV-2 viral particles using direct, reagent-free electrochemical sensing. *J. Am. Chem. Soc.* **2021**, *143*, 1722–1727. [CrossRef] [PubMed]
41. Torrente-Rodríguez, R.M.; Lukas, H.; Tu, J.; Min, J.; Yang, Y.; Xu, C.; Rossiter, H.B.; Gao, W. SARS-CoV-2 RapidPlex: A graphene-based multiplexed telemedicine platform for rapid and low-cost COVID-19 diagnosis and monitoring. *Matter* **2020**, *3*, 1981–1998. [CrossRef] [PubMed]
42. Li, T.; Wang, L.; Wang, H.; Li, X.; Zhang, S.; Xu, Y.; Wei, W. Serum SARS-COV-2 nucleocapsid protein: A sensitivity and specificity early diagnostic marker for SARS-COV-2 infection. *Front. Cell. Infect. Microbiol.* **2020**, *10*, 470. [CrossRef]

43. Li, J.; Lillehoj, P.B. Microfluidic magneto immunosensor for rapid, high sensitivity measurements of SARS-CoV-2 nucleocapsid protein in serum. *ACS Sens.* **2021**, *6*, 1270–1278. [CrossRef]
44. Bourouiba, L. Turbulent gas clouds and respiratory pathogen emissions: Potential implications for reducing transmission of COVID-19. *JAMA* **2020**, *323*, 1837–1838. [CrossRef]
45. Amendola, L.; Saurini, M.T.; Di Girolamo, F.; Arduini, F. A rapid screening method for testing the efficiency of masks in breaking down aerosols. *Microchem. J.* **2020**, *157*, 104928. [CrossRef]
46. Bianco, G.M.; Marrocco, G. Sensorized facemask with moisture-sensitive RFID antenna. *IEEE Sens. Lett.* **2021**, *5*, 1–4. [CrossRef]
47. Xue, Q.; Kan, X.; Pan, Z.; Li, Z.; Pan, W.; Zhou, F.; Duan, X. An intelligent face mask integrated with high density conductive nanowire array for directly exhaled coronavirus aerosols screening. *Biosens. Bioelectron.* **2021**, *186*, 113286. [CrossRef] [PubMed]
48. Lippi, G.; Simundic, A.; Plebani, M. Potential preanalytical and analytical vulnerabilities in the laboratory diagnosis of coronavirus disease 2019 (COVID-19). *Clin. Chem. Lab. Med.* **2020**, *58*, 1070–1076. [CrossRef] [PubMed]
49. Mao, K.; Zhang, H.; Yang, Z. An integrated biosensor system with mobile health and wastewater-based epidemiology (iBMW) for COVID-19 pandemic. *Biosens. Bioelectron.* **2020**, *169*, 112617. [CrossRef] [PubMed]

MDPI
St. Alban-Anlage 66
4052 Basel
Switzerland
Tel. +41 61 683 77 34
Fax +41 61 302 89 18
www.mdpi.com

Biosensors Editorial Office
E-mail: biosensors@mdpi.com
www.mdpi.com/journal/biosensors

MDPI

www.ingramcontent.com/pod-product-compliance
Lightning Source LLC
LaVergne TN
LVHW070627100526
838202LV00012B/744